Lifestyle and Chronic Pain

Lifestyle and Chronic Pain

Editors

Jo Nijs
Felipe J J Reis

MDPI • Basel • Beijing • Wuhan • Barcelona • Belgrade • Manchester • Tokyo • Cluj • Tianjin

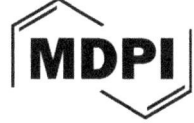

Editors
Jo Nijs
Physiotherapy, Human
Physiology & Anatomy
Vrije Universiteit Brussel
Brussels
Belgium

Felipe J J Reis
Physical Therapy
Instituto Federal do
Rio de Janeiro (IFRJ)
Rio de Janeiro
Brazil

Editorial Office
MDPI
St. Alban-Anlage 66
4052 Basel, Switzerland

This is a reprint of articles from the Special Issue published online in the open access journal *Journal of Clinical Medicine* (ISSN 2077-0383) (available at: www.mdpi.com/journal/jcm/special_issues/Pain).

For citation purposes, cite each article independently as indicated on the article page online and as indicated below:

LastName, A.A.; LastName, B.B.; LastName, C.C. Article Title. *Journal Name* **Year**, *Volume Number*, Page Range.

ISBN 978-3-0365-3578-4 (Hbk)
ISBN 978-3-0365-3577-7 (PDF)

© 2022 by the authors. Articles in this book are Open Access and distributed under the Creative Commons Attribution (CC BY) license, which allows users to download, copy and build upon published articles, as long as the author and publisher are properly credited, which ensures maximum dissemination and a wider impact of our publications.

The book as a whole is distributed by MDPI under the terms and conditions of the Creative Commons license CC BY-NC-ND.

Contents

About the Editors vii

Preface to "Lifestyle and Chronic Pain" ix

Astrid Lahousse, Eva Roose, Laurence Leysen, Sevilay Tümkaya Yilmaz, Kenza Mostaqim and Felipe Reis et al.
Lifestyle and Pain following Cancer: State-of-the-Art and Future Directions
Reprinted from: *J. Clin. Med.* **2021**, *11*, 195, doi:10.3390/jcm11010195 1

Annelie Gutke, Karin Sundfeldt and Liesbet De Baets
Lifestyle and Chronic Pain in the Pelvis: State of the Art and Future Directions
Reprinted from: *J. Clin. Med.* **2021**, *10*, 5397, doi:10.3390/jcm10225397 21

Emily F. Law, Agnes Kim, Kelly Ickmans and Tonya M. Palermo
Sleep Health Assessment and Treatment in Children and Adolescents with Chronic Pain: State of the Art and Future Directions
Reprinted from: *J. Clin. Med.* **2022**, *11*, 1491, doi:10.3390/jcm11061491 49

Katherine Brain, Tracy L. Burrows, Laura Bruggink, Anneleen Malfliet, Chris Hayes and Fiona J. Hodson et al.
Diet and Chronic Non-Cancer Pain: The State of the Art and Future Directions
Reprinted from: *J. Clin. Med.* **2021**, *10*, 5203, doi:10.3390/jcm10215203 61

Thomas Bilterys, Carolie Siffain, Ina De Maeyer, Eveline Van Looveren, Olivier Mairesse and Jo Nijs et al.
Associates of Insomnia in People with Chronic Spinal Pain: A Systematic Review and Meta-Analysis
Reprinted from: *J. Clin. Med.* **2021**, *10*, 3175, doi:10.3390/jcm10143175 85

Lirios Dueñas, Marta Aguilar-Rodríguez, Lennard Voogt, Enrique Lluch, Filip Struyf and Michel G. C. A. M. Mertens et al.
Specific versus Non-Specific Exercises for Chronic Neck or Shoulder Pain: A Systematic Review
Reprinted from: *J. Clin. Med.* **2021**, *10*, 5946, doi:10.3390/jcm10245946 107

Sevilay Tümkaya Yılmaz, Anneleen Malfliet, Ömer Elma, Tom Deliens, Jo Nijs and Peter Clarys et al.
Diet/Nutrition: Ready to Transition from a Cancer Recurrence/Prevention Strategy to a Chronic Pain Management Modality for Cancer Survivors?
Reprinted from: *J. Clin. Med.* **2022**, *11*, 653, doi:10.3390/jcm11030653 129

Jente Bontinck, Marlies den Hollander, Amanda L. Kaas, Jeroen R. De Jong and Inge Timmers
Individual Patterns and Temporal Trajectories of Changes in Fear and Pain during Exposure In Vivo: A Multiple Single-Case Experimental Design in Patients with Chronic Pain
Reprinted from: *J. Clin. Med.* **2022**, *11*, 1360, doi:10.3390/jcm11051360 145

Hye-Mi Noh, Yi Hwa Choi, Soo Kyung Lee, Hong Ji Song, Yong Soon Park and Namhyun Kim et al.
Association between Dietary Protein Intake, Regular Exercise, and Low Back Pain among Middle-Aged and Older Korean Adults without Osteoarthritis of the Lumbar Spine
Reprinted from: *J. Clin. Med.* **2022**, *11*, 1220, doi:10.3390/jcm11051220 163

Barbara Kleinmann and Tilman Wolter
Opioid Consumption in Chronic Pain Patients: Role of Perceived Injustice and Other Psychological and Socioeconomic Factors
Reprinted from: *J. Clin. Med.* **2022**, *11*, 647, doi:10.3390/jcm11030647 . . . . **175**

Lisa Goudman, Ann De Smedt, Marc Noppen and Maarten Moens
Is Central Sensitisation the Missing Link of Persisting Symptoms after COVID-19 Infection?
Reprinted from: *J. Clin. Med.* **2021**, *10*, 5594, doi:10.3390/jcm10235594 . . . . **189**

Jani Mikkonen, Ville Leinonen, Hannu Luomajoki, Diego Kaski, Saana Kupari and Mika Tarvainen et al.
Cross-Cultural Adaptation, Reliability, and Psychophysical Validation of the Pain and Sleep Questionnaire Three-Item Index in Finnish
Reprinted from: *J. Clin. Med.* **2021**, *10*, 4887, doi:10.3390/jcm10214887 . . . . **201**

Carina F. Pinheiro, Anamaria S. Oliveira, Tenysson Will-Lemos, Lidiane L. Florencio, César Fernández-de-las-Peñas and Fabiola Dach et al.
Neck Active Movements Assessment in Women with Episodic and Chronic Migraine
Reprinted from: *J. Clin. Med.* **2021**, *10*, 3805, doi:10.3390/jcm10173805 . . . . **223**

About the Editors

Jo Nijs

Jo Nijs is professor at the Vrije Universiteit Brussel (Brussels, Belgium), physiotherapist/manual therapist at the University Hospital Brussels, holder of a Chair on oncological physiotherapy funded by the Berekuyl Academy, the Netherlands, and part of the Visiting Professor program of the University of Gothenburg (Sweden). Jo runs the Pain in Motion international research group. The primary aim of his research is improving care for patients with chronic pain. At the age of 45, he has (co-)authored 282 peer reviewed publications (including papers in high impact journals such as The Lancet, JAMA Neurology and The Lancet Rheumatology), obtained €12 million grant income, supervised 21 PhD projects to completion and served >300 times as an invited speaker at national and international meetings in 25 countries (including 36 keynotes). He trained >3k clinicians in 100 courses held in 12 countries spread over 4 continents. His work has been cited >9k times (h-index: 55), with 26 citations per article (ISI Web of Knowledge). Jo is ranked 2nd in the world among chronic pain researchers (1st in Europe), received the 2017 Excellence in Research Award from the JOSPT (USA), and the 2020 Francqui Collen Chair awarded by the University of Hasselt, Belgium.

Felipe J J Reis

Felipe Reis is Professor at the Instituto Federal do Rio de Janeiro, Brasil, visiting researcher at McGill University and visiting professor at Pain in Motion Research Group (PAIN), Department of Physiotherapy, Human Physiology and Anatomy, Vrije Universiteit Brussel, Belgium. I earned my PhD degree in Medical Sciences (2012) at Universidade Federal do Rio de Janeiro. My research interests are: the integration of pain, emotion and cognition, and pain education. I serve as the chair of the IASP Special Interest Group Pain, Mind and Movement. Currently, I am responsible for coordinating an international research group (Pesquisa em Dor). In the last years, this group provided the integration of researchers from several countries and has developed pain education resources for adults and children in different languages.

Preface to "Lifestyle and Chronic Pain"

The Key Role of Lifestyle Factors in Sustaining Chronic Pain: Towards Precision Pain Medicine

Chronic pain has a tremendous personal and socioeconomic impact and remains a challenge for many clinicians. Cumulating evidence shows that lifestyle factors such as physical (in)activity, stress, poor sleep, unhealthy diet, and smoking are associated with chronic pain severity and sustainment across all age categories (1). Precision medicine refers to the ability to classify patients into subgroups that differ in their susceptibility to, biology, or prognosis of a particular disease, or in their response to a specific treatment, and thus to tailor treatment to the individual patient characteristics (2). A paradigm shift from a tissue- and disease-based approach towards individually tailored multimodal lifestyle interventions should lead to improved outcomes and decrease the psychological and socioeconomic burden of chronic pain. Such an approach fits well into the global move towards precision pain medicine for patients with chronic pain (3). For all these reasons, this special issue of Journal of Clinical Medicine is dedicated to Lifestyle and Chronic Pain.

The Special Issue includes featured state of the art papers addressing key lifestyle factors of importance to patients having persistent pain and written by leading experts and key opinion leaders in the field. For instance, an exciting state of the art review proposes to clinicians working with patients with chronic pelvic pain to make use of the window of opportunity to prevent a potential transition from localized or periodic pain in the pelvis (e.g., pain during pregnancy and after delivery) towards persistent chronic pain, by promoting a healthy lifestyle (4). In addition, original contributions to this Special Issue include literature reviews (systematic literature reviews with meta analyses and narrative reviews) and exciting original research (trials, cohort studies, experimental lab work, case-control studies) focussed on lifestyle and chronic pain. For instance, an exciting study reports that graded exposure in vivo treatment in patients with chronic low back pain and complex regional pain syndrome type I was accompanied by reductions in fear that preceded pain relief (5). In 164 patients with chronic pain, opioid use was more closely related to perceived injustice and depression, but not anxiety and stress (6). In more than 70% of patients post COVID-19 infection (total n=567), symptoms of central sensitisation were present (7). The authors suggest that patient education and multimodal rehabilitation to target nociplastic pain can be considered in patients post COVID-19 infection with long-lasting symptoms of central sensitisation (7).

In patients with episodic and chronic migraines, less mobility and less velocity of neck movements, without differences in muscle activity, was observed, with neck disability and kinesiophobia being negative and weakly associated with cervical movement (8). This brings us to physical activity as a key lifestyle factor in patients with chronic pain, and the potential of exercise therapy and physical activity interventions to address this factor. A systematic literature review included in this Special Issue discusses the available evidence (including short- and long-term effects) supporting specific versus general exercise therapy for patients with chronic neck and shoulder pain (9).

Sleep is another key lifestyle factor in many patients with chronic pain (10), which was addressed by several papers included in the Special Issue. A state of the art review provided recommendations for best practices in the clinical assessment and treatment approaches to promote sleep health in children and adolescents with chronic pain (11). A systematic literature review with meta-analyses provides an overview of the associates of insomnia in people with chronic spinal pain, highlighting several significant associates of insomnia (12). This review is helpful in gaining a better understanding of the characteristics and potential origin of insomnia in patients with chronic spinal pain, including identifying patients with chronic spinal pain who are likely to have insomnia (12). Finally, an original research report presents the cross-cultural translation and validation of the Pain and Sleep Questionnaire three-item index (PSQ-3) (13), allowing implementation of the PSQ-3 In Finland, potentially leading to better understanding of the direct effects of pain on sleep in Finish patients with chronic pain (13).

Diet is another key lifestyle factor that is gaining scientific momentum in relation to chronic pain (treatment) (14, 15). This Special Issue contributes to this global move with an original research report that studied 2,367 middle-aged and older adults, and found that low protein intake and lack of regular exercise are associated with high odds for low back pain in women (16). In addition, a review describes the current state of the art regarding nutrition in patients with chronic (non-cancer) pain, highlighting why nutrition is critical within a person-centred approach to pain management, and providing recommendations to guide clinicians in doing so (17). In addition, another review included in this Special Issue focusses on patients with post-cancer pain, and argues that diet/nutrition might be ready to transition from a cancer recurrence/prevention strategy towards a chronic pain management modality for cancer survivors (18). The importance of evidence-based pain management in cancer survivors is another global trend thoroughly addressed in this Special Issue, with another state of the art review discussing how multiple modifiable lifestyle factors, such as stress, insomnia, diet, obesity, smoking, alcohol consumption and physical activity, play a role in shaping the pain experience after cancer, and how available treatment programs for cancer survivors can be improved by including an individually-tailored lifestyle management approach (19).

Together, this Special Issue contributes substantially to the paradigm shift towards a lifestyle approach for patients having non-cancer and cancer-related chronic pain!

References

1. Nijs J, D'Hondt E, Clarys P, Deliens T, Polli A, Malfliet A, Coppieters I, Willaert W, Tumkaya Yilmaz S, Elma Ö, Ickmans K. Lifestyle and Chronic Pain across the Lifespan: An Inconvenient Truth? Pm r. 2020;12(4):410-419.

2. National Research Council Committee on AFfDaNToD. The National Academies Collection: Reports funded by National Institutes of Health. Toward Precision Medicine: Building a Knowledge Network for Biomedical Research and a New Taxonomy of Disease. Washington (DC): National Academies Press (US) Copyright ©2011, National Academy of Sciences.; 2011.

3. Nijs JG, SZ; Clauw, DJ; Fernández-de-las-Peñas, C; Kosek, E; Ickmans, K; Fernández Carnero, J; Polli, A; Kapreli, E; Huysmans, E; Cuesta-Vargas, AI; Mani, R; Lundberg, M; Leysen, L; Rice, D; Sterling, M; Curatolo, M. . Central sensitisation in chronic pain conditions: Latest discoveries and their potential for precision medicine. The Lancet Rheumatology 2021;3:e383-392.

4. Gutke A, Sundfeldt K, De Baets L. Lifestyle and Chronic Pain in the Pelvis: State of the Art and Future Directions. Journal of Clinical Medicine. 2021;10(22):5397.

5. Bontinck J, den Hollander M, Kaas AL, De Jong JR, Timmers I. Individual Patterns and Temporal Trajectories of Changes in Fear and Pain during Exposure In Vivo: A Multiple Single-Case Experimental Design in Patients with Chronic Pain. J Clin Med. 2022;11(5).

6. Kleinmann B, Wolter T. Opioid Consumption in Chronic Pain Patients: Role of Perceived Injustice and Other Psychological and Socioeconomic Factors. Journal of Clinical Medicine. 2022;11(3):647.

7. Goudman L, De Smedt A, Noppen M, Moens M. Is Central Sensitisation the Missing Link of Persisting Symptoms after COVID-19 Infection? Journal of Clinical Medicine. 2021;10(23):5594.

8. Pinheiro CF, Oliveira AS, Will-Lemos T, Florencio LL, Fernández-de-las-Peñas C, Dach F,

Bevilaqua-Grossi D. Neck Active Movements Assessment in Women with Episodic and Chronic Migraine. Journal of Clinical Medicine. 2021;10(17):3805.

9. Dueñas L, Aguilar-Rodríguez M, Voogt L, Lluch E, Struyf F, Mertens MGCAM, Meulemeester KD, Meeus M. Specific versus Non-Specific Exercises for Chronic Neck or Shoulder Pain: A Systematic Review. Journal of Clinical Medicine. 2021;10(24):5946.

10. Nijs J, Mairesse O, Neu D, Leysen L, Danneels L, Cagnie B, Meeus M, Moens M, Ickmans K, Goubert D. Sleep Disturbances in Chronic Pain: Neurobiology, Assessment, and Treatment in Physical Therapist Practice. Phys Ther. 2018;98(5):325-335.

11. Law EF, Kim A, Ickmans K, Palermo TM. Sleep Health Assessment and Treatment in Children and Adolescents with Chronic Pain: State of the Art and Future Directions. Journal of Clinical Medicine. 2022;11(6):1491.

12. Bilterys T, Siffain C, De Maeyer I, Van Looveren E, Mairesse O, Nijs J, Meeus M, Ickmans K, Cagnie B, Goubert D, Danneels L, Moens M, Malfliet A. Associates of Insomnia in People with Chronic Spinal Pain: A Systematic Review and Meta-Analysis. J Clin Med. 2021;10(14).

13. Mikkonen J, Leinonen V, Luomajoki H, Kaski D, Kupari S, Tarvainen M, Selander T, Airaksinen O. Cross-Cultural Adaptation, Reliability, and Psychophysical Validation of the Pain and Sleep Questionnaire Three-Item Index in Finnish. Journal of Clinical Medicine. 2021;10(21):4887.

14. Elma Ö, Yilmaz ST, Deliens T, Coppieters I, Clarys P, Nijs J, Malfliet A. Do Nutritional Factors Interact with Chronic Musculoskeletal Pain? A Systematic Review. J Clin Med. 2020;9(3).

15. Nijs J, Tumkaya Yilmaz S, Elma Ö, Tatta J, Mullie P, Vanderweeën L, Clarys P, Deliens T, Coppieters I, Weltens N, Van Oudenhove L, Huysmans E, Malfliet A. Nutritional intervention in chronic pain: an innovative way of targeting central nervous system sensitization? Expert Opin Ther Targets. 2020;24(8):793-803.

16. Noh HM, Choi YH, Lee SK, Song HJ, Park YS, Kim N, Cho J. Association between Dietary Protein Intake, Regular Exercise, and Low Back Pain among Middle-Aged and Older Korean Adults without Osteoarthritis of the Lumbar Spine. J Clin Med. 2022;11(5).

17. Brain K, Burrows TL, Bruggink L, Malfliet A, Hayes C, Hodson FJ, Collins CE. Diet and Chronic Non-Cancer Pain: The State of the Art and Future Directions. Journal of Clinical Medicine. 2021;10(21):5203.

18. Tümkaya Yılmaz S, Malfliet A, Elma Ö, Deliens T, Nijs J, Clarys P, De Groef A, Coppieters I. Diet/Nutrition: Ready to Transition from a Cancer Recurrence/Prevention Strategy to a Chronic Pain Management Modality for Cancer Survivors? J Clin Med. 2022;11(3).

19. Lahousse A, Roose E, Leysen L, Yilmaz ST, Mostaqim K, Reis F, Rheel E, Beckwée D, Nijs J. Lifestyle and Pain following Cancer: State-of-the-Art and Future Directions. Journal of Clinical Medicine. 2022;11(1):195.

Jo Nijs and Felipe J J Reis
Editors

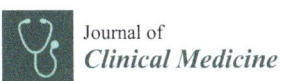

Review

Lifestyle and Pain following Cancer: State-of-the-Art and Future Directions

Astrid Lahousse [1,2,3,4,*], Eva Roose [2,3,4], Laurence Leysen [1,2,3,4], Sevilay Tümkaya Yilmaz [2,3], Kenza Mostaqim [2,3,4], Felipe Reis [3,5,6], Emma Rheel [2,3,7], David Beckwée [2,4] and Jo Nijs [2,3,8,9]

1. Research Foundation–Flanders (FWO), 1000 Brussels, Belgium; Laurence.leysen@vub.be
2. Department of Physiotherapy, Human Physiology and Anatomy, Faculty of Physical Education and Physiotherapy, Vrije Universiteit Brussel, 1090 Brussels, Belgium; Eva.Charlotte.S.Roose@vub.be (E.R.); sevilay.tumkaya.yilmaz@vub.be (S.T.Y.); kenza.mostaqim@vub.be (K.M.); Emma.Rheel@vub.be (E.R.); David.Beckwee@vub.be (D.B.); jo.nijs@vub.be (J.N.)
3. Pain in Motion Research Group (PAIN), Department of Physiotherapy, Human Physiology and Anatomy, Faculty of Physical Education and Physiotherapy (KIMA), Vrije Universiteit Brussel, 1090 Brussels, Belgium; felipe.reis@ifrj.edu.br
4. Rehabilitation Research (RERE) Research Group, Department of Physiotherapy, Human Physiology and Anatomy, Faculty of Physical Education and Physiotherapy (KIMA), Vrije Universiteit Brussel, 1090 Brussels, Belgium
5. Physical Therapy Department, Instituto Federal do Rio de Janeiro (IFRJ), Rio de Janeiro 20270-021, Brazil
6. Postgraduation Program-Clinical Medicine Department of Universidade Federal do Rio de Janeiro (UFRJ), Rio de Janeiro 21941-901, Brazil
7. Department of Experimental-Clinical and Health Psychology, Ghent University, 9000 Gent, Belgium
8. Department of Physical Medicine and Physiotherapy, University Hospital Brussels, 1090 Brussels, Belgium
9. Unit of Physiotherapy, Department of Health and Rehabilitation, Institute of Neuroscience and Physiology, University of Gothenburg, 405 30 Gothenburg, Sweden
* Correspondence: astrid.lucie.lahousse@vub.be; Tel.: +32-(0)-247-745-27

Abstract: This review discusses chronic pain, multiple modifiable lifestyle factors, such as stress, insomnia, diet, obesity, smoking, alcohol consumption and physical activity, and the relationship between these lifestyle factors and pain after cancer. Chronic pain is known to be a common consequence of cancer treatments, which considerably impacts cancer survivors' quality of life when it remains untreated. Improvements in lifestyle behaviour are known to reduce mortality, comorbid conditions (i.e., cardiovascular diseases, other cancer, and recurrence) and cancer-related side-effects (i.e., fatigue and psychological issues). An inadequate stress response plays an important role in dysregulating the body's autonomic, endocrine, and immune responses, creating a problematic back loop with pain. Next, given the high vulnerability of cancer survivors to insomnia, addressing and treating those sleep problems should be another target in pain management due to its capacity to increase hyperalgesia. Furthermore, adherence to a healthy diet holds great anti-inflammatory potential for relieving pain after cancer. Additionally, a healthy diet might go hand in hand with weight reduction in the case of obesity. Consuming alcohol and smoking have an acute analgesic effect in the short-term, with evidence lacking in the long-term. However, this acute effect is outweighed by other harms on cancer survivors' general health. Last, informing patients about the benefits of an active lifestyle and reducing a sedentary lifestyle after cancer treatment must be emphasised when considering the proven benefits of physical activity in this population. A multimodal approach addressing all relevant lifestyle factors together seems appropriate for managing comorbid conditions, side-effects, and chronic pain after cancer. Further research is needed to evaluate whether modifiable lifestyle factors have a beneficial influence on chronic pain among cancer survivors.

Keywords: cancer survivor; chronic pain; lifestyle; diet; obesity; physical activity; stress; sleep

1. Introduction

Cancer has overtaken vascular diseases as the leading cause of death in high-income countries [1]. On top of that, it is expected that the global cancer burden will grow 47% by 2040 [2]. Despite these appalling numbers, cancer survivorship has fortunately increased to 70% in developed countries, mainly due to early detections and treatment advances [3].

Different definitions for cancer survivor (CS) exist, but according to a systematic review of Marzorati et al., (2017), the most widely used definition is: "being a CS, starts on the day of diagnosis and continues until the end of life" [4]. Three cancer survivorship phases can be distinguished: "acute survivorship" (i.e., early-stage or time during curative treatment), "permanent survivorship" (i.e., living with cancer or also called the palliative stage), and "extended survivorship" (i.e., cured but not free of suffering) [4]. This article focuses on the extended survivorship phase since it is difficult for cancer survivors (CSs) to recognize themselves as 'cured' if they continue to suffer after treatment completion [4]. Unfortunately, in this phase, an important proportion of these CSs will face unwanted and debilitating adverse effects that arise or persist beyond primary treatment, which is frightening and should therefore be dealt with seriously [5].

Chronic pain is one of these and occurs in 40% of CSs [6]. Chronic pain is defined by the International Association for the Study of Pain (IASP) as pain that persists or recurs for longer than three months [7]. Unrelieved pain can have considerable adverse consequences on a CSs' quality of life [6]. Therefore, providing CSs with optimal pain treatments is essential to reduce their psychological, physical, and socio-economic impact [6]. Although several initiatives attempted to increase awareness about (post) cancer pain (e.g., the Global Year Against Cancer Pain in 2008 promoted by IASP), chronic pain in CSs remains undertreated, misunderstood, and highly prevalent [6].

Nowadays, the National Comprehensive Cancer Network guidelines [8] advise pharmacological and non-pharmacological treatments for pain during cancer treatment, but after treatment, a decrease of pain medication is recommended to avoid the risk of addiction, misuse, and adverse effects such as opioid-induced hyperalgesia and sleeping disruptions. Unfortunately, shifting towards non-pharmacological treatments remains challenging for many oncologists since they are used to treat patients with acute pain associated with cancer or its therapy [9]. However, the aggressive and curative treatments, including surgery, chemo-, radio- and or maintenance therapy, are not the only factors contributing to the transition of acute to chronic pain. Other factors such as young age at diagnosis, depression, anxiety, low education, and negative lifestyle behaviour (e.g., high body mass index (BMI), low physical activity levels, high alcohol consumption, etc.) might have an impact as well [10–12]. Unfortunately, not all these factors are treatable or modifiable. However, new evidence on healthy lifestyle behaviour demonstrates promising results on pain, quality of life, cancer recurrence, psychological well-being [13–16]. A healthy lifestyle is defined as actions or method one initiate to achieve optimum health and lower the risk of disease or early death [17], which underlines the need to target (pain) multimodally and tailor treatment according to the CS's needs [18]. Therefore, the purpose of this paper is to review and update knowledge on chronic pain and modifiable lifestyle factors in CSs and to discuss the beneficial impact of modifiable lifestyle factors on chronic pain after cancer (Figure 1).

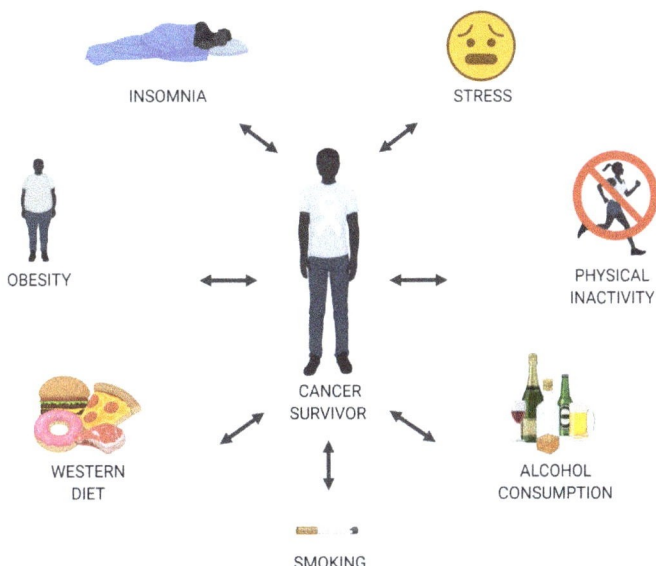

Figure 1. Discussed modifiable lifestyle factors in cancer survivors and might contribute to chronic pain after cancer (Creates with BioRender.com (accessed on: 26 November 2021)).

2. Methods

The best evidence regarding lifestyle behaviour and chronic pain in CSs was retrieved in PubMed and Web of Science up to September 2021. Relevant articles were selected by combining the following keywords: CS, chronic pain, lifestyle factors, risk factors, smoking, dietary intake, physical activity, obesity, medication, distress, stress, sleep disorders. To be included, articles had to meet the following criteria: (1) display original data in CSs; (2) address the aims of this review; (3) be published as full articles; and (4) written in English, Dutch, German or French. The following criteria were applied for exclusion: (1) articles reporting animal studies; and (2) studies with the following study design: case reports, congress proceedings, abstracts, letters to the editor, opinions or editorials.

3. State-of-the-Art

3.1. Pain

Chronic cancer-related pain represented in the International Classification of Diseases (ICD-11) differs from the pain of other chronic pain populations [19]. Chronic pain in CSs is caused by damage of primary cancer, its metastasis or its treatment, inducing chronic secondary pain syndromes such as musculoskeletal and neuropathic pains [7]. That can persist over time if no adequate pain management was provided initially [7].

Glare et al., (2014) published a comprehensive overview of the types of treatment-related cancer pain arising after the curative treatments [19]. For example, post-operative syndromes might occur after surgery, such as phantom pain after amputation, post-mastectomy pain and other complications [19]. Furthermore, chemo- and radiotherapy can also cause adverse effects. Chemotherapy, for example, can cause symmetrical painful numbness, burning, and tingling in both hands and feet. On top of that, it could also lead to osteoporosis, osteonecrosis, arthralgias, and myalgia. Radiotherapy can lead to serious adverse effects caused by ionising radiation, inducing reactive oxygen species (ROS) production, and DNA and regulatory proteins damage to targeted cells. These provoke apoptosis and increased inflammation in the exposed cells and the neighbouring cells by radiation-induced bystander effects, possibly leading to plexopathies and osteoradionecrosis [19,20]. Maintenance therapy like aromatase inhibitors can produce arthralgia and myalgia [19]. In addition to these adverse effects, health care providers have to evaluate new arising or aggravating pain complaints with caution because these can indicate a recurrence or a second malignant tumour [19].

Despite the existing guidelines, chronic pain remains underrecognized and mistreated in the extended survivorship phase [5]. Under recognition might be due to: (1) patients' belief that pain is inevitable and uncontrollable, causing them not to report pain to their physicians; and/or (2) physicians' poor knowledge of pain assessment methods [21]. Mistreatment of pain, on the other hand, might be due to: (1) suboptimal communication between CSs and physicians; (2) non-adherence of the patients due to misconception of pain medication; and/or (3) lack of knowledge or confidence of the physicians in applying pain management guidelines in the clinical field [22]. Moreover, CSs typically are insufficiently informed about the origin of their pain, the possibilities of pain relief, and how they can access support when needed, which might affect their happiness of having survived and beaten cancer [23–25].

Over the last decade, the education provided to CSs made a shift from a biomedical pain management, falling short in explaining persistent pain, to a biopsychosocial pain management [26]. This is in concordance with recent findings of the multidimensional aspect of pain [23]. Psychosocial factors, such as cognitive appraisals and expectations, are cornerstones in the patient's pain experience and might bring patients in a downward spiral if not considered [27]. The underlying mechanism can be explained by the fact that psychological factors and pain sensations share similar brain activity, such as the prefrontal cortex, thalamus, hypothalamus, and amygdala and might subsequently affect the descending nociceptive pathways of the periaqueductal grey and rostro-ventral medulla [28]. So, depressive mood, anxiety, and cognitions play an essential role in pain modulation, and the understanding of its mechanism is primordial for appropriate assessment and treatment [10,28]. One cognitive appraisal that gained attention in the past years is perceived injustice (PI) [29,30]. It is demonstrated that people experiencing PI, attribute blame to others for their suffering, have the tendency to interpret their losses as severe and irreparable, and experience a sense of unfairness [29] (*e.g., someone who never smoked yet was diagnosed with lung cancer*). A systematic review showed significant associations between PI and worse pain-related outcomes, including more intense pain, more disability, and worse mental health [31]. These along with lower quality of life are seen in breast CSs with higher PI scores, and PI rather than pain catastrophizing mediates the relationship between pain and quality of life [32]. A more intense expression in terms of their suffering and loss is seen due to increased maladaptive pain behaviour. In turn, this increases the likelihood of being prescribed opioids [29,33]. People displaying more maladaptive pain behaviour affect clinicians' decision to prescribe opioids [34]. Considering the known long-term adverse effects of long-term opioid use [9] and the possibility of developing opiate-induced hyperalgesia [35], PI seems to be a new perspective that should be further investigated in the future.

Other factors that also play a vital role in chronic pain after cancer are associated with patients' healthy lifestyle behaviour. Addressing modifiable lifestyle factors is essential to prevent recurrence of cancer, adverse effects, mortality, as well as improving quality of life and pain relief [36,37]. These factors' impacts and their relationship with pain in CSs are discussed in detail in the following sections of this paper (Figure 2).

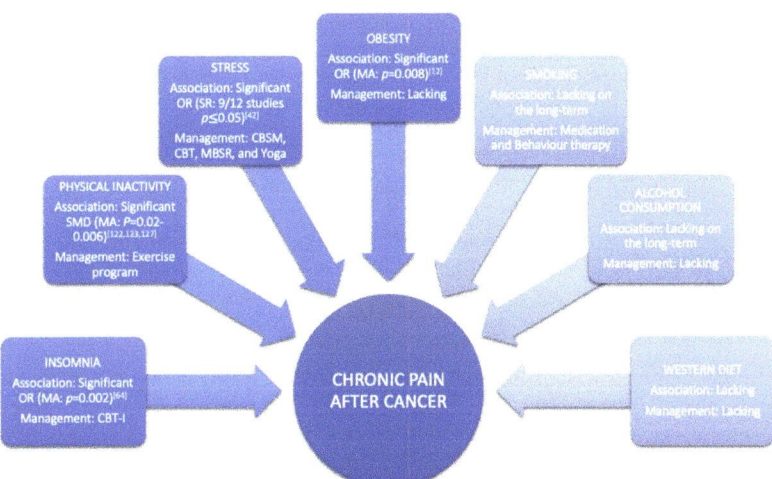

Figure 2. Evidence of modifiable lifestyle factors contributing to chronic pain in cancer survivors. Abbreviations: CBT(-I): Cognitive behavioural therapy (Insomnia); CBSM: Cognitive Behavioural Stress Management; MA: Meta-analysis; MBSR: Mindfulness-based Stress Reduction; OR: Odds Ratio.

3.2. Lifestyle Behaviour

3.2.1. Stress

Stress has been categorised as "the health epidemic of the 21st century" by the World Health Organization (WHO) [38]. It has been defined as a state, whether an actual or perceived event disturbs the physiological homeostasis or the psychological well-being [39,40]. About 12.6% of CSs will develop a lifetime cancer-related post-traumatic stress disorder [41]. Additionally, during survivorship, a substantial proportion of CSs are confronting lingering adverse events and/or experiencing an intense fear of recurrence, both causing anxiety and major distress [42]. Cancer-related distress is defined as a state during which CS cannot deal with their cancer, treatment, or adverse effects due to interference of a multifactorial unpleasant psychological, social, spiritual, or physical event. Distress can transfer normal feelings to disabling problems such as panic attacks, depression, anxiety, existential crises [43]. The presence of chronic stress or distress sustains the overproduction of pro-inflammatory cytokines, which in turn induces fatigue, sleep disorders, depression, and symptoms of sickness [44]. The other stress-related mechanisms behind a heightened inflammation level are higher stress-induced sympathetic activity or a dysregulated hypothalamic-pituitary-adrenal axis (and associated cortisol dysbalance as a characteristic feature of long-term stress exposure) [44,45]. New insights also point out that distress in CSs changes the function and/or structure of some areas of the brain, such as the thalamus, amygdala, prefrontal cortex, hippocampus, subgenual area, hypothalamus, basal ganglia and insula, which are mainly the same areas associated with chronic pain [28,46]. Understanding these changes may open new treatment perspectives and enhance the quality of provided interventions for distress among CSs.

Early screening of distress might enhance treatment response [42,47]. As stated in the systematic review of Syrowatka et al., (2017), several predictors for distress after cancer could be identified according to the provided treatment, sociodemographic characteristics, comorbidities, and modifiable lifestyle factors (Table 1, Figure 2) [42]. Interestingly, pain is one of the manageable risk factors for distress creating a problematic back loop because distress, in turn, promotes pain by dysregulating the autonomic, endocrine, and immune response [44,48]. This vicious cycle can be interrupted by cognitive behavioural stress management (CBSM) consisting of aspects of cognitive behavioural therapy (CBT) [49–51] or, more precisely, coping skills for stress management combined with relaxation training [45,52–54]. According to recent published systematic reviews and meta-analyses, CBT has a beneficial effect on cortisol secretion, distress, anxiety, depression, emotional well-being, and negative thoughts in CSs [49–51]. Mindfulness-based stress reduction (MBSR) and yoga have also shown promising results on distress in CSs (Figure 2) [52–54].

3.2.2. Sleep

Insomnia is one the most frequently experienced survivorship concerns and is characterised by difficulty with sleep initiation, duration, consolidation, and quality, resulting in daytime impairments and distress. These difficulties have to occur at least three times a week for more than one month [55]. Insomnia affects more than 30% of CSs years after treatment ending [56–58]. The two-fold higher prevalence rate in comparison to the general population can be attributed to the emotional consequences of cancer diagnosis, the direct effects of cancer treatment, and its side-effects [56]. Among cancer patients, prevalence numbers of insomnia are the highest in breast and gynaecologic cancers compared to prostate cancer [56]. Breast CSs are particularly vulnerable to insomnia due to fear of recurrence, endocrine therapy, and other hormonal changes related to breast cancer treatment [59–61]. Due to hormonal changes, about 85% of breast CSs will report hot flushes, night sweats and arthralgia, resulting in multiple awakenings throughout the night [62,63]. Moreover, breast CSs with hot flushes and (joint) pain are respectively 2.25 (95% CI 1.64–3.08) and 2.31 (95% CI 1.36–3.92) more likely to develop sleep problems (Table 1, Figure 2) [64]. On the other hand, in non-cancer populations, insomnia forms a higher risk for developing future chronic pain disorders compared to chronic pain leading to new insomnia cases [65]. Sleep problems lower pain thresholds and exacerbate response to painful stimuli by dysregulating the immune system, hypothalamus-pituitary-adrenal axis, monoaminergic pathways, and endogenous substances (adenosine, nitric oxide, melatonin, and orexin), which will, for example, increase the pro-inflammatory state [66].

Based on compelling efficacy data, CBT for insomnia (CBT-I) is the gold standard treatment for insomnia (Figure 2) [67]. CBT-I addresses cognitive and behavioural factors that perpetuate insomnia using a multi-component treatment that includes sleep hygiene, stimulus control, sleep restriction, cognitive therapy and relaxation training [68]. The efficacy of CBT-I in CSs was investigated by a systematic review of Johnson et al., (2016) [57] in which they demonstrated that CBT-I improves insomnia symptom severity, sleep efficiency, sleep onset latency, and wake after sleep onset in CSs. The same research question was investigated specifically in breast CSs by a recent review of Ma et al., (2021) [69], in which moderate to large treatment effects were found with clinically significant effects lasting up to one year after therapy for insomnia symptom severity, sleep efficiency and sleep onset latency. Even though solid evidence has shown that CBT-I improves sleep in CSs [57], it remains underused and not readily available in the community or clinical settings [70]. Barriers on the provider level are a shortage of CBT-I specialists and a lack of physician training about sleep [71,72]. On the patient level, barriers include limited understanding of the consequences of insomnia, limited awareness of available treatment options and lack of treatment adherence due to the possible burdensome treatment format [73,74]. There is no doubt about the effectiveness of CBT-I in CSs. However, future studies are needed to investigate the optimal integration of the CBT-I components before adding to the pain management.

3.2.3. Diet

Dietary Intake

Dietary recommendations have only recently been brought into the picture for CSs treatment; therefore, the literature is sparse and limited to breast CSs. However, nutritional guidelines have been introduced by the National Cancer Institute, American Cancer Society, Academy of Nutrition to encourage CSs to start a healthy and prudent diet [13,75]. Unfortunately, the adherence is low because CSs have no guarantee that their prognosis will improve by adopting a healthy diet [76]. According to a meta-analysis of cohort studies, a Western diet, which is characterised by a high consumption of eggs, red meats, and processed foods, is associated with a higher risk of mortality (odds ratio = 1.51; 95% CI 1.24–1.85) and cancer recurrence (odds ratio = 1.34; 95% CI 0.61–2.92) in CSs [77]. However, weak evidence suggests that CSs may be able to reduce their mortality and cancer recurrence rate by switching to a healthy diet that consists of fruits, vegetables, fish, and whole grains after diagnosis [78]. A healthy diet is usually rich in anti-oxidative, anti-inflammatory, endothelial protective, metabolic substances, which affect tumour growth and promote cancer apoptosis [79]. As advised by different associations, nutritional counselling should be provided by registered dietitians specialised in oncology [13].

Furthermore, ongoing research shows that food could have both an adverse and a beneficial influence on chronic pain. A recent systematic review revealed that studies examining whether diet influences chronic pain in CSs are essentially lacking (Table 1) [80]. Nevertheless, evidence in breast CSs points out some significant relation between pain and nutrition. A network meta-analysis for therapeutic options for aromatase inhibitor-associated arthralgia in breast cancer has suggested that omega-3 fatty acids might be effective in reducing pain severity scores and pointed out the need for further evaluation for omega-3 fatty acids as well as vitamin D (Table 1) [81]. Additionally, a cross-sectional study showed clearly that breast CSs who were well-nourished or anabolic according to category A of the patient-generated subjective global assessment (PG-SGA) had fewer pain symptoms than those who were malnourished category B of PG-SGA [82].

As discussed earlier, nutritional sciences are only now beginning to address chronic pain in CSs. However, why should "diet" be advised in chronic pain management to CSs? Knowing the benefits and drawbacks of various diets for survivors with chronic pain could be the key to finding a clear answer. The most important vision of implementing a specific diet in pain management is based on using regulatory effects of nutrition on several pain mechanisms with no or bare minimum side effects. This could provide a long-term, sustainable, and cost-effective pain management alternative for CSs. Therefore, in the future, interdisciplinary collaboration across researchers and clinicians is needed to unravel the role of nutrition in pain-related mechanisms and its implications on pain reduction in CSs. Currently, the lack of evidence supporting the added value of dietary interventions for chronic pain management in CSs precludes to advise its use (Figure 2).

Obesity

Obesity is a condition characterised by an increase in body fat [83,84]. At the neurobiological level, obesity is considered to cause pain through various mechanisms, including inflammation and hormone imbalance [85]. At the mechanical level, obesity can also cause pain by structural overloading [84,86], which can lead to altered body posture and joint misuse [87]. The latest review in taxane- and platinum-treated CSs demonstrated a good-to-moderate relationship between obesity and higher severity or incidence of chemotherapy-induced peripheral neuropathy (CIPN), with moderate evidence showing diabetes did not increase incidence or severity of CIPN [88]. Furthermore, a systematic review with meta-analyses of Leysen et al., (2017) demonstrated that breast CSs with a BMI > 30 have a higher risk (odds ratio = 1.34, 95% CI 1.08–1.67) of developing pain (Table 1, Figure 2) [12]. However, more research is needed to determine the long-term impact of obesity among the expanding population of CSs [89]. Studies looking at the link between changes in body mass index, fat mass, inflammatory markers, and chronic pain might help us better comprehend the relationship between these variables in the CS population. Additionally, well-designed, high-quality randomised controlled trials on the effect of combined weight loss/pain therapies are required to inform patients and clinicians on how to personalise the approach to reduce chronic pain prevalence, intensity, or severity in CSs through obesity management (Figure 2).

3.2.4. Smoking

Smoking tobacco and, to a lesser extent, e-cigarettes is well-known to negatively influence cancer's prognosis and forms a major risk factor for various cancer types and several other chronic diseases [90–92]. Smoking cessation has a favourable effect on treatment efficacy, psychological well-being and general quality of life [93]. The National Comprehensive Cancer Network offers a guideline for smoking cessation, consisting of pharmacotherapy (e.g., nicotine replacement therapy or varenicline) and behaviour therapy (Figure 2) [47,94]. This program is more successful when initiated at the time of diagnosis because an early start avoids more adverse effects [90]. Patients who continue to smoke have a higher likelihood of facing post-operative complications due to (wound) infections, failed reconstruction and tissue necrosis, which could lead to prolonged hospitalisation [95,96]. Unfortunately, a big proportion of young CSs continue to smoke after their diagnosis. Approximately 25.2% of CSs aged 18 to 44 years were current smokers compared to 15.8% in the general population [97]. Thus, during the survivor phase, additional support should be provided to target patients' barriers to smoking cessation to prevent cancer recurrence.

Pain might be one of the barriers to smoking cessation in CSs [98]. An observational study by Aigner et al., (2016) demonstrated that when patients experience higher pain levels, they usually smoke a larger number of cigarettes during these days and initiate fewer attempts to quit smoking [98]. This can be explained by the fact that nicotine produces an acute analgesic effect, making it much harder for them to stop due to the rewarding sensation they experience [99]. Despite its short-term analgesic effect, tobacco smoking sustains pain in the long-term [93]. This underlines the importance of incorporating anti-smoking medications in CSs with pain to avoid relapse during nicotine withdrawal [99]. Moreover, pain management should be added to the counselling aspect to enhance the patient's knowledge, which in turn, might improve their adherence to the whole smoking cessation program [98]. Furthermore, the 5As (Ask, Advise, Assess, Assist, Arrange) approach, which assesses the willingness of the patient to quit smoking, is no longer recommended since studies have demonstrated that smokers who did not feel ready to quit smoking at the same rate as those who wanted to [100]. The model with the most promising results might be "opt-out", during which health care providers offer counselling and pharmacotherapy to all smokers, which is more ethical [101]. However, research on how to integrate this approach in current cancer care for CSs is needed.

3.2.5. Alcohol Consumption

Similar to smoking, alcohol consumption is a preventable risk factor for liver, oesophageal, colorectal, breast, head, neck, and many other cancers [102]. It is established that excessive or binge drinking enhances the likelihood of cancer recurrence, bad prognosis, or death [77]. Despite this, up to now, no evidence supports or refutes that drinking with moderation ($\leq$1 drink for women and $\leq$2 drinks for men per day) is associated with a lower risk of cancer [103–105]. On top of this, some studies show a reduction in risk due to moderate alcohol intake, which might be explained by confounders, and/or the anti-cancer effect of polyphenols (present in wine) [106] or phytoestrogen and polysaccharides (present in beer) that lower free testosterone, inducing prostate cancer [107,108]. However, these small benefits are quickly outweighed by other harms of alcohol consumption. Furthermore, a growing trend in alcohol intake among CSs is observed, but no explanation for this trend could be found [109]. Nevertheless, alcohol consumption can initiate people to smoke or smoke even more [109]. Combining both multiplies their adverse effects because alcohol slows down the body's capacity to eliminate the carcinogenic chemicals of smoking [97,109,110]. These findings highlight the importance of increasing CSs' awareness about these lifestyle factors.

The impact of alcohol use on pain is poorly investigated in CSs, but according to one systematic review of two cohort studies, the risk of developing pain can be reduced by alcohol use (Table 1) [12]. This finding might be misleading due to the fact that alcohol has an acute analgesic effect [111]. In non-cancer populations, studies demonstrated that this analgesic effect diminishes over time, and there is an association between chronic pain and alcohol consumption [112]. This pain might be evoked by developing alcoholic neuropathy, musculoskeletal disorders, or alcohol withdrawal [112]. Conversely, chronic pain increases the risk of alcohol abuse [113]. Nevertheless, psychosocial factors are also highly present in patients with alcohol abuse and can be attributed to abnormalities in the reward system of the brain [114]. Additionally, a recently published study demonstrated that chronic pain patients with high levels of pain catastrophising are more likely to be heavy drinkers [115]. General advice on alcohol consumption after cancer is currently not possible due to the high variability of results in different CSs. Therefore, health care providers should tailor their advice according to cancer types and patients [116]. Within that view, an overview of recommendations regarding individualised alcohol consumption for each CS type could support clinicians in doing so, yet such evidence-based recommendations are currently lacking (Figure 2).

3.2.6. Physical Activity

Being physically active after a cancer diagnosis improves CSs' survival rate by 30% [117–119], which underlines that healthy behaviour during the extended survival phase is essential [117]. The American College of Sports Medicine, American Cancer Society and the US Department of Health and Human Services developed exercise guidelines that advise every CS to engage weekly in 75 min of vigorous-intensity or 150 min of moderate-intensity aerobic physical activity [90,120,121]. For instance, the evidence demonstrated that supervised physical activity reduces cancer-related fatigue, depression, and increases quality of life, cardiovascular and musculoskeletal fitness in CSs [14–16]. Additional beneficial effects of physical activity were also seen on musculoskeletal pain and stiffness in breast CSs taking aromatase inhibitors for a long period (Table 1, Figure 2) [81,122,123]. However, only few CSs attain the recommended physical activity levels, with pain being an important limiting factor [116,124]. Inappropriate beliefs regarding the expected outcome of physical activity represent a major barrier for CSs to engage in physical activity programs. For example, some breast CSs fear that resistance exercises can aggravate cancer-related lymphedema, which is proven to be wrong as resistance exercises are perfectly safe in this group and do not increase lymphedema [125], others might fear that exercise can exacerbate their pain, which was refuted by systematic reviews with meta-analyses in CSs and a Cochrane review in chronic non-cancer pain populations, demonstrating that physical activity has a small positive effect on pain (Table 1, Figure 2) [123,126,127]. Despite all this evidence, patients' adherence to physical activity remains low and remains a bottleneck in current care [128]. Therefore, how to reduce a sedentary lifestyle in CSs with chronic pain should be more thoroughly investigated and implemented in guidelines, and patients should be better informed about the benefits of an active lifestyle [128].

Identifying predictors of adherence will offer the possibility to provide personalised guidance to CSs who are less likely to adhere to exercise, which will undoubtedly lead to better treatment outcomes [129]. According to a systematic review, behavioural (i.e., motivation) and sociodemographic predictors (i.e., distance and social support of the family or therapists) should be addressed [130]. To improve CSs' exercise motivation or lifestyle behaviours, motivational interviewing can be used [131]. During this patient-centred approach, five different stages can be distinguished: pre-contemplation, contemplation, preparation, action, and maintenance. In each stage, behaviour changes will be tackled differently [130,131]. A Cochrane review concluded that exercise interventions with determined goals, graded activity, and behaviour change reached the highest adherence in CSs [118]. Behavioural graded activity is such an intervention that combines these three components and aims (i.e., determined goals, graded activity, and behaviour change) to target patients' difficulties and complaints during their daily living [132]. This approach might enhance patients' willingness to adhere to healthy behaviour compared to other exercise interventions. Additionally, in recent years, alternative therapies such as mindfulness-based approaches, hypnosis and yoga gained importance and demonstrated significant beneficial effects on quality of life, psychological distress, anxiety, depression, fear of cancer recurrence, fatigue, sleep, and pain [133–135]. Obviously, mindfulness-based approaches and yoga fit into the 'stress management' category as well, and therefore potentially serve two lifestyle factors (i.e., stress and physical therapy). However, more research is needed to find the optimal approach for higher long-term adherence to an active lifestyle in CSs.

Table 1. Evidence of lifestyle factors on pain in cancer survivors. Abbreviations: AIA: Aromatase Inhibitor-associated Arthralgia; C: Cohort; CI: Confidence Interval; CIPN: Chemotherapy-Induced Peripheral Neurotoxicity; CS: Cross-sectional Study; ES: Effect Size; I^2: Heterogeneity; MD: Mean Difference; OR: Odds Ratio; p: p-value; RCT: Randomized Controlled Trial; SMD: Standardized Mean Difference; SORT: Strength of Recommendation Taxonomy.

Lifestyle Factor	First Author, Year Published, Study Type	Included Population	Number of Included Studies (n_1) and Participants (n_2)	Detail of Lifestyle Factor/Intervention Assessed	Main Results in Context of the Specified State-of-the-Art	Level of Evidence [136]
Alcohol consumption	Leysen et al., 2017, Systematic review with meta-analysis [12]	Breast Cancer Survivors	$n_1 = 2$ (1 CS and 1 C) and $n_2 = 2519$	Alcohol use	Alcohol (OR 0.94, 95% CI [0.47, 1.89], $p = 0.86$, $I^2 = 67\%$) was not a predictor for pain, Inconsistent and low evidence	3b
Diet	Kim et al., 2018, Systematic review of systematic reviews [81]	Breast Cancer Survivors with AIA	$n_1 = 3$ (systematic review of RCT), and $n_{2\_Omega-3} = 817$, and $n_{2\_VD} = 453$	Omega-3 Fatty Acids, and Vitamin D	Significant effects were found for omega-3 fatty acids (MD -2.10, 95% CI [-3.23, -0.97]), and vitamin D (MD 0.63, 95% CI [0.13, 1.13]) on pain, Low evidence	1a
	Yilmaz et al., 2021, Systematic review [80]	Cancer Survivors	$n_1 = 2$ (uncontrolled clinical trial) and $n_2 = 77$	Nutritional supplements: vitamin C, chondroitin, and glucosamine	Lack of evidence	2a
Obesity	Leysen et al., 2017, Systematic review with meta-analysis [12]	Breast Cancer Survivors	$n_1 = 7$ (4 CS and 3 C) and $n_2 = 5573$	BMI	BMI > 30 (OR 1.34, 95% CI [1.08, 1.67], $p = 0.008$, $I^2 = 33\%$,) was a predictor for pain, Consistent and low evidence	3b
	Timmins et al., 2021, Systematic review [88]	Cancer Survivors	$n_1 = 16$ (3 CS, 11 C, and 2 retrospective chart review) and $n_2 = 14{,}033$	Obesity	According to the SORT: the association between obesity and CIPN was good-to-moderate patient-centred evidence	3b

Table 1. Cont.

Lifestyle Factor	First Author, Year Published, Study Type	Included Population	Number of Included Studies (n_1) and Participants (n_2)	Detail of Lifestyle Factor/Intervention Assessed	Main Results in Context of the Specified State-of-the-Art	Level of Evidence [136]
Physical Activity	Boing et al., 2020, Systematic review with meta-analysis [123]	Breast Cancer Survivors with AIA	$n_1 = 3$ (2 RCT, 1 pilot study), and $n_2 = 118$	Exercise	Significant effect was found on pain (SMD −0.55, 95 % CI [−1.11, −0.00], $p = 0.05$ $I^2 = 80\%$), Low Evidence	1b
	Kim et al., 2018, Systematic review of systematic reviews [81]	Breast Cancer Survivors with AIA	$n_1 = 2$ (systematic review of RCT), and $n_2 = 262$	Aerobic Exercise	No significant effect was found on pain (MD −0.80, 95% CI [−1.33, 0.016]), Low evidence	1a
	Lavín-Pérez et al., 2021, Systematic review with meta-analysis [127]	Cancer Survivors	$n_1 = 7$ (RCT), and $n_2 = 355$	Exercise (HIT)	Significant effect was found on pain (SMD −0.18, 95% CI [−0.34, −0.02], $p = 0.02$, $I^2 = 4\%$), Moderate evidence	1a
	Lu et al., 2020, Systematic review with meta-analysis [122]	Breast Cancer Survivors with AIA	$n_1 = 6$ (RCT), and $n_2 = 416$	Exercise	Significant effect was found on pain (SMD −0.46, 95% CI [−0.79, −0.13], $p = 0.006$, $I^2 = 63\%$), Moderate evidence	1a
	Timmins et al., 2021, Systematic review [88]	Cancer Survivors	$n_1 = 5$ (2 C and 3 CS), and $n_2 = 3950$	Low physical activity	According to the SORT: the association between physical inactivity and CIPN was of moderate evidence	3b
Sleep	Leysen et al., 2019, Systematic review with meta-analysis [64]	Breast Cancer Survivors	$n_1 = 4$ (2 CS and 2 C) and $n_2 = 1907$	Sleep Disturbances	Pain was a predictor for sleep disturbances (OR 1.68, 95% CI [1.19, 2.37], $p = 0.05$, $I^2 = 55\%$, after subgroup analysis OR 2.31, 95% CI [1.36, 3.92], $p = 0.002$, $I^2 = 27\%$)	3b
Smoking	Leysen et al., 2017, Systematic review with meta-analysis [12]	Breast Cancer Survivors	$n_1 = 2$ (1 CS and 1 C) and $n_2 = 2519$	Smoking status	Smoking (OR 0.75, 95% CI [0.62, 0.92], $p = 0.005$, $I^2 = 0\%$) was not a predictor for pain, Consistent and low evidence	3b

Table 1. Cont.

Lifestyle Factor	First Author, Year Published, Study Type	Included Population	Number of Included Studies (n_1) and Participants (n_2)	Detail of Lifestyle Factor/Intervention Assessed	Main Results in Context of the Specified State-of-the-Art	Level of Evidence [136]
Stress	Syrowatka et al., 2017, Systematic review [42]	Breast Cancer Survivors	n_1 = 12 (6 CS and 6 C) and n_2 = 7842	Distress	Pain was significantly associated with distress: 9/12 studies (75%)	3b
Intervention	Chang et al., 2020, Systematic review with meta-analysis [54]	Breast Cancer Survivors	n_1 = 5 (RCT) and n_2 = 827	Mindfulness-Based interventions	No significant effect was found on pain (SMD −0.39, 95% CI, [−0.81, 0.03], p = 0.07, I^2 = 85%), Moderate evidence	1a
	Cillessen et al., 2019, Systematic review with meta-analysis [133]	Cancer Patients and Survivors	n_1 = 4 (RCT) and n_2 = 587	Mindfulness-Based interventions	Significant effect was found on pain (ES 0.2, 95% CI [0.04, 0.36], p = 0.16, I^2 = 0%), Moderate evidence	1a
	Martinez-Miranda [26]	Breast Cancer Survivors	n_1 = 2 (RCT) and n_2 = 134	Patient Education	No significant effect was found on pain (SMD −0.05, 95% CI [−0.26, 0.17], p = 0.67, I^2 = 0%, Low evidence	1a
	Silva et al., 2019, Systematic review [137]	Cancer Survivors	n_1 = 4 (4 quasi-experimental studies), and n_2 = 522	Promoting healthy behaviour by mHealth apps	Effect found on pain was inconsistent and of low quality of evidence	2b

4. Future Directions for Scientists

First, it is recommended that researchers make a clear distinction between CSs' phases when initiating and reporting studies in CSs. Currently, the term CS is too globally used, making it difficult to compare or combine results of studies due to their high heterogeneity. An individual in palliative care has different needs than an individual that is cured of cancer; however, both are CSs according to the most widely used definition [4]. A distinction between the different phases has been described by Mullan et al., in 1985 [138]. Unfortunately, these terms are not frequently used in the literature [138] even though a clear distinction between phases could help clinicians to communicate more easily and to provide the appropriate care to patients' needs according to their phase in the survival of cancer.

Second, most studies were performed on Caucasian breast CSs with high socio-economic status. This population is more likely to have a higher adherence and willingness to change their lifestyle habits [139]. However, to reach a better understanding of barriers for lifestyle changes, research needs to be performed among CS populations with diverse socio-economic backgrounds. This way, oncological care for CSs can be more tailored to patients of different gender, race, and socio-economic capacities.

Third, future studies regarding lifestyle factors in CSs should more thoroughly account for possible confounders. Indeed, research studying a particular lifestyle factor should not only be adjusted for age, gender, education, and so forth, but also for other established lifestyle factors, which might be a considerable confounder. Furthermore, the effects of lifestyle factors in CSs are most often observed over a short period, preventing to draw conclusions regarding long-term impact of lifestyle factors in CSs. More research is warranted to observe the long-term effects of pain management and healthy lifestyle interventions in CSs.

5. Future Directions for Clinicians

The literature indicates that implementing healthy lifestyle habits in CSs has low compliance rates [140]. A barrier that might cause low adherence to healthy lifestyle behaviours is the burdensome treatment format of most behavioural interventions [73,74]. Therefore, stepped care models might provide clinicians with a possible solution to improve the feasibility and deliver care efficiently [141]. In existing stepped care models, the first step is typically a form of self-management therapy (e.g., recommendations) with the possibility to progress to the highest step of six to eight individual sessions with a specialist, if needed [142,143]. For example, a recent study in CSs demonstrated that more than 50% of CSs with insomnia benefit form a one-hour group-delivered session that empowers CSs by teaching them about sleep health and provides specific information on how to adapt their sleep behaviours [142]. Interestingly, they found that CSs who had experienced sleep problems for a shorter period and perceived less burden from their sleep problems were most likely to benefit from the one-hour program, suggesting that it is crucial to identify CS with sleep problems as soon as possible to enhance the efficacy of low-intensity interventions [142]. However, further research is warranted before implementing stepped care for the other lifestyle factors. In addition, systematic reviews demonstrated promising findings for virtual therapy, suggesting that virtual interventions might be a possible option to enhance access to care, which solves the distance issue [69,137,144].

Furthermore, to reduce the treatment burden, clinicians should perform early screenings and identify negative predictors to improve patients' self-efficacy to sustain a healthy lifestyle. Developing evidence-based guidelines, including algorithms with practical triage and referral plans to other healthcare professionals, will improve survivorship care. Enhancing the productivity of oncological care by 2025 is of utmost importance because there will be a shortage of oncologists due to the growing cancer population [145]. Besides that, many clinicians have difficulties providing the ideal pain management plan and delivering health promotion guidance due to a lack of knowledge [22]. Supplementary support and educational interventions should be organized for health care providers to enhance their expertise and confidence in this field.

Another recommendation for future clinical practice is considering the use of pain neuroscience education as a way to decrease the threatening nature of pain, catastrophic thinking and fear-avoidance beliefs in CSs [146]. Cancer patients indicate themselves that they have insufficient knowledge regarding pain during or after cancer, what the possibilities of pain relief are and how they can access support when needed [24,25]. When comparing pain knowledge between CSs, healthy controls and caregivers, CSs had the lowest pain knowledge of the three groups [147]. Education about pain is underused in the field of oncology and non-existent in the survivorship phase [148]. Pain neuroscience education can clear the path for more active approaches to pain management, including providing lifestyle interventions. Manuals with guidelines for clinicians on how to explain pain following cancer [146], including accounting for perceived injustice during pain neuroscience education [149], are available to support clinicians in doing so.

Lastly, this state-of-the-art paper underlines once more the complexity of managing chronic pain in CSs. As discussed previously, adopting a healthy lifestyle might have a beneficial influence on the chronic pain of CSs. Unfortunately, there is currently a lack of research about the effectiveness of modifiable lifestyle factors on pain. Moreover, pain in CSs should be targeted on cognitive, behavioural, sensory and emotional levels due to its complexity [18]. Therefore, all pain interventions should be multidisciplinary and personalized for each CS [19].

6. Conclusions

Emerging evidence shows that CSs find it challenging to receive optimal treatment plans for their burdens, and support or reinforcement to maintain a healthy lifestyle. Therefore, it is crucially important to prepare clinicians well, so they can provide guidance along and after primary treatment. For chronic pain in CSs, it is primordial to identify factors that contribute to the transition of acute to chronic pain in CSs because chronic pain remains underrecognized and mistreated in this population. Furthermore, a proper definition between CSs' phases should be developed for optimal research and treatment. In the clinical field, new psychosocial factors and modifiable lifestyle factors should be targeted to improve pain relief in CSs.

Modifiable lifestyle factors and their impact on pain have been discussed in depth in this paper and are, for instance, stress, insomnia, diet, obesity, smoking, alcohol consumption and physical activity. First, an inappropriate stress response promotes pain by dysregulating the autonomic, endocrine, and immune response creating a problematic back loop because pain is a manageable risk factor for distress. The stress response can be managed by CBSM, CBT, MBSR and yoga. Second, sleep and pain also form a vicious cycle (sleep problems exacerbate response to nociceptive stimuli and pain can disturb sleep quality) that CBT-I can break. Third, guidelines recommend prudent diets in CSs. However, more research is needed to unravel the role of nutrition and obesity in CSs. Fourth, alcohol consumption and smoking are both negative lifestyle behaviours that impact patients' general health. Smoking cessation should consist of behaviour therapy and medication. Last, physical activity demonstrates its beneficial impact in several systematic reviews. However, the adherence is low and new treatment strategies such as motivational interviewing or BGA should be investigated in CSs to increase treatment outcomes in the long-term.

In the future, there will be an insufficient number of professionals (oncologists) due to the growing cancer population [150,151]. Therefore, it is a priority that researchers refine current treatment plans and define the benefits of modifiable lifestyle factors and their impact on chronic pain in CSs.

Author Contributions: Conceptualization, A.L., E.R. (Eva Roose), L.L., S.T.Y., K.M., F.R., E.R. (Emma Rheel), D.B., and J.N.; methodology, A.L. and J.N.; software, A.L.; validation, A.L., E.R. (Eva Roose), L.L., S.T.Y., K.M., F.R., E.R. (Emma Rheel), D.B., and J.N.; investigation, A.L., E.R. (Eva Roose), L.L., S.T.Y., and J.N.; writing—original draft preparation, A.L., E.R. (Eva Roose), L.L., S.T.Y., K.M., F.R., E.R. (Emma Rheel), D.B., and J.N.; writing—review and editing, A.L., L.L., S.T.Y., F.R., and J.N.; visualization, A.L.; funding acquisition, A.L., E.R. (Eva Roose), L.L., S.T.Y., E.R. (Emma Rheel), and J.N. All authors have read and agreed to the published version of the manuscript.

Funding: A.L. is a research fellow funded by the Research Foundation Flanders (Fonds Wetenschappelijk Onderzoek-FWO), Belgium (grant number 11B1920N). E.R. is funded by Stand Up to Cancer (Kom op tegen Kanker-KOTK), a Belgian cancer charity (project code ANI251). L.L. is a postdoctoral research fellow appointed on 2 funded projects, one by the Research Foundation Flanders (FWO) (grant number G040919N) and one by Stand up to Cancer (KOTK-project code ANI251). S.T.Y. is funded by the Ministry of National Education of the Turkish State as scholarship student for her Ph.D. research program. J.N. and E.R. are holders of a chair on oncological rehabilitation funded by the Berekuyl Academy/European College for Decongestive Lymphatic Therapy, the Netherlands.

Institutional Review Board Statement: Not applicable.

Informed Consent Statement: Not applicable.

Data Availability Statement: Not applicable.

Acknowledgments: We thank K. Ickmans (Vrije Universiteit Brussel) for creating Figure 1 with BioRender.com.

Conflicts of Interest: The authors declare no conflict of interest. The funders had no role in the design of the study; in the collection, analyses, or interpretation of data; in the writing of the manuscript, or in the decision to publish the results.

References

1. Mahase, E. Cancer ovet alertakes CVD to become leading cause of death in high income countries. *BMJ* **2019**, *366*, l5368. [CrossRef]
2. Sung, H.; Ferlay, J.; Siegel, R.; Laversanne, M.; Soerjomataram, I.; Jemal, A.; Bray, F. Global Cancer Statistics 2020: GLOBOCAN Estimates of Incidence and Mortality Worldwide for 36 Cancers in 185 Countries. *CA Cancer J. Clin.* **2021**, *71*, 209–249. [CrossRef] [PubMed]
3. Viale, P.H. The American Cancer Society's facts & figures: 2020 edition. *J. Adv. Pract. Oncol.* **2020**, *11*, 135.
4. Marzorati, C.; Riva, S.; Pravettoni, G. Who Is a Cancer Survivor? A Systematic Review of Published Definitions. *J. Cancer Educ.* **2017**, *32*, 228–237. [CrossRef] [PubMed]
5. Pachman, D.R.; Barton, D.L.; Swetz, K.M.; Loprinzi, C.L. Troublesome symptoms in cancer survivors: Fatigue, insomnia, neuropathy, and pain. *J. Clin. Oncol.* **2012**, *30*, 3687–3696. [CrossRef] [PubMed]
6. Van den Beuken-van Everdingen, M.H.; Hochstenbach, L.M.; Joosten, E.A.; Tjan-Heijnen, V.C.; Janssen, D.J. Update on Prevalence of Pain in Patients With Cancer: Systematic Review and Meta-Analysis. *J. Pain Symptom Manag.* **2016**, *51*, 1070–1090.e9. [CrossRef]
7. Bennett, M.I.; Kaasa, S.; Barke, A.; Korwisi, B.; Rief, W.; Treede, R.D. The IASP classification of chronic pain for ICD-11: Chronic cancer-related pain. *Pain* **2019**, *160*, 38–44. [CrossRef]
8. Tevaarwerk, A.; Denlinger, C.S.; Sanft, T.; Ansbaugh, S.M.; Armenian, S.; Baker, K.S.; Broderick, G.; Day, A.; Demark-Wahnefried, W.; Dickinson, K.; et al. Survivorship, Version 1.2021: Featured Updates to the NCCN Guidelines. *J. Natl. Compr. Cancer Netw.* **2021**, *19*, 676–685. [CrossRef] [PubMed]
9. Paice, J.A.; Portenoy, R.; Lacchetti, C.; Campbell, T.; Cheville, A.; Citron, M.; Constine, L.S.; Cooper, A.; Glare, P.; Keefe, F. Management of Chronic Pain in Survivors of Adult Cancers: American Society of Clinical Oncology Clinical Practice Guideline. *J. Clin. Oncol.* **2016**, *34*, 3325–3345. [CrossRef]
10. Moloney, N.A.; Pocovi, N.C.; Dylke, E.S.; Graham, P.L.; De Groef, A. Psychological Factors Are Associated with Pain at All Time Frames After Breast Cancer Surgery: A Systematic Review with Meta-Analyses. *Pain Med.* **2021**, *22*, 915–947. [CrossRef]
11. Wang, L.; Guyatt, G.H.; Kennedy, S.A.; Romerosa, B.; Kwon, H.Y.; Kaushal, A.; Chang, Y.; Craigie, S.; de Almeida, C.P.B.; Courban, R.J.; et al. Predictors of persistent pain after breast cancer surgery: A systematic review and meta-analysis of observational studies. *CMAJ* **2016**, *188*, E352–E361. [CrossRef]
12. Leysen, L.; Beckwée, D.; Nijs, J.; Pas, R.; Bilterys, T.; Vermeir, S.; Adriaenssens, N. Risk factors of pain in breast cancer survivors: A systematic review and meta-analysis. *Support. Care Cancer* **2017**, *25*, 3607–3643. [CrossRef]
13. Demark-Wahnefried, W.; Rogers, L.Q.; Alfano, C.M.; Thomson, C.A.; Courneya, K.S.; Meyerhardt, J.A.; Stout, N.L.; Kvale, E.; Ganzer, H.; Ligibel, J.A. Practical clinical interventions for diet, physical activity, and weight control in cancer survivors. *CA Cancer J. Clin.* **2015**, *65*, 167–189. [CrossRef]
14. Meneses-Echávez, J.F.; González-Jiménez, E.; Ramírez-Vélez, R. Effects of supervised exercise on cancer-related fatigue in breast cancer survivors: A systematic review and meta-analysis. *BMC Cancer* **2015**, *15*, 77. [CrossRef]
15. Kessels, E.; Husson, O.; van der Feltz-Cornelis, C.M. The effect of exercise on cancer-related fatigue in cancer survivors: A systematic review and meta-analysis. *Neuropsychiatr. Dis. Treat.* **2018**, *14*, 479–494. [CrossRef] [PubMed]
16. Fuller, J.T.; Hartland, M.C.; Maloney, L.T.; Davison, K. Therapeutic effects of aerobic and resistance exercises for cancer survivors: A systematic review of meta-analyses of clinical trials. *Br. J. Sports Med.* **2018**, *52*, 1311. [CrossRef] [PubMed]
17. Bobyrov, V. *Bases of Bioethics and Biosafety: Study Guide for Stud. of Higher Med. Est*; Ho a Ka: Vinnytsia, Ukraine, 2012.
18. Maindet, C.; Burnod, A.; Minello, C.; George, B.; Allano, G.; Lemaire, A. Strategies of complementary and integrative therapies in cancer-related pain-attaining exhaustive cancer pain management. *Support. Care Cancer* **2019**, *27*, 3119–3132. [CrossRef] [PubMed]
19. Glare, P.A.; Davies, P.S.; Finlay, E.; Gulati, A.; Lemanne, D.; Moryl, N.; Oeffinger, K.C.; Paice, J.A.; Stubblefield, M.D.; Syrjala, K.L. Pain in cancer survivors. *J. Clin. Oncol.* **2014**, *32*, 1739. [CrossRef]
20. Brown, M.R.; Ramirez, J.D.; Farquhar-Smith, P. Pain in cancer survivors. *Br. J. Pain* **2014**, *8*, 139–153. [CrossRef]
21. Sun, V.; <monospace> </monospace>Borneman, T.; Piper, B.; Koczywas, M.; Ferrell, B. Barriers to pain assessment and management in cancer survivorship. *J. Cancer Surviv.* **2008**, *2*, 65–71. [CrossRef]
22. Chow, R.; Saunders, K.; Burke, H.; Belanger, A.; Chow, E. Needs assessment of primary care physicians in the management of chronic pain in cancer survivors. *Support. Care Cancer* **2017**, *25*, 3505–3514. [CrossRef]
23. Oldenmenger, W.H.; Geerling, J.I.; Mostovaya, I.; Vissers, K.C.; de Graeff, A.; Reyners, A.K.; van der Linden, Y.M. A systematic review of the effectiveness of patient-based educational interventions to improve cancer-related pain. *Cancer Treat. Rev.* **2018**, *63*, 96–103. [CrossRef]
24. Binkley, J.M.; Harris, S.R.; Levangie, P.K.; Pearl, M.; Guglielmino, J.; Kraus, V.; Rowden, D. Patient perspectives on breast cancer treatment side effects and the prospective surveillance model for physical rehabilitation for women with breast cancer. *Cancer* **2012**, *118*, 2207–2216. [CrossRef]
25. McGuire, D.B. Occurrence of cancer pain. *J. Natl. Cancer Inst. Monogrphs* **2004**, *2004*, 51–56. [CrossRef] [PubMed]
26. Martínez-Miranda, P.; Casuso-Holgado, M.J.; Jiménez-Rejano, J.J. Effect of patient education on quality-of-life, pain and fatigue in breast cancer survivors: A systematic review and meta-analysis. *Clin. Rehabil.* **2021**, *35*, 1722–1742. [CrossRef] [PubMed]

27. Boland, E.G.; Ahmedzai, S.H. Persistent pain in cancer survivors. *Curr. Opin. Support Palliat. Care* **2017**, *11*, 181–190. [CrossRef] [PubMed]
28. Ong, W.Y.; Stohler, C.S.; Herr, D.R. Role of the Prefrontal Cortex in Pain Processing. *Mol. Neurobiol.* **2019**, *56*, 1137–1166. [CrossRef]
29. Sullivan, M.J.; Scott, W.; Trost, Z. Perceived injustice: A risk factor for problematic pain outcomes. *Clin. J. Pain.* **2012**, *28*, 484–488. [CrossRef]
30. Sullivan, M.J.; Davidson, N.; Garfinkel, B.; Siriapaipant, N.; Scott, W. Perceived injustice is associated with heightened pain behavior and disability in individuals with whiplash injuries. *Psychol. Inj. Law* **2009**, *2*, 238–247. [CrossRef]
31. Carriere, J.S.; Donayre Pimentel, S.; Yakobov, E.; Edwards, R.R. A Systematic Review of the Association Between Perceived Injustice and Pain-Related Outcomes in Individuals with Musculoskeletal Pain. *Pain Med.* **2020**, *21*, 1449–1463. [CrossRef]
32. Leysen, L.; Cools, W.; Nijs, J.; Adriaenssens, N.; Pas, R.; van Wilgen, C.P.; Bults, R.; Roose, E.; Lahousse, A.; Beckwée, D. The mediating effect of pain catastrophizing and perceived injustice in the relationship of pain on health-related quality of life in breast cancer survivors. *Support. Care Cancer* **2021**, *29*, 5653–5661. [CrossRef] [PubMed]
33. Carriere, J.S.; Martel, M.O.; Kao, M.C.; Sullivan, M.J.; Darnall, B.D. Pain behavior mediates the relationship between perceived injustice and opioid prescription for chronic pain: A Collaborative Health Outcomes Information Registry study. *J. Pain Res.* **2017**, *10*, 557–566. [CrossRef]
34. Turk, D.C.; Okifuji, A. What factors affect physicians' decisions to prescribe opioids for chronic noncancer pain patients? *Clin. J. Pain* **1997**, *13*, 330–336. [CrossRef]
35. Paice, J.A. Chronic treatment-related pain in cancer survivors. *Pain* **2011**, *152*, S84–S89. [CrossRef]
36. Derksen, J.W.G.; Beijer, S.; Koopman, M.; Verkooijen, H.M.; van de Poll-Franse, L.V.; May, A.M. Monitoring potentially modifiable lifestyle factors in cancer survivors: A narrative review on currently available methodologies and innovations for large-scale surveillance. *Eur. J. Cancer* **2018**, *103*, 327–340. [CrossRef]
37. Gopalakrishna, A.; Longo, T.A.; Fantony, J.J.; Van Noord, M.; Inman, B.A. Lifestyle factors and health-related quality of life in bladder cancer survivors: A systematic review. *J Cancer Surviv.* **2016**, *10*, 874–882. [CrossRef]
38. Fink, G. *Stress: Concepts, Cognition, Emotion, and Behavior*; Academic Press Elsevier: Cambridge, MA, USA, 2007.
39. Tsigos, C.; Kyrou, I.; Kassi, E.; Chrousos, G.P. Stress: Endocrine Physiology and Pathophysiology. In *Endotext*; Feingold, K.R., Anawalt, B., Boyce, A., Chrousos, G., de Herder, W.W., Dhatariya, K., Dungan, K., Hershman, J.M., Hofland, J., Kalra, S., et al., Eds.; MDText.com: South Dartmouth, MA, USA, 2000.
40. National Research Council Committee on, R. and A. Alleviation of Distress in Laboratory, The National Academies Collection: Reports funded by National Institutes of Health. In *Recognition and Alleviation of Distress in Laboratory Animals*; National Academies Press: Washington, DC, USA, 2008.
41. Abbey, G.; Thompson, S.B.N.; Hickish, T.; Heathcote, D. A meta-analysis of prevalence rates and moderating factors for cancer-related post-traumatic stress disorder. *Psychooncology* **2015**, *24*, 371–381. [CrossRef]
42. Syrowatka, A.; Motulsky, A.; Kurteva, S.; Hanley, J.A.; Dixon, W.G.; Meguerditchian, A.N.; Tamblyn, R. Predictors of distress in female breast cancer survivors: A systematic review. *Breast Cancer Res. Treat* **2017**, *165*, 229–245. [CrossRef]
43. Riba, M.B.; Donovan, K.A.; Andersen, B.; Braun, I.; Breitbart, W.S.; Brewer, B.W.; Buchmann, L.O.; Clark, M.M.; Collins, M.; Corbett, C.; et al. NCCN Clinical Practice Guidelines in Oncology: Distress Management, v3.2019. *Natl. Compr. Cancer Network.* **2019**, *17*, 1229–1249. Available online: https://www.nccn.org/professionals/physician_gls/pdf/distress.pdf (accessed on 14 December 2021). [CrossRef] [PubMed]
44. Fagundes, C.; LeRoy, A.; Karuga, M. Behavioral Symptoms after Breast Cancer Treatment: A Biobehavioral Approach. *J. Pers. Med.* **2015**, *5*, 280–295. [CrossRef] [PubMed]
45. Liu, Y.Z.; Wang, Y.X.; Jiang, C.L. Inflammation: The Common Pathway of Stress-Related Diseases. *Front. Hum. Neurosci.* **2017**, *11*, 316. [CrossRef]
46. Reis, J.C.; Antoni, M.H.; Travado, L. Emotional distress, brain functioning, and biobehavioral processes in cancer patients: A neuroimaging review and future directions. *CNS Spectr.* **2020**, *25*, 79–100. [CrossRef]
47. National Comprehensive Cancer Netwerk. Survivorship 2021 (Version 3. 2021). 2021. Available online: https://www.nccn.org/login?ReturnURL=https://www.nccn.org/professionals/physician_gls/pdf/survivorship.pdf (accessed on 8 September 2021).
48. Thornton, L.M.; Andersen, B.L.; Blakely, W.P. The pain, depression, and fatigue symptom cluster in advanced breast cancer: Covariation with the hypothalamic-pituitary-adrenal axis and the sympathetic nervous system. *Health Psychol.* **2010**, *29*, 333–337. [CrossRef]
49. Addison, S.; Shirima, D.; Aboagye-Mensah, E.B.; Dunovan, S.G.; Pascal, E.Y.; Lustberg, M.B.; Arthur, E.K.; Nolan, T.S. Effects of tandem cognitive behavioral therapy and healthy lifestyle interventions on health-related outcomes in cancer survivors: A systematic review. *J. Cancer Surviv.* **2021**, 1–24. [CrossRef]
50. Traeger, L.; Penedo, F.J.; Benedict, C.; Dahn, J.R.; Lechner, S.C.; Schneiderman, N.; Antoni, M.H. Identifying how and for whom cognitive-behavioral stress management improves emotional well-being among recent prostate cancer survivors. *Psychooncology* **2013**, *22*, 250–259. [CrossRef]
51. Tang, M.; Liu, X.; Wu, Q.; Shi, Y. The Effects of Cognitive-Behavioral Stress Management for Breast Cancer Patients: A Systematic Review and Meta-analysis of Randomized Controlled Trials. *Cancer Nurs.* **2020**, *43*, 222–237. [CrossRef]

52. Danhauer, S.C.; Addington, E.L.; Cohen, L.; Sohl, S.J.; Van Puymbroeck, M.; Albinati, N.K.; Culos-Reed, S.N. Yoga for symptom management in oncology: A review of the evidence base and future directions for research. *Cancer* **2019**, *125*, 1979–1989. [CrossRef]
53. Matchim, Y.; Armer, J.M.; Stewart, B.R. Mindfulness-based stress reduction among breast cancer survivors: A literature review and discussion. *Oncol. Nurs. Forum* **2011**, *38*, E61–E71. [CrossRef]
54. Chang, Y.C.; Yeh, T.L.; Chang, Y.M.; Hu, W.Y. Short-term Effects of Randomized Mindfulness-Based Intervention in Female Breast Cancer Survivors: A Systematic Review and Meta-analysis. *Cancer. Nurs.* **2021**, *44*, E703–E714. [CrossRef]
55. Roth, T. Insomnia: Definition, prevalence, etiology, and consequences. *J. Clin. Sleep Med.* **2007**, *3*, S7–S10. [CrossRef]
56. Savard, J.; Ivers, H.; Villa, J.; Caplette-Gingras, A.; Morin, C.M. Natural course of insomnia comorbid with cancer: An 18-month longitudinal study. *J. Clin. Oncol.* **2011**, *29*, 3580–3586. [CrossRef]
57. Johnson, J.A.; Rash, J.A.; Campbell, T.S.; Savard, J.; Gehrman, P.R.; Perlis, M.; Carlson, L.E.; Garland, S.N. A systematic review and meta-analysis of randomized controlled trials of cognitive behavior therapy for insomnia (CBT-I) in cancer survivors. *Sleep Med. Rev.* **2016**, *27*, 20–28. [CrossRef]
58. Miller, K.D.; Siegel, R.L.; Lin, C.C.; Mariotto, A.B.; Kramer, J.L.; Rowland, J.H.; Stein, K.D.; Alteri, R.; Jemal, A. Cancer treatment and survivorship statistics, 2016. *CA Cancer J. Clin.* **2016**, *66*, 271–289. [CrossRef]
59. Hall, D.L.; Mishel, M.H.; Germino, B.B. Living with cancer-related uncertainty: Associations with fatigue, insomnia, and affect in younger breast cancer survivors. *Support. Care Cancer* **2014**, *22*, 2489–2495. [CrossRef]
60. Carpenter, J.S.; Elam, J.L.; Ridner, S.H.; Carney, P.H.; Cherry, G.J.; Cucullu, H.L. Sleep, fatigue, and depressive symptoms in breast cancer survivors and matched healthy women experiencing hot flashes. *Oncol. Nurs. Forum* **2004**, *31*, 591–5598. [CrossRef]
61. Savard, J.; Davidson, J.R.; Ivers, H.; Quesnel, C.; Rioux, D.; Dupere, V.; Lasnier, M.; Simard, S.; Morin, C.M. The association between nocturnal hot flashes and sleep in breast cancer survivors. *J. Pain Symptom Manag.* **2004**, *27*, 513–522. [CrossRef]
62. Gupta, P.; Sturdee, D.W.; Palin, S.L.; Majumder, K.; Fear, R.; Marshall, T.; Paterson, I. Menopausal symptoms in women treated for breast cancer: The prevalence and severity of symptoms and their perceived effects on quality of life. *Climacteric* **2006**, *9*, 49–58. [CrossRef]
63. Desai, K.; Mao, J.J.; Su, I.; Demichele, A.; Li, Q.; Xie, S.X.; Gehrman, P.R. Prevalence and risk factors for insomnia among breast cancer patients on aromatase inhibitors. *Support. Care Cancer* **2013**, *21*, 43–51. [CrossRef]
64. Leysen, L.; Lahousse, A.; Nijs, J.; Adriaenssens, N.; Mairesse, O.; Ivakhnov, S.; Bilterys, T.; Van Looveren, E.; Pas, R.; Beckwée, D. Prevalence and risk factors of sleep disturbances in breast cancersurvivors: Systematic review and meta-analyses. *Support. Care Cancer* **2019**, *27*, 4401–4433. [CrossRef]
65. Finan, P.H.; Goodin, B.R.; Smith, M.T. The association of sleep and pain: An update and a path forward. *J. Pain* **2013**, *14*, 1539–1552. [CrossRef]
66. Haack, M.; Simpson, N.; Sethna, N.; Kaur, S.; Mullington, J. Sleep deficiency and chronic pain: Potential underlying mechanisms and clinical implications. *Neuropsychopharmacology* **2020**, *45*, 205–216. [CrossRef]
67. Qaseem, A.; Kansagara, D.; Forciea, M.A.; Cooke, M.; Denberg, T.D. Management of Chronic Insomnia Disorder in Adults: A Clinical Practice Guideline From the American College of Physicians. *Ann. Intern. Med.* **2016**, *165*, 125–133. [CrossRef] [PubMed]
68. Perlis, M.L.; Jungquist, C.; Smith, M.T.; Posner, D. *Cognitive Behavioral Treatment of Insomnia: A Session-by-Session Guide*; Springer Science and Business Media: New York, NY, USA, 2008.
69. Ma, Y.; Hall, D.L.; Ngo, L.H.; Liu, Q.; Bain, P.A.; Yeh, G.Y. Efficacy of cognitive behavioral therapy for insomnia in breast cancer: A meta-analysis. *Sleep Med. Rev.* **2021**, *55*, 101376. [CrossRef]
70. Zhou, E.S.; Partridge, A.H.; Syrjala, K.L.; Michaud, A.L.; Recklitis, C.J. Evaluation and treatment of insomnia in adult cancer survivorship programs. *J. Cancer Surviv.* **2017**, *11*, 74–79. [CrossRef] [PubMed]
71. Mindell, J.A.; Bartle, A.; Wahab, N.A.; Ahn, Y.; Ramamurthy, M.B.; Huong, H.T.; Kohyama, J.; Ruangdaraganon, N.; Sekartini, R.; Teng, A.; et al. Sleep education in medical school curriculum: A glimpse across countries. *Sleep Med.* **2011**, *12*, 928–931. [CrossRef] [PubMed]
72. Thomas, A.; Grandner, M.; Nowakowski, S.; Nesom, G.; Corbitt, C.; Perlis, M.L. Where are the Behavioral Sleep Medicine Providers and Where are They Needed? A Geographic Assessment. *Behav. Sleep Med.* **2016**, *14*, 687–698. [CrossRef]
73. Stinson, K.; Tang, N.K.; Harvey, A.G. Barriers to treatment seeking in primary insomnia in the United Kingdom: A cross-sectional perspective. *Sleep* **2006**, *29*, 1643–1646. [CrossRef]
74. Matthews, E.E.; Arnedt, J.T.; McCarthy, M.S.; Cuddihy, L.J.; Aloia, M.S. Adherence to cognitive behavioral therapy for insomnia: A systematic review. *Sleep Med. Rev.* **2013**, *17*, 453–464. [CrossRef]
75. American Cancer Society. *Cancer Treatment & Survivorship Facts & Figures 2019–2021*; American Cancer Society: Atlanta, GA, USA, 2019; Available online: https://www.cancer.org/content/dam/cancer-org/research/cancer-facts-and-statistics/cancer-treatment-and-survivorship-facts-and-figures/cancer-treatment-and-survivorship-facts-and-figures-2019-2021.pdf (accessed on 20 September 2021).
76. Zhang, F.F.; Liu, S.; John, E.M.; Must, A.; Demark-Wahnefried, W. Diet quality of cancer survivors and noncancer individuals: Results from a national survey. *Cancer* **2015**, *121*, 4212–4221. [CrossRef]
77. Schwedhelm, C.; Boeing, H.; Hoffmann, G.; Aleksandrova, K.; Schwingshackl, L. Effect of diet on mortality and cancer recurrence among cancer survivors: A systematic review and meta-analysis of cohort studies. *Nutr. Rev.* **2016**, *74*, 737–748. [CrossRef]

78. Jochems, S.H.J.; Van Osch, F.H.M.; Bryan, R.T.; Wesselius, A.; van Schooten, F.J.; Cheng, K.K.; Zeegers, M.P. Impact of dietary patterns and the main food groups on mortality and recurrence in cancer survivors: A systematic review of current epidemiological literature. *BMJ Open* **2018**, *8*, e014530. [CrossRef] [PubMed]
79. Schwingshackl, L.; Schwedhelm, C.; Galbete, C.; Hoffmann, G. Adherence to Mediterranean Diet and Risk of Cancer: An Updated Systematic Review and Meta-Analysis. *Nutrients* **2017**, *9*, 1063. [CrossRef] [PubMed]
80. Yilmaz, S.T.; Elma, Ö.; Deliens, T.; Coppieters, I.; Clarys, P.; Nijs, J.; Malfliet, A. Nutrition/Dietary Supplements and Chronic Pain in Patients with Cancer and Survivors of Cancer: A Systematic Review and Research Agenda. *Pain Physician* **2021**, *24*, 335–344. [PubMed]
81. Kim, T.H.; Kang, J.W.; Lee, T.H. Therapeutic options for aromatase inhibitor-associated arthralgia in breast cancer survivors: A systematic review of systematic reviews, evidence mapping, and network meta-analysis. *Maturitas* **2018**, *118*, 29–37. [CrossRef]
82. Mohammadi, S.; Sulaiman, S.; Koon, P.B.; Amani, R.; Hosseini, S.M. Association of nutritional status with quality of life in breast cancer survivors. *Asian Pac. J. Cancer Prev.* **2013**, *14*, 7749–7755. [CrossRef]
83. Fu, M.R.; Axelrod, D.; Guth, A.; McTernan, M.L.; Qiu, J.M.; Zhou, Z.; Ko, E.; Magny-Normilus, C.; Scagliola, J.; Wang, Y. The Effects of Obesity on Lymphatic Pain and Swelling in Breast Cancer Patients. *Biomedicines* **2021**, *9*, 818. [CrossRef]
84. Blazek, K.; Favre, J.; Asay, J.; Erhart-Hledik, J.; Andriacchi, T. Age and obesity alter the relationship between femoral articular cartilage thickness and ambulatory loads in individuals without osteoarthritis. *J. Orthop. Res.* **2014**, *32*, 394–402. [CrossRef]
85. Rogers, A.H.; Kauffman, B.Y.; Garey, L.; Asmundson, G.J.; Zvolensky, M.J. Pain-Related Anxiety among Adults with Obesity and Chronic Pain: Relations with Pain, Opioid Misuse, and Mental Health. *Behav. Med.* **2020**, 1–9. [CrossRef]
86. Singh, D.; Park, W.; Hwang, D.; Levy, M.S. Severe obesity effect on low back biomechanical stress of manual load lifting. *Work* **2015**, *51*, 337–348. [CrossRef]
87. Fabris de Souza, S.A.; Faintuch, J.; Valezi, A.C.; Sant'Anna, A.F.; Gama-Rodrigues, J.J.; de Batista Fonseca, I.C.; de Melo, R.D. Postural changes in morbidly obese patients. *Obes. Surg.* **2005**, *15*, 1013–1016. [CrossRef]
88. Timmins, H.C.; Mizrahi, D.; Li, T.; Kiernan, M.C.; Goldstein, D.; Park, S.B. Metabolic and lifestyle risk factors for chemotherapy-induced peripheral neuropathy in taxane and platinum-treated patients: A systematic review. *J. Cancer Surviv.* **2021**, 1–15. [CrossRef]
89. Parekh, N.; Chandran, U.; Bandera, E.V. Obesity in cancer survival. *Annu. Rev. Nutr.* **2012**, *32*, 311–342. [CrossRef]
90. Miller, K.D.; Nogueira, L.; Mariotto, A.B.; Rowland, J.H.; Yabroff, K.R.; Alfano, C.M.; Jemal, A.; Kramer, J.L.; Siegel, R.L. Cancer treatment and survivorship statistics, 2019. *CA Cancer J. Clin.* **2019**, *69*, 363–385. [CrossRef]
91. Bracken-Clarke, D.; Kapoor, D.; Baird, A.M.; Buchanan, P.J.; Gately, K.; Cuffe, S.; Finn, S.P. Vaping and lung cancer—A review of current data and recommendations. *Lung Cancer* **2021**, *153*, 11–20. [CrossRef]
92. Strick, K. E-cigarettes: Time to realign our approach? *Lancet* **2019**, *394*, 1297.
93. Lucchiari, C.; Masiero, M.; Botturi, A.; Pravettoni, G. Helping patients to reduce tobacco consumption in oncology: A narrative review. *Springerplus* **2016**, *5*, 1136. [CrossRef]
94. De Moor, J.S.; Elder, K.; Emmons, K.M. Smoking prevention and cessation interventions for cancer survivors. *Semin. Oncol. Nurs.* **2008**, *24*, 180–192. [CrossRef] [PubMed]
95. Santa Mina, D.; Brahmbhatt, P.; Lopez, C.; Baima, J.; Gillis, C.; Trachtenberg, L.; Silver, J.K. The Case for Prehabilitation Prior to Breast Cancer Treatment. *PM&R* **2017**, *9*, S305–S316.
96. Sørensen, L.T.; Hørby, J.; Friis, E.; Pilsgaard, B.; Jørgensen, T. Smoking as a risk factor for wound healing and infection in breast cancer surgery. *Eur. J. Surg. Oncol.* **2002**, *28*, 815–820. [CrossRef] [PubMed]
97. Cancer Trends Progress Report National Cancer Institute. Available online: https://www.progressreport.cancer.gov/after/smoking (accessed on 20 September 2021).
98. Aigner, C.J.; Cinciripini, P.M.; Anderson, K.O.; Baum, G.P.; Gritz, E.R.; Lam, C.Y. The Association of Pain With Smoking and Quit Attempts in an Electronic Diary Study of Cancer Patients Trying to Quit. *Nicotine Tob. Res.* **2016**, *18*, 1449–1455. [CrossRef] [PubMed]
99. Ditre, J.W.; Heckman, B.W.; Zale, E.L.; Kosiba, J.D. Acute analgesic effects of nicotine and tobacco in humans: A meta-analysis. *Pain* **2016**, *157*, 1373–1381. [CrossRef]
100. Davidson, S.M.; Boldt, R.G.; Louie, A.V. How can we better help cancer patients quit smoking? The London Regional Cancer Program experience with smoking cessation. *Curr. Oncol.* **2018**, *25*, 226–230. [CrossRef]
101. Richter, K.P.; Ellerbeck, E.F. It's time to change the default for tobacco treatment. *Addiction* **2015**, *110*, 381–386. [CrossRef] [PubMed]
102. Bagnardi, V.; Rota, M.; Botteri, E.; Tramacere, I.; Islami, F.; Fedirko, V.; Scotti, L.; Jenab, M.; Turati, F.; Pasquali, E.; et al. Alcohol consumption and site-specific cancer risk: A comprehensive dose-response meta-analysis. *Br. J. Cancer* **2015**, *112*, 580–593. [CrossRef] [PubMed]
103. Cao, Y.; Willett, W.C.; Rimm, E.B.; Stampfer, M.J.; Giovannucci, E.L. Light to moderate intake of alcohol, drinking patterns, and risk of cancer: Results from two prospective US cohort studies. *BMJ* **2015**, *351*, h4238. [CrossRef] [PubMed]
104. Bagnardi, V.; Rota, M.; Botteri, E.; Tramacere, I.; Islami, F.; Fedirko, V.; Scotti, L.; Jenab, M.; Turati, F.; Pasquali, E.; et al. Light alcohol drinking and cancer: A meta-analysis. *Ann. Oncol.* **2013**, *24*, 301–308. [CrossRef] [PubMed]
105. Myung, S.K. Erroneous conclusions about the association between light alcohol drinking and the risk of cancer: Comments on Bagnardi et al.'s meta-analysis. *Ann. Oncol.* **2016**, *27*, 2138. [CrossRef]

106. Xia, E.Q.; Deng, G.F.; Guo, Y.J.; Li, H.B. Biological activities of polyphenols from grapes. *Int. J. Mol. Sci.* **2010**, *11*, 622–646. [CrossRef]
107. Ali, A.M.; Schmidt, M.K.; Bolla, M.K.; Wang, Q.; Gago-Dominguez, M.; Castelao, J.E.; Carracedo, A.; Garzón, V.M.; Bojesen, S.E.; Nordestgaard, B.G.; et al. Alcohol consumption and survival after a breast cancer diagnosis: A literature-based meta-analysis and collaborative analysis of data for 29,239 cases. *Cancer Epidemiol. Biomark. Prev.* **2014**, *23*, 934–945. [CrossRef]
108. Watts, E.L.; Appleby, P.N.; Perez-Cornago, A.; Bueno-de-Mesquita, H.B.; Chan, J.M.; Chen, C.; Cohn, B.A.; Cook, M.B.; Flicker, L.; Freedman, N.D.; et al. Low Free Testosterone and Prostate Cancer Risk: A Collaborative Analysis of 20 Prospective Studies. *Eur. Urol.* **2018**, *74*, 585–594. [CrossRef]
109. Sanford, N.N.; Sher, D.J.; Xu, X.; Ahn, C.; D'Amico, A.V.; Aizer, A.A.; Mahal, B.A. Alcohol use among patients with cancer and survivors in the United States 2000–2017. *J. Natl. Compr. Cancer Netw.* **2020**, *18*, 69–79. [CrossRef] [PubMed]
110. Hashibe, M.; Brennan, P.; Chuang, S.C.; Boccia, S.; Castellsague, X.; Chen, C.; Curado, M.P.; Dal Maso, L.; Daudt, A.W.; Fabianova, E.; et al. Interaction between tobacco and alcohol use and the risk of head and neck cancer: Pooled analysis in the International Head and Neck Cancer Epidemiology Consortium. *Cancer Epidemiol. Biomark. Prev.* **2009**, *18*, 541–550. [CrossRef] [PubMed]
111. Thompson, T.; Oram, C.; Correll, C.U.; Tsermentseli, S.; Stubbs, B. Analgesic effects of alcohol: A systematic review and meta-analysis of controlled experimental studies in healthy participants. *J. Pain* **2017**, *18*, 499–510. [CrossRef] [PubMed]
112. Zale, E.L.; Maisto, S.A.; Ditre, J.W. Interrelations between pain and alcohol: An integrative review. *Clin. Psychol. Rev.* **2015**, *37*, 57–71. [CrossRef] [PubMed]
113. Boissoneault, J.; Lewis, B.; Nixon, S.J. Characterizing chronic pain and alcohol use trajectory among treatment-seeking alcoholics. *Alcohol* **2019**, *75*, 47–54. [CrossRef] [PubMed]
114. Maleki, N.; Oscar-Berman, M. Chronic Pain in Relation to Depressive Disorders and Alcohol Abuse. *Brain Sci.* **2020**, *10*, 826. [CrossRef]
115. Nieto, S.J.; Green, R.; Grodin, E.N.; Cahill, C.M.; Ray, L.A. Pain catastrophizing predicts alcohol craving in heavy drinkers independent of pain intensity. *Drug Alcohol Depend.* **2021**, *218*, 108368. [CrossRef]
116. Rock, C.L.; Doyle, C.; Demark-Wahnefried, W.; Meyerhardt, J.; Courneya, K.S.; Schwartz, A.L.; Bandera, E.V.; Hamilton, K.K.; Grant, B.; McCullough, M.; et al. Nutrition and physical activity guidelines for cancer survivors. *CA Cancer J. Clin.* **2012**, *62*, 243–274. [CrossRef]
117. Friedenreich, C.M.; Stone, C.R.; Cheung, W.Y.; Hayes, S.C. Physical Activity and Mortality in Cancer Survivors: A Systematic Review and Meta-Analysis. *JNCI Cancer Spectr.* **2020**, *4*, pkz080. [CrossRef]
118. Turner, R.R.; Steed, L.; Quirk, H.; Greasley, R.U.; Saxton, J.M.; Taylor, S.J.; Rosario, D.J.; Thaha, M.A.; Bourke, L. Interventions for promoting habitual exercise in people living with and beyond cancer. *Cochrane Database Syst. Rev.* **2018**, *9*. [CrossRef]
119. Garcia, D.O.; Thomson, C.A. Physical activity and cancer survivorship. *Nutr. Clin. Pract.* **2014**, *29*, 768–779. [CrossRef]
120. Wolin, K.Y.; Schwartz, A.L.; Matthews, C.E.; Courneya, K.S.; Schmitz, K.H. Implementing the exercise guidelines for cancer survivors. *J. Support. Oncol.* **2012**, *10*, 171–177. [CrossRef]
121. Runowicz, C.D.; Leach, C.R.; Henry, N.L.; Henry, K.S.; Mackey, H.T.; Cowens-Alvarado, R.L.; Cannady, R.S.; Pratt-Chapman, M.L.; Edge, S.B.; Jacobs, L.A.; et al. American Cancer Society/American Society of Clinical Oncology Breast Cancer Survivorship Care Guideline. *J. Clin. Oncol.* **2016**, *34*, 611–635. [CrossRef]
122. Lu, G.; Zheng, J.; Zhang, L. The effect of exercise on aromatase inhibitor-induced musculoskeletal symptoms in breast cancer survivors: A systematic review and meta-analysis. *Support. Care Cancer* **2020**, *28*, 1587–1596. [CrossRef] [PubMed]
123. Boing, L.; Vieira, M.C.S.; Moratelli, J.; Bergmann, A.; Guimarães, A.C.A. Effects of exercise on physical outcomes of breast cancer survivors receiving hormone therapy—A systematic review and meta-analysis. *Maturitas* **2020**, *141*, 71–81. [CrossRef]
124. Ballard-Barbash, R.; Friedenreich, C.M.; Courneya, K.S.; Siddiqi, S.M.; McTiernan, A.; Alfano, C.M. Physical activity, biomarkers, and disease outcomes in cancer survivors: A systematic review. *J. Natl. Cancer Inst.* **2012**, *104*, 815–840. [CrossRef] [PubMed]
125. Hasenoehrl, T.; Palma, S.; Ramazanova, D.; Kölbl, H.; Dorner, T.E.; Keilani, M.; Crevenna, R. Resistance exercise and breast cancer-related lymphedema-a systematic review update and meta-analysis. *Support Care Cancer* **2020**, *28*, 3593–3603. [CrossRef] [PubMed]
126. Geneen, L.J.; Moore, R.A.; Clarke, C.; Martin, D.; Colvin, L.A.; Smith, B.H. Physical activity and exercise for chronic pain in adults: An overview of Cochrane Reviews. *Cochrane Database Syst. Rev.* **2017**, *1*, Cd011279. [PubMed]
127. Lavín-Pérez, A.M.; Collado-Mateo, D.; Mayo, X.; Liguori, G.; Humphreys, L.; Copeland, R.J.; Jiménez, A. Effects of high-intensity training on the quality of life of cancer patients and survivors: A systematic review with meta-analysis. *Sci. Rep.* **2021**, *11*, 15089. [CrossRef]
128. Ijsbrandy, C.; Ottevanger, P.B.; Gerritsen, W.R.; van Harten, W.H.; Hermens, R. Determinants of adherence to physical cancer rehabilitation guidelines among cancer patients and cancer centers: A cross-sectional observational study. *J. Cancer Surviv.* **2021**, *15*, 163–177. [CrossRef]
129. Kampshoff, C.S.; Jansen, F.; van Mechelen, W.; May, A.M.; Brug, J.; Chinapaw, M.J.; Buffart, L.M. Determinants of exercise adherence and maintenance among cancer survivors: A systematic review. *Int. J. Behav. Nutr. Phys. Act.* **2014**, *11*, 80. [CrossRef]
130. Ormel, H.L.; van der Schoot, G.G.F.; Sluiter, W.J.; Jalving, M.; Gietema, J.A.; Walenkamp, A.M.E. Predictors of adherence to exercise interventions during and after cancer treatment: A systematic review. *Psychooncology* **2018**, *27*, 713–724. [CrossRef]
131. Spencer, J.C.; Wheeler, S.B. A systematic review of Motivational Interviewing interventions in cancer patients and survivors. *Patient Educ. Couns.* **2016**, *99*, 1099–1105. [CrossRef]

132. Veenhof, C.; Köke, A.J.; Dekker, J.; Oostendorp, R.A.; Bijlsma, J.W.; van Tulder, M.W.; van den Ende, C.H. Effectiveness of behavioral graded activity in patients with osteoarthritis of the hip and/or knee: A randomized clinical trial. *Arthritis Rheum.* **2006**, *55*, 925–934. [CrossRef]
133. Cillessen, L.; Johannsen, M.; Speckens, A.E.M.; Zachariae, R. Mindfulness-based interventions for psychological and physical health outcomes in cancer patients and survivors: A systematic review and meta-analysis of randomized controlled trials. *Psychooncology* **2019**, *28*, 2257–2269. [CrossRef]
134. Duan, L.; Xu, Y.; Li, M. Effects of Mind-Body Exercise in Cancer Survivors: A Systematic Review and Meta-Analysis. *Evid. Based Complement. Altern. Med.* **2020**, *2020*, 7607161. [CrossRef]
135. Mendoza, M.E.; Capafons, A.; Gralow, J.R.; Syrjala, K.L.; Suárez-Rodríguez, J.M.; Fann, J.R.; Jensen, M.P. Randomized controlled trial of the Valencia model of waking hypnosis plus CBT for pain, fatigue, and sleep management in patients with cancer and cancer survivors. *Psychooncology* **2017**, *26*, 1832–1838. [CrossRef]
136. The Joanna Briggs Institute Levels of Evidence and Grades of RecommendationWorking Party Joanna Briggs Institute Levels of Evidence and Grades of Recommendation. 2014. Available online: https://jbi.global/sites/default/files/2019-05/JBI-Levels-of-evidence_2014_0.pdf (accessed on 22 November 2021).
137. Hernandez Silva, E.; Lawler, S.; Langbecker, D. The effectiveness of mHealth for self-management in improving pain, psychological distress, fatigue, and sleep in cancer survivors: A systematic review. *J. Cancer Surviv.* **2019**, *13*, 97–107. [CrossRef]
138. Mullan, F. Seasons of survival: Reflections of a physician with cancer. *N. Engl. J. Med.* **1985**, *313*, 270–273. [CrossRef] [PubMed]
139. Paxton, R.J.; Jones, L.A.; Chang, S.; Hernandez, M.; Hajek, R.A.; Flatt, S.W.; Natarajan, L.; Pierce, J.P. Was race a factor in the outcomes of the Women's Health Eating and Living Study? *Cancer* **2011**, *117*, 3805–3813. [CrossRef] [PubMed]
140. Blanchard, C.M.; Courneya, K.S.; Stein, K. Cancer survivors' adherence to lifestyle behavior recommendations and associations with health-related quality of life: Results from the American Cancer Society's SCS-II. *J. Clin. Oncol.* **2008**, *26*, 2198–2204. [CrossRef]
141. Bower, P.; Gilbody, S. Stepped care in psychological therapies: Access, effectiveness and efficiency. Narrative literature review. *Br. J. Psychiatry* **2005**, *186*, 11–17. [CrossRef]
142. Zhou, E.S.; Michaud, A.L.; Recklitis, C.J. Developing efficient and effective behavioral treatment for insomnia in cancer survivors: Results of a stepped care trial. *Cancer* **2020**, *126*, 165–173. [CrossRef]
143. Lynch, F.A.; Katona, L.; Jefford, M.; Smith, A.B.; Shaw, J.; Dhillon, H.M.; Ellen, S.; Phipps-Nelson, J.; Lai-Kwon, J.; Milne, D.; et al. Feasibility and Acceptability of Fear-Less: A Stepped-Care Program to Manage Fear of Cancer Recurrence in People with Metastatic Melanoma. *J. Clin. Med.* **2020**, *9*, 2969. [CrossRef] [PubMed]
144. Roberts, A.L.; Fisher, A.; Smith, L.; Heinrich, M.; Potts, H.W.W. Digital health behaviour change interventions targeting physical activity and diet in cancer survivors: A systematic review and meta-analysis. *J. Cancer Surviv.* **2017**, *11*, 704–719. [CrossRef] [PubMed]
145. Yang, W.; Williams, J.H.; Hogan, P.F.; Bruinooge, S.S.; Rodriguez, G.I.; Kosty, M.P.; Bajorin, D.F.; Hanley, A.; Muchow, A.; McMillan, N.; et al. Projected supply of and demand for oncologists and radiation oncologists through 2025: An aging, better-insured population will result in shortage. *J. Oncol. Pract.* **2014**, *10*, 39–45. [CrossRef] [PubMed]
146. Nijs, J.; Wijma, A.J.; Leysen, L.; Pas, R.; Willaert, W.; Hoelen, W.; Ickmans, K.; Wilgen, C.P.V. Explaining pain following cancer: A practical guide for clinicians. *Braz. J. Phys. Ther.* **2019**, *23*, 367–377. [CrossRef]
147. Lexmond, W.; Jäger, K. *Psychomteric Properties of the Dutch Version of the Revised Neurophysiology of Pain Questionnaire*; Vrije Universiteit Brussel: Brussels, Belgium, 2019; p. 36.
148. Bennett, M.I.; Bagnall, A.M.; Closs, S.J. How effective are patient-based educational interventions in the management of cancer pain? Systematic review and meta-analysis. *Pain* **2009**, *143*, 192–199. [CrossRef]
149. Nijs, J.; Roose, E.; Lahousse, A.; Mostaqim, K.; Reynebeau, I.; De Couck, M.; Beckwee, D.; Huysmans, E.; Bults, R.; van Wilgen, P.; et al. Pain and Opioid Use in Cancer Survivors: A Practical Guide to Account for Perceived Injustice. *Pain Physician* **2021**, *24*, 309–317.
150. Levit, L.A.; Balogh, E.; Nass, S.J.; Ganz, P. *Delivering High-Quality Cancer Care: Charting a New Course for a System in Crisis*; National Academies Press: Washington, DC, USA, 2013.
151. Bluethmann, S.M.; Mariotto, A.B.; Rowland, J.H. Anticipating the "Silver Tsunami": Prevalence Trajectories and Comorbidity Burden among Older Cancer Survivors in the United States. *Cancer Epidemiol. Biomark. Prev.* **2016**, *25*, 1029–1036. [CrossRef]

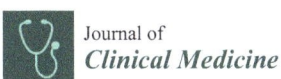

Review

Lifestyle and Chronic Pain in the Pelvis: State of the Art and Future Directions

Annelie Gutke [1,*], Karin Sundfeldt [2,3] and Liesbet De Baets [4]

1. Department of Health and Rehabilitation, Institute of Neuroscience and Physiology, Sahlgrenska Academy, University of Gothenburg, 40350 Gothenburg, Sweden
2. Department of Obstetrics and Gynecology, Institute of Clinical Sciences, Sahlgrenska Academy, University of Gothenburg, 40350 Gothenburg, Sweden; karin.sundfeldt@obgyn.gu.se
3. Department of Gynecology, Sahlgrenska University Hospital, 41346 Gothenburg, Sweden
4. Pain in Motion Research Group (PAIN), Department of Physiotherapy, Human Physiology and Anatomy, Faculty of Physical Education & Physiotherapy, Vrije Universiteit Brussel, 1050 Brussel, Belgium; liesbet.de.baets@vub.be
* Correspondence: annelie.gutke@gu.se

Abstract: During their lifespan, many women are exposed to pain in the pelvis in relation to menstruation and pregnancy. Such pelvic pain is often considered normal and inherently linked to being a woman, which in turn leads to insufficiently offered treatment for treatable aspects related to their pain experience. Nonetheless, severe dysmenorrhea (pain during menstruation) as seen in endometriosis and pregnancy-related pelvic girdle pain, have a high impact on daily activities, school attendance and work ability. In the context of any type of chronic pain, accumulating evidence shows that an unhealthy lifestyle is associated with pain development and pain severity. Furthermore, unhealthy lifestyle habits are a suggested perpetuating factor of chronic pain. This is of specific relevance during lifespan, since a low physical activity level, poor sleep, or periods of (di)stress are all common in challenging periods of women's lives (e.g., during menstruation, during pregnancy, in the postpartum period). This state-of-the-art paper aims to review the role of lifestyle factors on pain in the pelvis, and the added value of a lifestyle intervention on pain in women with pelvic pain. Based on the current evidence, the benefits of physical activity and exercise for women with pain in the pelvis are supported to some extent. The available evidence on lifestyle factors such as sleep, (di)stress, diet, and tobacco/alcohol use is, however, inconclusive. Very few studies are available, and the studies which are available are of general low quality. Since the role of lifestyle on the development and maintenance of pain in the pelvis, and the value of lifestyle interventions for women with pain in the pelvis are currently poorly studied, a research agenda is presented. There are a number of rationales to study the effect of promoting a healthy lifestyle (early) in a woman's life with regard to the prevention and management of pain in the pelvis. Indeed, lifestyle interventions might have, amongst others, anti-inflammatory, stress-reducing and/or sleep-improving effects, which might positively affect the experience of pain. Research to disentangle the relationship between lifestyle factors, such as physical activity level, sleep, diet, smoking, and psychological distress, and the experience of pain in the pelvis is, therefore, needed. Studies which address the development of management strategies for adapting lifestyles that are specifically tailored to women with pain in the pelvis, and as such take hormonal status, life events and context, into account, are required. Towards clinicians, we suggest making use of the window of opportunity to prevent a potential transition from localized or periodic pain in the pelvis (e.g., dysmenorrhea or pain during pregnancy and after delivery) towards persistent chronic pain, by promoting a healthy lifestyle and applying appropriate pain management.

Keywords: chronic pelvic pain; endometriosis; pelvic girdle pain; lifestyle factors; pain management; physical activity/exercise; (di)stress; sleep; diet; smoking

Citation: Gutke, A.; Sundfeldt, K.; De Baets, L. Lifestyle and Chronic Pain in the Pelvis: State of the Art and Future Directions. *J. Clin. Med.* **2021**, *10*, 5397. https://doi.org/10.3390/jcm10225397

Academic Editors: Jo Nijs, Felipe Reis and Laxmaiah Manchikanti

Received: 12 October 2021
Accepted: 16 November 2021
Published: 19 November 2021

Publisher's Note: MDPI stays neutral with regard to jurisdictional claims in published maps and institutional affiliations.

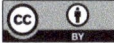

Copyright: © 2021 by the authors. Licensee MDPI, Basel, Switzerland. This article is an open access article distributed under the terms and conditions of the Creative Commons Attribution (CC BY) license (https://creativecommons.org/licenses/by/4.0/).

1. Introduction

During their lifespans, women are at a high risk for experiencing pain complaints in the pelvic region due to gynecologic and obstetric reasons. Indeed, hormonal changes in the menstruation cycle are typically associated with pain in the pelvis [1]. Most women experience pain for one or more days of the menstruation period, for which pain killers or hormonal contraceptive pills are the first-choice treatment. However, this pharmacological treatment is not sufficient for pain reduction in an important subgroup of women [2], resulting in recurrent or persistent pelvic pain, such in women who experience endometriosis-related pelvic pain [3]. Severe dysmenorrhea (pain during the menstrual period) is a cardinal symptom of endometriosis and is known to have a high social impact as it is often associated with absence from school or work [1]. Apart from endometriosis-related pelvic pain, pain in the pelvis also occurs in relation to pregnancy and childbirth [4]. Such pregnancy-related pelvic girdle pain (PGP) is suggested to relate to both hormonal, musculoskeletal and biomechanical changes [4,5]. The pain intensity is often severe enough to hinder pregnant women or women in the postpartum period to participate in activities of daily living, including work [4,6–8]. Since pharmacological treatment is not the first choice for pain management for many pregnant or breast-feeding women, other conservative approaches, such as physical therapy, are generally applied [4,9]. However, this care is not considered successful in appropriately alleviating pain in a subgroup of women with PGP, or is not consistently offered to women with PGP [10].

Indeed, women experiencing pain in the pelvis (endometriosis-related pelvic pain and pregnancy-related PGP) are not consistently guided towards appropriate treatment for their pain complaint. It is even more disturbing that these women are often told that their experienced pain should be considered 'normal', and inextricably linked to being a woman [3,11]. Apart of being unethical, such a message also contributes to the fact that many women seek too little help for a pain complaint that may be treatable [10]. This might result in the fact that an initial pain experience, e.g., experienced during menstruation or pregnancy or immediately following childbirth, evolves towards persistent pain in the pelvis.

To improve this current practice, knowledge on adequate treatment approaches for reducing pain in women with pain in the pelvis is required. It is furthermore believed that adequate strategies to prevent an increase in pain during periods of life in which a hormone or pregnancy-related pain can be foreseen, are of even greater importance. In this context, the effect of lifestyle changes on pain has received more attention in recent years. There are many possible causes for pain in the pelvis, and in this review we focus on two common disorders related to specific painful events during lifespan of women to point out the possibility to prevent development of chronic pain. However, to understand why a healthy lifestyle might be effective in reducing pain in women with endometriosis-related pelvic pain and pregnancy-related PGP, more information about the pathophysiology of these conditions is first provided.

1.1. Endometriosis-Related Chronic Pelvic Pain

Endometriosis is, with a reported prevalence around 10%, a very common condition among women of childbearing age, and one of the most common structural causes of chronic pelvic pain [3,12]. It is classically defined as an estrogen-dependent, chronic inflammatory condition in which the endometrium of the uterus grows outside the uterus by implantation of endometrial cells and creates an inflammatory response of the surrounding tissue. Both superficial lesions on the peritoneum, ovarian endometriosis and a more aggressive deep infiltrating type that may obstruct the intestines or bladder, have been reported [13]. In this context, increasing evidence suggests that endometriosis should be considered a systemic disease, not only restricted to the pelvis [3]. Indeed, endometriosis is reported to co-exist with other conditions such as irritable bowel syndrome, mental health disorders, central sensitization and pain conditions (fibromyalgia, migraine), and immunological conditions (e.g., rheumatoid arthritis, multiple sclerosis) [13,14]. Given these multiple facets of endometriosis, its diagnosis is currently very challenging [13], resulting commonly in a delay in diagnosis of multiple years [3,13,15,16].

Variable clinical symptoms are related to endometriosis. Typical pain symptoms in women with endometriosis are (a)cyclic pelvic pain, dysmenorrhea and pain at ovulation [3,13,15]. This may be combined with radiating pain to the lower back, groin and thighs, as well as deep intercourse pain [3]. Bladder problems, difficulties in emptying the bowel and infertility can be attributed to endometriosis as well [17]. Given these debilitating symptoms, endometriosis might affect a woman's physical, mental and social well-being, her quality of life and her work ability [18]. These, in turn, are related to higher levels of psychological distress. Furthermore, poorer sleep quality, endometriosis-related fatigue and physical deconditioning are reported in women suffering from endometriosis [19].

Current first-line treatment for endometriosis is conservative pharmacological care, and surgical procedures when pharmacological options are ineffective or with deep infiltrating endometriosis. However, for a large group of women, endometriosis recurs after surgical treatment or are ineffective, as evident from the large rate of (50%) [3]. In this context, the link between the grade of laparoscopic detected lesions and level of symptoms is also inconsistent [3]. This emphasizes the value of looking beyond tissue-related aspects and to look for treatment options addressing the mechanisms underlying symptom development. Therefore, it seems valuable to take a closer look into the lifestyle of women suffering symptomatic endometriosis. As endometriosis is considered an inflammatory and estrogen-dependent disease, targeting lifestyle factors that influence these factors can open the path for multiple conservative treatment options for women with endometriosis-related pelvic pain (e.g., dietary intervention, physical activity, sleep management). Thereby, the anti-inflammatory effect of a healthy lifestyle might positively influence pain perception given the association between inflammatory mediators and peripheral as well as central sensitization [20].

1.2. Pregnancy-Related Pelvic Girdle Pain

Pregnancy-related PGP is reported by 50% of pregnant women globally [4,5,10]. PGP is classified by its pain location, i.e., between the posterior iliac crest and the gluteal fold, most commonly around the sacroiliac joints and/or pubic bone, sometimes with radiating pain in the thighs, with onset close to, or within three weeks of delivery [5]. For the classification of PGP, it is recommended that the pain is reproduced during clinical pain provocations tests and that it is associated with, and time-dependent on, weight bearing activities. Typical symptoms of PGP, both during and after pregnancy are a decrease in endurance in standing, walking, and sitting (often within 30 min of activity) [4,21] which lead to limitations in daily functioning [6–8], and at work [4,22]. Since PGP is mostly related to pregnancy, it is expected to disappear when pregnancy-related changes disappear after birth [6], which is true for the majority of women [23]. However up to 11 years after pregnancy, 10% of women report persistent and per definition chronic PGP [8]. The etiology of PGP is multifactorial. One suggested cause of PGP is inefficient neuromuscular control [4,5] related to hormonal changes during pregnancy. However, a systematic review of evidence on whether this results in pelvic instability causing PGP is low [24]. In women with PGP, higher prevalence rates of prenatal anxiety and depressive symptoms are reported in comparison to pregnant women without pain [25,26]. This co-occurrence of pain with anxiety and depression continues in women with chronic PGP, who also seem to have less general self-efficacy than women who recovered from PGP after pregnancy [8]. Furthermore, from a recent cohort study [27], lack of physical activity was added as a predisposing factor for pain in the lumbo-pelvic area in pregnancy together with the hitherto reported previous history of pain in the lumbo-pelvic area, low job satisfaction, and increased weight during pregnancy [4].

In general, the evidence is low for the effectiveness of interventions for PGP [4,9]. As PGP treatment, acupuncture shows the most coherent findings in the literature [4,9,28]. Other suggested treatment strategies are the application of a pelvic belt and exercises [4,9].

In recent years, a cognitive behavioral approach and self-management strategies have been proposed for women with PGP [29]. In the above-described context, it seems valuable to take a closer look into the lifestyle factors of women suffering from PGP.

1.3. Lifestyle Factors in Chronic Pain in the Pelvis

Within the chronic pain field, there is cumulating evidence that unhealthy lifestyle factors such as physical inactivity, increased psychological distress, poor sleep, unhealthy diet, and smoking are associated with chronic pain severity and sustainment [30–32]. A proposed mechanism underlying the association between lifestyle and pain in this regard is related to inflammatory mediators. For example, it is known that in chronic pain patients, disturbed sleep modulates the endogenous inhibitory pain control system, produces changes in the hypothalamic-pituitary-adrenal axis and induces aberrant inflammatory reactions [33]. Specifically in relation to pregnancy, an increase in inflammatory biomarkers in sleep-deprived pregnant women in comparison to non-pregnant has been reported [34]. Even after pregnancy, an inflammatory response with increased cytokine levels is associated with short sleep duration [35].

Within the field of pain in the pelvis, the scientific literature points towards the role of lifestyle on pain. Being overweight/obese or experiencing emotional distress during pregnancy have been associated with less recovery at 3–6 months after pregnancy when the natural course of PGP is over [36]. In women with chronic PGP, level of physical activity, exercises, sleep quality and distress are associated with pain perception [8]. Regarding lifestyle factors and endometriosis, poor sleep quality is reported to be associated with pelvic pain [37].

An increased understanding of the role of exercise, insomnia, diet, and other lifestyle factors on the perception of pain in women with pain in the pelvis is assumed to provide treatment opportunities to optimize current care. Of even greater importance, such understanding on the role of lifestyle factors in the development and maintenance of pain in the pelvis, can provide invaluable knowledge on how we might develop prevention strategies for severe pain in the pelvis. This is of utmost importance, since it can be theorized that painful experiences early in a woman's life that are not handled according to the best of knowledge, might be a reason why higher rates of chronic pain in women as compared to men are reported [38,39]. Therefore, in the early stages, when pain in the pelvis can be expected, there is a window of opportunity to take the right preventive actions, with good pain management strategies, and possibly by advocating a healthy lifestyle.

This review aims to give an overview of the best evidence on the role of lifestyle factors in the development or maintenance of pain in the pelvis in women related to common painful events during their lifespan. Since very few studies are published in the field, a systematic review was not considered feasible. A best-evidence review was considered the appropriate format to explore the field and to present a research agenda. A best-evidence synthesis of the effect of lifestyle interventions on women with pain in the pelvis is provided. The best evidence knowledge is reviewed in a way such that clinicians can integrate the evidence into their daily clinical routine. In addition, the state-of-the-art overview also serves clinical researchers in building upon the best evidence for designing future trials, implementation studies, and to develop new innovative studies.

2. State-of-the-Art

For this best-evidence review, the following lifestyle factors were defined a priori: physical (in)activity, exercise, sleep, psychological distress, food intake, tobacco use, smoking and alcohol consumption. With regard to the interventions for these lifestyle factors, only active interventions such as exercise, psychologically informed approaches, cognitive behavioral therapy, dietary interventions (focusing on altering food uptake) and multimodal approaches, were considered. Studies on surgical procedures, pharmaceutical treatment in isolation (including supplements e.g., vitamin supplements), Chinese medicine and passive treatments such as acupuncture, in isolation, were not eligible.

A nonsystematic search of scientific studies was performed in MEDLINE (PubMed), and web-of-science from their inception to August 2021, using the following search terms: ((endometriosis OR pelvic girdle pain OR lumbopelvic pain) AND (physical activity OR exercise* OR insomnia OR sleep OR stress OR diet OR nutrition OR smoking OR tobacco OR alcohol). The searches were conducted by two researchers (AG and LDB) independently. To minimize selection bias and to ensure high quality evidence was selected, systematic reviews and meta-analyses in accordance with PRISMA guidelines were preferred. If these were not available, narrative, and critical reviews were selected. Recent high-quality prospective studies and randomized clinical trials (RCTs) not already included in systematic reviews were also included, as well as information from large population-based cohorts.

Physical activity and exercise were defined as any bodily movement generated by skeletal muscles resulting in energy expenditure above resting levels [40]. The use of the terms 'physical activity' and 'exercise' in the included studies was not consistently in accordance with published definitions [40], and the terms were sometimes used interchangeably. Therefore, this review was not able to differentiate between interventions for either of them.

To retrieve all relevant articles within the area of PGP, a search was done for both PGP and lumbopelvic pain (LPP), since the latter term is often used when the studies do not distinguish between PGP and combined pain from the lumbar and pelvic areas [41]. Some authors have used the term low back pain (LBP) for pain in the lumbar area and evaluated the subgroup with LBP separately e.g., Weis et al., [42], which is also presented separately in our review.

3. Endometriosis-Related Chronic Pelvic Pain and Lifestyle Factors

Seven systematic reviews were found that were prepared and outlined in accordance with the PRISMA guidelines. Of these reviews, four provided a narrative synthesis of their data due to study heterogeneity (design, research questions, outcomes, interventions, etc.). Three studies performed a meta-analysis. Characteristics of the included systematic reviews and meta-analyses, together with their main results and level of evidence (if applicable) are outlined in Table 1.

In the text that follows, the results of the systematic reviews and meta-analyses are described, together with the results of narrative/critical reviews and recent original studies.

Table 1. Best evidence for lifestyle factors for women with endometriosis according to systematic reviews following PRISMA.

Lifestyle Factor	First Author Year Published Type of Data Synthesis	Included Population	Number of Papers Included and Number of Participants in Original Research	Detail of Lifestyle Factor/Intervention Assessed	Quality of Studies (Tool and Results)	Main Results in Context of the Specified State-of-the-Art Objectives	Summary of Evidence
Physical activity and/or Exercise	Hansen et al., 2021 [43] Systematic review, narrative synthesis of data	Women of reproductive age with a laparoscopically confirmed diagnosis of endometriosis	Two RCTs ($n = 39$ and 40) Two cohort studies ($n = 20$ and 26) One case-control study ($n = 81$) One cross-sectional survey study ($n = 484$)	Any type of exercise	Cochrane risk of bias Tool for RCTs: 'Unclear' in at least 4 of 7 domains. Low risk of selection and attrition bias ROBINS-I quality assessment scale for case-control and cohort studies: moderate to critical risk of bias in at least 4 of 7 domains in 3 studies. 1 study with low risk of bias on 4 domains and no information on 2 domains	RCTs: no significant effect on pain Cohort studies: no consistent outcome: one positive impact on pain, one no impact on pain Case control study and survey: one no impact and one negative impact on pain	No indication for beneficial effect of exercise on pain in women with endometriosis
Physical activity and/or Exercise	Ricci et al., 2016 [44] Systematic review and meta-analysis	Women with a clinical and/or histological based diagnosis of endometriosis. However, all but one study included participants with laparoscopic confirmed endometriosis	Three cohort studies (n between 1481 and 2703) Six case-control studies (n cases between 50 and 268)	Recent and past recreational PA, evaluated in different ways: hours of PA per week, metabolic equivalents (MET)-h/week, author-defined low or high intensity activity	Newcastle-Ottawa quality assessment scale, 3 domains (selection —max. score 4; comparability—max. score 2; exposure—max. score 3) case-control studies: between 2–4 on selection; 0–2 on comparability; 1–2 on exposure cohort studies: between 2–3 on selection; 2 on comparability; 1–2 on outcome	When adjusted estimates of odds ratios were provided, PA was protective against endometriosis. However, the overall estimate was not statistically significant when including all retrieved articles. Studies on the association between PA during adolescence and endometriosis are inconsistent, and meta-analysis' results are inconclusive	Inconclusive results on relation between risk of endometriosis and PA

Table 1. Cont.

Lifestyle Factor	First Author Year Published Type of Data Synthesis	Included Population	Number of Papers Included and Number of Participants in Original Research	Detail of Lifestyle Factor/Intervention Assessed	Quality of Studies (Tool and Results)	Main Results in Context of the Specified State-of-the-Art Objectives	Summary of Evidence
Diet	Huijs and Nap 2020 [45] Systematic review, narrative synthesis of data	Women with surgically or magnetic resonance imaging/ultrasound confirmed endometriosis	Four RCTs (n between 39–240) Four non-randomized clinical trials (n between 4–60) One retrospective study ($=59$) Once case series ($n = 8$) Two case reports ($n = 2$ and 1)	Nutrient or diet	GRADE criteria: low to very low Risk of bias Imprecision, inconsistency, indirectness and/or publication bias were found in all included studies	In nine studies, nutrients were added to patients' diets, and in seven of these a positive effect was found. In three studies, nutrients were avoided, with positive effects on endometriosis associated symptoms	Dietary interventions may potentially have an influence on symptoms in women with endometriosis, but no clinical recommendations can be provided yet.
Diet	Nirgianakis et al., 2021 [46] Systematic review, narrative synthesis of data	Women diagnosed with endometriosis—no details described	Nine human studies, Two RCTs ($n = 19$ and 37) Two controlled studies ($n = 30$ and 35) Four uncontrolled before-after studies (n between 47 and 295) once qualitative study ($n = 12$)	Dietary intervention, including supplementation with selected dietary components, exclusion of selected dietary components, and complete diet modification.	Quality in Prognostic Studies tool for observational research Cochrane risk-of-bias tool for RCTs Moderate to high risk of bias	All included studies assessed a different dietary intervention, with most of them finding a positive effect on endometriosis.	No subcategories of patients who are more likely to benefit from a dietary intervention can be defined. No specific dietary interventions that ameliorate certain endometriosis-associated symptoms can be identified.

Table 1. *Cont.*

Lifestyle Factor	First Author Year Published Type of Data Synthesis	Included Population	Number of Papers Included and Number of Participants in Original Research	Detail of Lifestyle Factor/Intervention Assessed	Quality of Studies (Tool and Results)	Main Results in Context of the Specified State-of-the-Art Objectives	Summary of Evidence
Diet	Qi et al., 2021 [47] Systematic review and meta-analysis	Women with a clinical and/or laparoscopic confirmed endometriosis. All but two case-control studies included women with laparoscopic confirmed endometriosis.	Two cohort studies (*n* = 581 and 1385) Five case-control studies (*n* between 78 and 504)	Dairy intake	Newcastle–Ottawa Scale, 3 domains (selection —max. score 4; comparability—max score 2; exposure—max. score 3) All studies scored 6 stars or higher and were considered high-quality studies.	Total dairy intake is inversely associated with the risk of endometriosis Risk of endometriosis tended to decrease when dairy products intake was over 21 servings/week (RR 0.87, 95% CI 0.76–1.00; *p* = 0.04). When more than 18 servings of high-fat dairy products per week are consumed, a reduced risk of endometriosis (RR 0.86, 95% CI 0.76–0.96) is reported. Stratified-analyses based on specific dairy product categories: Evidence for reduced risk of endometriosis: a high cheese intake (RR 0.86, 95%CI 0.74–1.00). No Evidence for reduced risk of endometriosis: High intake of whole milk (RR 0.90, 95% CI 0.72–1.12), reduced-fat/skim milk (RR 0.83, 95% CI 0.50–1.73), ice cream (RR 0.83, 95% CI 0.50–1.73), and yogurt (RR 0.83, 95% CI 0.62–1.11) Evidence for higher risk of endometriosis: Higher butter intake (1.27, 95% CI 1.03–1.55).	Dairy products intake is associated with a reduction in endometriosis, with significant effects when the average daily intake is three servings or more. When analyzed according to the specific type of dairy product, it is suggested that women with higher high-fat dairy and cheese intake have a reduced risk of endometriosis

Table 1. Cont.

Lifestyle Factor	First Author Year Published Type of Data Synthesis	Included Population	Number of Papers Included and Number of Participants in Original Research	Detail of Lifestyle Factor/Intervention Assessed	Quality of Studies (Tool and Results)	Main Results in Context of the Specified State-of-the-Art Objectives	Summary of Evidence
(Di)-stress	Evans et al., 2019 [48] Systematic review, narrative synthesis of data	Women with medically confirmed endometriosis (such as via a previous laparoscopy)- no further details	Three RCTs (n between 28 and 50) One qualitative study ($n = 28$) One controlled study ($n = 64$) Two single arm studies ($n = 26$ and 10) One retrospective cohort study ($n = 47$) Two case series ($n = 5$ and 2)	Physical therapy with cognitive behavioral therapy, yoga, biofeedback, mindfulness and psychotherapy, psychotherapy combined with acupuncture, and progressive muscle relaxation	Four criteria of the Cochrane Risk of Bias tool for RCTs (adequate generation of allocation sequence, concealment of allocation to conditions, assessor masking, dealing with incomplete data): For RCTs, mostly low risk of bias, apart from attrition bias and selection bias For non-randomized trials (including single-arm studies), observational cohort studies and case reports, the relevant National Institutes of Health quality assessment tool was used with a final quality rating of 'Good', 'Fair' or 'Poor.': Fair risk of bias in all non-randomized trials Critical Appraisal Skills Programme for qualitative studies (10 questions which can be answered "Yes", "Can't Tell", or "No.", with "Yes" implying a low risk of bias): Low risk of bias	89% of studies report improvement in pain	Based on the included mainly pilot studies, it is suggested that psychological and mind-body interventions show promise in alleviating pain in women with endometriosis
Tobacco use	Bravi et al., 2014 [49] Systematic review and meta-analysis	Women with histologically confirmed and/or clinically based diagnosis of endometriosis.	Nine cohort studies (n between 19 and 3110) Twenty-nine case-control studies (n between 28 and 947)	Tobacco smoking	Newcastle-Ottawa Scale, 3 domains (selection –max. score 4; comparability—max score 2; exposure –max. score 3) Cohort studies: 2 studies 6, rest lower Case control: 3 more than 6, other below 6 Most studies have high risk of bias	Considering ever smokers or, separately, former smokers, current smokers, moderate smokers and heavy smokers, no statistically significant association is found with risk of endometriosis	There is no association between smoking and risk of endometriosis

RR: risk ratio; SMD: standardized mean difference; CI: 95% confidence interval; SR: systematic reviews; RCT: randomized controlled trials; PA: physical activity.

3.1. Physical Activity and Exercise

Two systematic reviews reported on endometriosis and physical activity/exercise. Hansen and colleagues (2021) studied the recent evidence on the impact of exercise on pain perception in women with endometriosis [43]. No general positive effect of exercise on pain could be concluded. However, the included studies were generally of high risk of bias. Ricci et al. (2016) studied the role of physical activity on the risk for endometriosis [44]. In their meta-analysis, women with endometriosis performing recent physical activity, and women performing physical activity in the past, were included. The pooled estimate of adjusted odds ratios for current exercise indicated a significantly protective effect of exercise, but the overall estimates did not reach levels of significance. Furthermore, the review did not specify the influence of physical activity on pain symptoms. The aforementioned results are in line with the results of the earlier published narrative review of Bonocher et al. (2014) that assessed the relationship between physical exercise and the prevalence and/or improvement of symptoms associated with endometriosis [50].

The data available are inconclusive regarding the benefits of physical exercise on the risk of endometriosis, and no firm data exist on the added value of physical activity on pain in women with endometriosis.

3.2. Psychological Distress

One systematic review was found that assessed the effectiveness of psychological and mind-body interventions to improve pain, psychological distress, sleep and fatigue in women with endometriosis [48]. The studies assessed the value of yoga, mindfulness, relaxation training, cognitive behavioral therapy combined with physical therapy, Chinese medicine combined with psychotherapy, and biofeedback. No firm conclusions could be drawn given the high variety of interventions and designs. Most studies were considered pilot studies. However, the results of the studies suggested that psychological and mind-body interventions are promising avenues to decrease pain, anxiety, depression, distress, and fatigue in women with endometriosis.

3.3. Sleep

No systematic nor narrative reviews on the role of insomnia on pain in women with endometriosis were found, nor on the effectiveness of sleep interventions on pain symptoms in women with endometriosis. No recent original prospective cohort studies or intervention studies regarding this topic were found.

Arion et al., (2020) performed a quantitative analysis of sleep quality in women with surgically confirmed endometriosis to assess which variables were associated with poorer sleep [51]. Based on regression analyses, the following factors were independently associated with poorer sleep: functional quality of life, more depressive symptoms and painful bladder syndrome. In a former cross-sectional study on the sleep quality of women with endometriosis and the relation between sleep quality and pressure pain thresholds, sleep quality was significantly poorer in women with endometriosis compared to women without endometriosis [52]. Furthermore, the pressure pain threshold in the greater trochanter and abdomen was significantly lower in women with endometriosis when compared to women without endometriosis, which is indicative of an increased central sensitivity; however, there was no difference in pain intensity between women with and without endometriosis.

3.4. Diet

Huijs and Nap (2020) performed a literature search to gain insights into the role of nutrients on the symptoms of women with surgically or magnetic resonance imaging/ultrasound confirmed endometriosis [45]. Using the GRADE criteria, the quality of the evidence in this review turned out to be low to very low. It was suggested that the intake of additional fatty acids, antioxidants and a combination of vitamins and minerals could have a positive effect on endometriosis-associated symptoms.

Nirgianakis et al., (2021) performed a systematic review on the effectiveness of dietary interventions in the treatment of endometriosis [46]. Changes in endometriosis-associated symptoms measured with pain scales or patient-reported quality of life outcomes were the outcomes of interest in this systematic review. Different dietary interventions were assessed, including: supplementation of vitamin D; supplementation of vitamins A, C, and E; supplementation of omega-3/6, quercetin, vitamin B3, 5-methyltetrahydrofolate calcium salt, turmeric, and parthenium; Mediterranean diet; low-FODMAP diet; low nickel diet; gluten-free diet, and individual diet changes. Most studies identified a positive effect of the dietary intervention on endometriosis symptoms. However, all studies were of moderate and/or high-risk risk of bias limiting the validity of the results. Furthermore, it was not possible based on the available evidence to identify certain subcategories of patients, which would be more likely to benefit from a dietary intervention. In addition, it was not possible, based on the current literature, to identify specific dietary interventions that would ameliorate certain endometriosis-associated symptoms. Therefore, it was concluded that more, and especially higher quality original studies, are needed to draw conclusions on the effectiveness of dietary intervention on pain in women with endometriosis.

Recently, Qi et al., (2021) performed a systematic review and dose-response meta-analysis to investigate the association between dairy products and the risk of endometriosis, and to evaluate the amount of dairy intake affecting the risk of endometriosis [47], though the effect on pain perception was not taken into consideration. Based on the meta-analysis results, the authors concluded that the intake of dairy products was associated with a reduction in endometriosis when the average daily intake was three servings or more. When analyzed according to the specific type of dairy product, it was suggested that females with a higher high-fat dairy and cheese intake were at lower risk of endometriosis. Regarding butter intake, it was suggested that high intake was related to an increased risk of endometriosis. All studies included in this meta-analysis were of high quality, as based on the Newcastle-Ottawa Scale [53].

Additionally, Helbig et al., (2021) performed a literature search for articles from 2000 onwards to answer the question whether diet influences the risk for and progression of endometriosis or whether it influences the postoperative condition [54]. This review did not take the effect of diet on pain symptoms into account. Based on the evidence, it was suggested that fish oil capsules in combination with vitamin B12 were associated with a positive effect on endometriosis symptoms (particularly of dysmenorrhea). It was reported that alcohol and increased consumption of red meat and trans-fats were associated with a negative effect on endometriosis. The results of the studies listed with regard to fruit and vegetables, dairy products, unsaturated fats, fibre, soy products and coffee were not clear.

In conclusion, no high-qualitative prospective data on the role of diet (which food products and in which amounts) in the development and maintenance of pain in women with endometriosis are available. Furthermore, no firm data exist on the added value of dietary interventions on pain in women with endometriosis, given the low study quality of currently existing trials.

3.5. Tobacco/Alcohol Use

One systematic review and meta-analysis studied the relation between tobacco smoking and endometriosis risk. No evidence for an association between tobacco smoking and risk of endometriosis was found [49]. When subgroups were considered, i.e., never smokers vs. former smokers, current smokers, moderate smokers or heavy smokers, no statistically significant associations were reported.

4. Pelvic Girdle Pain and Lifestyle Factors

Seven systematic reviews were found that evaluated lifestyle intervention for PGP prepared and outlined in accordance with the PRISMA guidelines. Of these reviews, five studies performed a meta-analysis. Characteristics of the included systematic reviews and meta-analyses, together with their main results and level of evidence are outlined in Table 2.

Table 2. Best evidence for lifestyle interventions for women with pelvic girdle pain according to systematic reviews following PRISMA.

Lifestyle Factor	First Author Year Published Type of Data Synthesis	Included Population PGP/LPP/LBP	Pregnancy/Postpartum Number of SR/RCT Number of Participants	Detail of Lifestyle Factor/Intervention Assessed	Quality of Studies (Tool and Results)	Main Results on Interventions	Summary of Evidence
Physical activity and/or Exercise	Weis et al., 2020 [55] SR and meta-analysis	PGP/LPP LBP	Pregnancy Six SRs based on nine RCTs PGP: Four SRs based on three RCTs LPP: Nine SRs based on four RCTs LBP: Five SRs based on seven RCTs	land or water-based exercise in group or individual	Modified version of Scottish Intercollegiate Guideline Network PGP: high-quality, low risk of bias (1 SR) acceptable-quality, moderate risk of bias (1 SR) low-quality, high risk of bias (2 SR) LPP: high-quality, low risk of bias (1 SR) acceptable-quality, moderate risk of bias (7 SR) LBP: high-quality, low risk of bias (1 SR) acceptable-quality, moderate risk of bias (3 SR) low-quality, high risk of bias (1 SR)	PGP: decreased pain intensity and disability LPP: improved function and reduced prevalence from most SRs LBP: 4/5 SRs reduced pain intensity and disability	PGP: inconclusive, evidence with favorable outcomes LPP: moderate strength evidence with unclear outcomes LBP: inconclusive, strength with favorable outcomes
Physical activity and/or Exercise	Weis et al., 2020 [42] SR and meta-analysis	PGP/LPP	Postpartum Two SRs based on six RCTs PGP: Two SRs based on four RCTs LPP: Two SRs based on two RCTs LBP: 0 SR	exercise in group or individual	Modified version of Scottish Intercollegiate Guideline Network PGP: Acceptable-quality, moderate risk of bias LPP: Acceptable-quality, moderate risk of bias	PGP: One of three SRs stated additional effect of exercises at reducing pain and disability. LPP: no firm conclusions could be drawn	PGP: moderate strength of evidence with unclear outcomes. LPP: inconclusive strength of evidence and unclear outcomes

Table 2. Cont.

Lifestyle Factor	First Author Year Published Type of Data Synthesis	Included Population PGP/LPP/LBP	Pregnancy/Postpartum Number of SR/RCT Number of Participants	Detail of Lifestyle Factor/Intervention Assessed	Quality of Studies (Tool and Results)	Main Results on Interventions	Summary of Evidence
Physical activity and/or Exercise	Davenport et al., 2019 [56] SR and meta-analysis	PGP/LPP LBP	Pregnancy and postpartum Thirty-two studies (n = 52,297) out of 23 RCTs (13 exercise only and 10 exercise +co-interventions) **pregnancy** -pooled estimates prevalence 12 RCTs (n = 1987) -pooled estimates severity 10 RCTs (n = 784). **postpartum** -pooled estimates prevalence 3 RCTs (n = 491) -severity 1 RCTs (n = 257)	result presented from 'exercise only' or 'exercise with co-intervention' (yoga, aerobic exercise, general muscle strengthening or muscle strengthening specific to one body region and combination of aerobic and resistance training)	GRADE criteria **pregnancy** Prevalence: very low-quality Serious risk of bias, serious directness of the interventions and serious imprecision. Severity: very low-quality Serious risk of bias, serious inconsistency, and serious indirectness of the interventions. **postpartum:** Prevalence: low-quality Serious indirectness of the interventions and serious imprecision. Severity: low quality Serious risk of bias and serious inconsistency.	**pregnancy** PGP/LPP/LBP: no reduced odds (OR 0.78, 95% CI 0.60, 1.02) lower pain severity (standardized mean difference −1.03, 95% CI −1.58, −0.48) **postpartum** PGP/LPP/LBP: no reduced odds (OR 0.89, 95% CI 0.51, 1.56) decreased severity of LBP ($p = 0.034$) (only 1 RCT)	**pregnancy** PGP/LPP/LBP: very low to moderate quality evidence **postpartum** PGP/LPP/LBP: low quality to moderate evidence low quality evidence
Physical activity and/or Exercise	Almousa et al., 2018 [57] SR	PGP	Pregnancy and postpartum Five RCTs + 1 follow up (n between 44 and 330) **pregnancy** Two RCTs (n = 426) **postpartum** Two RCTs (n = 125) + 1 follow up (n = 65) pregnancy and postpartum One RCT (n = 103)	stabilizing exercises	Pedro scale Scores range 5–8, i.e., 5 studies good-quality and 1 study fair-quality	**pregnancy** decrease pain (2 RCTs) and improved quality of life (1 RCT) **postpartum** contradictory results	insufficient evidence

Table 2. Cont.

Lifestyle Factor	First Author Year Published Type of Data Synthesis	Included Population PGP/LPP/LBP	Pregnancy/ Postpartum Number of SR/RCT Number of Participants	Detail of Lifestyle Factor/Intervention Assessed	Quality of Studies (Tool and Results)	Main Results on Interventions	Summary of Evidence
Physical activity and/or Exercise	Shiri et al., 2018 [58] SR and meta-analysis	PGP LBP	Pregnancy pooled 11 RCTs ($n = 2347$) PGP: Four RCTs ($n = 565$) LPP: Eight RCTs ($n = 1737$); out of only three RCTs ($n = 1168$) evaluating sick leave LBP: Seven RCTs ($n = 1175$) out of only two RCTs ($n = 349$) evaluating sick leave	exercise of different type and in different combinations	Cochrane Collaboration's tool. Low heterogeneity in meta-analyses * Low publication bias *	**PGP:** no protective effect (RR 0.99, 95% CI 0.81–1.21 **LPP:** no protective effect (RR 0.96, 95% CI 0.90–1.02) but prevented new episodes of sick leave (RR 0.79, 95% CI 0.64–0.99) **LBP:** reduced risk 9% (pooled RR 0.91, 95% CI 0.83–0.99) prevented new episodes of sick leave (RR 0.67, 95% CI 0.40–1.12)	Exercise appears to reduce risk of LBP and sick leave due to LPP but no clear evidence on PGP
Physical activity and/or Exercise	Liddle and Pennick 2015 [4] SR and meta-analysis	PGP/LPP LBP	pregnancy Thirty-four RCTs ($n = 5121$) PGP: Six RCTs ($n = 889$) pooled two RCTs ($n = 374$) LPP: Thirteen RCTs ($n = 2385$) pooled four RCTs ($n = 1176$) LBP: Fifteen RCTs ($n = 1847$) pooled seven RCTs ($n = 645$)	exercises on land/in water	Cochrane Collaboration's tool GRADE criteria Clinical heterogeneity precluded pooling results in many cases. Statistical heterogeneity was substantial in all but three meta-analyses, not improving following sensitivity analyses. Publication bias and selective reporting cannot be ruled out.	**PGP:** no effect on prevalence of PGP **LPP:** reduced prevalence and pain (RR 0.66; 95% CI 0.45 to 0.97) reduced sick leave (RR 0.76; 95% CI 0.62 to 0.94.) **LBP:** no effect on prevalence (RR 0.97; 95% CI 0.80 to 1.17) reduced pain (SMD −0.64; 95% CI −1.03 to −0.25) and reduced functional disability (SMD −0.56; 95% CI −0.89 to −0.23)	**PGP:** Low quality evidence **LPP:** Moderate-quality evidence **LBP:** Low-quality evidence

Table 2. Cont.

Lifestyle Factor	First Author Year Published Type of Data Synthesis	Included Population PGP/LPP/LBP	Pregnancy/ Postpartum Number of SR/RCT Number of Participants	Detail of Lifestyle Factor/Intervention Assessed	Quality of Studies (Tool and Results)	Main Results on Interventions	Summary of Evidence
Physical activity and/or Exercise	Tseng et al., 2015 [59] SR	LPP	postpartum Four RCTs n = 251	exercise programs to strengthen deep local muscles and global muscles in the lumbopelvic regions	Cochrane Collaboration's tool Pedro scale Scores range 4–8, i.e., three studies good-quality and one study fair quality. All studies except one were at low risk of bias on key domains such as sequence generation, allocation concealment, blinding of participants and personnel, completeness of outcome data for each main outcome, and selective reporting.	inconclusive on pain intensity and disability	no evidence

PGP: pelvic girdle pain; LPP: lumbopelvic pain; LBP: low back pain; RR: risk ratio; SMD: standardized mean difference; CI: 95% confidence interval; SR: systematic reviews; RCT: randomized controlled trials; * for details on risk of bias, refer to original study.

In the text that follows, the results of the systematic reviews and meta-analyses are described, together with the results of narrative/critical reviews and recent original studies.

4.1. Physical Activity and Exercise

Seven systematic reviews, performed according to PRISMA, reported on physical activity/exercise as management of PGP. Weis et al., (2020) conducted two systematic reviews on systematic reviews and RCTs to assess the effectiveness of chiropractic care options including exercises commonly used for pregnancy-related PGP, LPP and LBP during pregnancy [55] and postpartum [42]. For PGP in pregnancy, there was inconclusive evidence that an exercise program was more effective to decrease pain and disability compared with standard treatment [55]. For LPP, it was found that exercise had unclear outcomes on improvements in function (moderate strength evidence), and that exercise reduced the prevalence of LPP. This latter was reported in most included systematic reviews. For LBP, studies had inconclusive strength evidence with favorable outcomes on decreased pain and disability. From a systematic review focusing on the postpartum period [42], there was moderate evidence with no clear outcomes to suggest exercise as treatment for or prevention of PGP, since only one of three included systematic reviews stated the additional effect of exercises at reducing pain and disability. No firm conclusion could be drawn for LPP, but the authors reported some evidence which indicated that exercises could relieve LPP. There were no results for LBP postpartum. Davenport et al., (2019) performed a systematic review to investigate the relationship between the performance of prenatal exercises and PGP, LPP as well as LBP [56]. Based on very low-to-moderate quality evidence, prenatal exercise compared to no exercise during pregnancy did decrease pain severity in pregnancy and at postpartum but did not reduce the odds of suffering from PGP, LPP and LBP either in pregnancy or at postpartum.

Almousa et al., (2018) evaluated the effectiveness of stabilizing exercises in PGP during pregnancy and postpartum in a systematic review [57]. They concluded that there was limited evidence that stabilizing exercises decreased pain and improved quality of life during pregnancy and postpartum. Shiri et al., (2018) did a meta-analysis of RCTs to study the value of exercise in the prevention of PGP and LBP [58]. They concluded that exercise reduced the risk of LBP in pregnancy by 9% but that exercise had no effect on PGP or LPP. Additionally, exercise prevented new episodes of sick leave due to LPP. Liddle and Pennick (2015) performed a systematic review according to Cochrane Collaboration's tool to update the evidence on the effects of any intervention including exercise to prevent or treat PGP, LPP or LBP during pregnancy [4]. Low-quality evidence showed no significant difference in the prevalence of PGP or LBP from exercise. Low-quality evidence showed that any land-based exercise significantly reduced pain and disability from LBP. Moderate-quality evidence showed reduced the prevalence of LPP from 8–12 weeks of exercises.

Tseng et al., (2015) aimed to synthesize evidence from RCTs on the effectiveness of exercise on LPP in postpartum women [59]. Based on four RCTs they concluded that there was some evidence to indicate the effectiveness of exercise for relieving LPP but more trials were need to ascertain the most effective postpartum exercise programs.

Even though not proven to reduce the risk of developing PGP [56,58], a recent systematic review on physical activity and exercise in relation to pregnancy reported decreased severity of PGP and LPP [56]. Davenport et al. reported their intervention results separated as 'exercise only' or 'exercise plus co-intervention' [56], which could explain the somewhat different result to another recent systematic review that reported inconclusive, although favorable, evidence for exercises in pregnancy [55] as well as at postpartum [42]. These latest results confirm the most recent Cochrane review on exercise in pregnancy for LPP and LBP, but not the previous result of no effect for PGP [4]. The newer result, that exercise can reduce the severity of PGP, may be explained by more studies to build evidence on. Likewise, the number of studies to build the evidence on is probably the explanation of some other previously limited [57], inconclusive evidence [59] reported. The recent results confirm an earlier narrative review on LBP and PGP by Stuge (2015), where it was concluded that there is evidence of moderate quality that exercise reduced pain intensity but not prevalence [60].

Various types of exercises including general physical activity, low impact aerobic exercise such as walking, stabilizing exercises, resistance training, and other forms of exercises such as Yoga, or the combination of different exercises, have been evaluated for their effectiveness in PGP, LPP and LBP in the included systematic reviews. Systematic reviews usually include all exercise types together. Only one identified systematic review differentiated exercise only from exercise with co-interventions [56], but no significant difference between pooled estimates could be seen (pregnancy $p = 0.24$; postpartum $p = 0.70$). At this time, there is insufficient evidence to determine whether one type of exercise is superior to another or whether exercise should be combined with other interventions and, in that case, which co-intervention(s). One identified systematic review that focused on group training for LPP reported no effect as treatment of LPP among pregnant women but reported group training to be effective after pregnancy [61].

From four population-based cohort studies in Brazil, it was reported that 41.9% of 3827 pregnant women reported LBP of any type, and 10% of women during pregnancy reached recommended levels of physical activity [62]. The authors concluded that meeting the recommended levels of physical activity during pregnancy was associated with less activity limitation related to LBP during pregnancy. However, physical activity levels, either before (β coefficient: 0.07; 95% CI, -0.25 to 0.38) or during pregnancy (β coefficient: -0.07; 95% CI, -0.46 to 0.33), were not associated with pain intensity, care seeking, and postpartum LBP [62]. After pregnancy, physical activity level was continuously suboptimal for many women [63]. Recently, it was reported that sedentary behavior after birth was associated with persistent LPP in primiparas, but not multiparas [64]. The authors interpreted this to be a result of multiparas needing to be more active when raising an older child.

4.2. Psychological Distress

No systematic nor narrative reviews on the effectiveness of (di)stress interventions on pain symptoms in women with PGP were found.

In a recent systematic review on prognostic factors, experiencing emotional distress during pregnancy was associated with less recovery and severe pelvic girdle syndrome at 6 months after pregnancy, when the natural course of PGP is over ($n = 40,029$; Adjusted Odds Ratio (AOR) 1.3, 95% CI (1.1–1.5) [36]. The findings need to be taken with caution since quality of evidence according to GRADE was low to very low. Distress during pregnancy has also been associated with chronic PGP after delivery [65]. The conclusion is that there are indications that distress can affect PGP and its course and that this needs to be studied in more detail both within a prevention as well as a curative context.

4.3. Sleep

There was no identified systematic review regarding the effect of sleep management on PGP. Among pregnant women with pain in the lumbopelvic area, a high-pain group reported worse emotional health and poorer sleep quality than controls without pain [66]. Sleep disturbance has also been associated with persistent PGP and LPP at 4 months after pregnancy, even after adjustment for possible confounding variables such as BMI, parity, age, and history of LPP [67]. Sleep impairment related to quantity and adequacy of sleep has been associated with women with moderate disability from persistent PGP after pregnancy [68]. Different to these results, in a recent study the moderate or severe sleeping complaints associated with PGP disappeared after adjustment for depression [69]. This might be explained by the comorbidity of PGP and depression [26]. Many women experience disturbed sleep during pregnancy due to continuous hormonal-related changes of the body, need of nocturia and movement from the fetus. It is also known that around 50% of women get disturbed sleep during the first years of parenthood due to nighttime feeding and nocturnal awakening among infants [70,71].

To conclude, there is no evidence of sleep interventions for PGP. However, concerning the prevalence of sleep disturbance in relation to pregnancy and early childhood of women, there are indications of the importance of sleep as a lifestyle factor in women with chronic PGP.

4.4. Diet

There was no identified systematic review on the effectiveness of dietary interventions in the treatment of PGP. However, if an unhealthy diet leads to a high body mass index (BMI) there are some associations to consider. A systematic review reported an association between a BMI of 25 or more and having persistent PGP 12 weeks after pregnancy ($n = 179$; AOR 2.1, 95% CI 1.0–4.5) [36]. From the same study, it was reported that obese women (BMI 30 or more) had higher odds to have persistent pelvic girdle syndrome ($n = 27,025$; AOR 1.8, 95% CI 1.5–2.0) and severe pelvic girdle syndrome at 6 months ($n = 27,025$; AOR 1.6, 95% CI 1.1–2.4). Pre-pregnancy BMI > 25 was shown as a risk factor for chronic PGP in another recent systematic review [72]. Since interaction between factors could not be done in a multivariate analysis, the results should be taken with care [72].

Lifestyle intervention of physical activity in general in relation to pregnancy and postpartum are often focused on BMI as an outcome [73,74]. Effectiveness of a combination of diet and physical activity consistently showed a reduction in mean gestational weight gain during pregnancy and postnatal weight retention [75]. There were no reports on musculoskeletal pain of the studied groups, but from a coherent literature on PGP it is can be assumed that about 50% of the women had PGP in pregnancy and around 25% had persistent PGP after birth [4]. A major part of women used walking as physical activity intervention in the studies that reported types of physical activity [76,77]. Interesting to consider is whether professional individualized exercise advice would have further improved the outcomes.

Although no systematic review on PGP and diet was identified, there seems to be promising results of intervention for a combination of diet and physical activity in relation to pregnancy that needs further exploration of possible effects on chronic PGP.

4.5. Tobacco/Alcohol Use

There was no identified systematic review regarding the effect of tobacco or alcohol interventions on PGP.

In a systematic review on prognostic factors, Wuytack et al. reported an association with occasional smoking ($n = 38,865$; AOR 1.3, 95% CI 1.0–1.6), but not daily smoking, in women with pelvic girdle syndrome at 6 months postpartum [36].

5. Future Directions for Clinical Practice

In line with the World Health Organization's (WHO), a stronger focus towards a healthy lifestyle is recommended, i.e., being physically active for better health and for preventing noncommunicable diseases such as diabetes, cancer, and cardiovascular disease [78]. In the action plan for the prevention of long-term disability from LBP [79] and chronic pain in general across the lifespan [80], a positive health concept as an overarching strategic approach is emphasized. In this, a positive health concept entails, among others, learning to cope with a chronic health problem through self-management strategies. A healthier lifestyle promoting physical activity and staying active despite pain, maintaining a healthy weight, and promoting mental health, are in this context primary prevention strategies for chronic disability [79,80]. When specifically looking into the results of this state-of-the-art paper on lifestyle factors and their role in women with pain in the pelvis, only a few recommendations can be made based on the available literature. Regarding physical activity and exercise, encouraging women to be physically active and to exercise is supported to some extent. Nonetheless, because physical activity and exercises of different intensity, frequency, duration, and type were used in the available evidence, no specific recommendations regarding this point can be made. The available evidence on lifestyle factors such as sleep, (di)stress, diet, and tobacco/alcohol use for women with pain in the pelvis is inconclusive, since very few studies are available, and the studies which are available are of general low quality. Furthermore, most studies did not focus on the role of targeting lifestyle factors with the aim of improving pain in the pelvis. Therefore, no specific recommendations on the application of management strategies for these lifestyle factors can be provided.

We can, however, approach pain management in women with pain in the pelvis from a modern pain management point of view, which includes the management of lifestyle factors. Indeed, modern pain management implies change in the focus from pain reduction to pain management, i.e., managing thoughts and feelings related to pain (i.e., catastrophic worry), thereby influencing knowledge about pain [81–83] and providing opportunities for behavioral change towards a more active and healthier lifestyle. It also implies accurate self-management, which supports autonomy, and includes educational and supportive interventions to increase the skills and confidence for persons in pain to manage their health problems [84].

For women who are prone to pain experiences early in life, as related to menstruation [85] and pregnancy [4], learning healthy pain management is a priority. This includes the assessment and management of the individual woman with pain in the pelvis, taking into account her history, her present context and framing her messages into biopsycho-social and bio-inflammatory-psychological perspectives [29,86–90]. In this context, it is important for women who experience pain (cyclic pain from menstruation, local pregnancy-related pain, persistent pain at postpartum) to learn to approach activity despite pain. Indeed, physical activity has been described as a way to achieve exercise-induced analgesia [85,91] and as a strategy to promote self-efficacy (because of the experience of self-control [92], which is highly important given the relation between low self-efficacy and the development of disability [84]. In the context of pain in the pelvis, it has been shown that women with chronic PGP have less general self-efficacy than women who recovered from PGP after pregnancy [8]. From chronic pain science, it is known that physical activity additionally might have sleep improving [93], stress-reducing [94] and general anti-inflammatory effects [95], which are all relevant for optimal pain management [96]. Importantly, the intensity, volume, duration and type of activity that is most appropriate to reach these effects in women with pain in the pelvis are not firmly studied [97].

Nonetheless, it is known that pain is considered an important barrier against physical activity in women with pain in the pelvis [98]. For example, it is reported that women with PGP during pregnancy are less likely to exercise regularly [99]. Walking is the most chosen physical activity during pregnancy [77], but it is also the most painful physical activity when suffering from PGP [9]. Thus, decreased physical activity in pregnancy could be partly explained as a consequence of PGP. Importantly, women need to be guided into alternative physical activities and exercises when walking is painful. Therefore, in order to motivate women with pain in the pelvis to uptake physical activity despite tolerable levels of pain, and to reach a behavioral change, the use of a person-centred approach is essential [89]. A person-centred approach may increase the alliance between the care provider and the woman with pain in the pelvis, and subsequently lead to better adherence, improvements in general health and satisfaction [100]. It is important to approach the worries and concerns related to physical activity and exercise, e.g., how to interpret pain-increasing physical activity, which is different for a nociceptive versus nociplastic dominant pain mechanism. Pain neuroscience education is a known strategy that can reduce worries about pain by informing the individual mechanism of the experienced pain and is considered essential before starting physical activity interventions [81]. However, although it has been proven effective in several chronic pain populations, the evidence in women with chronic pain in the pelvis is still nonexistent [101].

Prevention of Chronic Pain in the Pelvis

During the woman's lifespan there are windows of opportunity to prevent the transition from localized and periodic pain in the pelvis (dysmenorrhea or from pregnancy) into chronic pain (Figure 1).

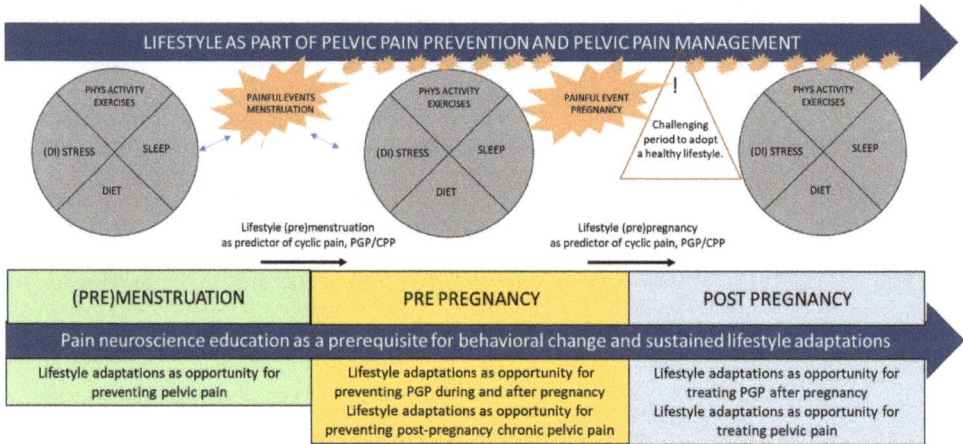

Figure 1. Women are exposed to pain in the pelvis during their lifespan in relation to hormonal changes and pregnancy. Lifestyle can influence the pain experience during the lifespan.

Pre-existing pro-inflammatory states increase the risk of chronification of pain [102]. During adolescence [103], and in relation to pregnancy [104], comorbid disorders of the urogenital systems are common and require attention. Early pain management with behavioral changes may reduce the risk of the transition towards chronic nociplastic pain in such cases, as was suggested from a systematic review (based on low to very low-quality evidence) [94].

Regarding the risk of chronic PGP, women at risk can be identified during pregnancy by a clinical assessment. The number of positive pain provocations tests is an established predictor of chronic PGP [8,105]. Pain provocation tests, as measures of increased pain sensitivity, have also been suggested as indicators of systematic inflammation [90]. Widespread pain, a characteristic feature of central sensitization [106], has been identified as the strongest predictor for a poor long-term outcome in women with PGP [107]. Moreover, it is reported that eleven years after PGP onset, women with chronic PGP show more concern and depression then women who recover from the PGP after pregnancy [8]. This observation supports the idea of cognitive-emotional sensitization in women with chronic PGP [108]. Therefore, clinical assessment in women with pregnancy-related PGP needs to contain at least pain provocation tests: a pain drawing to assess widespread pain and an evaluation of concern and depression [109,110]. This way, women at risk for chronic pain are identified and preventive interventions targeting the appropriate underlying mechanism might avoid the development of long-term pain [111].

The promotion of a healthy physical activity level during pregnancy, when women are extra prone to lifestyle changes [112], might improve health-promoting physical activity after childbirth [113]. Importantly, mothers' habits, including a healthy lifestyle, have demonstrated a positive effect on the offspring, as healthy role modelling behaviors for infants [74,87,112]. Current guidelines advise healthy pregnant women to follow the general guidelines of weekly, evenly distributed, physical activity which last 150 min, performed at a moderate intensity, plus two times per week resistance training [87]. Due to anatomical and physiological changes, as well as foetal requirements, some modification of exercise habits may be necessary. Reported barriers related to physical activity after pregnancy have been related to capability (e.g., limitation in healthcare providers' skills in providing lifestyle support), opportunity (support from partners) and motivation (e.g., identifying benefits of exercise) [74]. Therefore, it is important to focus on these barriers during pregnancy, and to find solutions on how to remove those obstacles [80]. In this context, it is known that women with PGP having a lack of knowledge and lack of support and knowledge from healthcare providers when seeking care, experience unmet needs [10,114,115]. Indeed, education and advice have been reported to positively influence pain, disability and/or sick leave [116].

It is common for pregnant women to seek knowledge and advice on the internet. However, it has been shown that bad advice flourishes and increases worries [117]. Therefore, women need guidance in what knowledge to trust and how to individualize it for their specific situation. This underlines the necessity for physical activity interventions and exercise regimes in pregnant women, guided by health care professionals with adequate education [86]. Indeed, expert advice and experiences on therapeutic exercise (with or without co-interventions) during pregnancy is proven effective [118]. In clinical practice, transcutaneous electric nerve stimulation and belts are common tools to support pain self-management, with some evidence to support their use in PGP [4,9]. They are generally seen as pain reduction tools but would rather be seen as tools to encourage appropriate physical activity, as they enable physical activity at a tolerable pain level.

Lastly and importantly, the promotion of a healthy lifestyle does not exclude the assessment of local nociception-inducing mechanisms in clinical examination and medical assessment, in order to identify and treat specific symptoms related to disorders causing pain in the pelvis.

6. Future Directions for Research

Women with pelvic pain due to severe dysmenorrhea are currently often told that their pain should be considered normal. In women with PGP during pregnancy or after delivery, pain is often considered a normal consequence of pregnancy and childbirth. Due to this narrow view on pain management, many women are undertreated for complaints that can be treatable. Since pain in the pelvis is associated with suffering, disability and a low health-related quality of life [115,119,120], there is an urgent need to better understand how to alleviate the suffering of women with pain in the pelvis, and to gain knowledge on adequate strategies to prevent (chronic) pain in the pelvis. This state-of-the-art review clearly shows that firm evidence on the role of lifestyle on pain, and on the effectiveness of lifestyle interventions on pain symptoms in women with pain in the pelvis, are essentially lacking. Therefore, we present a research agenda (Figure 2).

6.1. Pain Neuroscience Education: A Prerequisite for Sustained Lifestyle Adaptations in Women with Pain in the Pelvis?

It could be theorized that teaching women the science behind pain and the mechanisms related to pain in the pelvis (such as lifestyle factors) could be a strong protective factor for developing chronic pain in the pelvis throughout life and for intrinsically motivating them for a sustained engagement in a healthy lifestyle. Thereby, pain neuroscience education in the treatment of women with pelvic pain might provide women in pain with the necessary information to reach a sustained change towards a more active and healthier lifestyle. However, what pain neuroscience education in women with pelvic pain should look like, and whether it is effective in changing beliefs and behaviors, and subsequently in decreasing pain, should be a primary topic of research.

In this context, many questions related to pain education in women need to be considered. When during lifespan would it be optimal to educate women on pain which can appear in relation to menstruation or in relation to pregnancy and at postpartum? This question is of relevance as menstruation and pregnancy should not be medicalized, nor should be neglected. The delivery mode of pain education related to menstruation and pregnancy should also be considered. Can it be added to the curriculum in secondary school, or should the message be spread at a societal level to reach all stakeholders? In this context, it is also pertinent to study the societal and health care providers' ideas and beliefs about pain in the pelvis. A reflection on which women would need to be educated is another relevant topic in this regard; all women versus women experiencing painful menstruation or PGP, versus women who are mothers experience pelvic pain? Furthermore, the content of the education to achieve the highest impact on women should be explored. Information on all former topics can be studied using quantitative and qualitative research approaches. This way, the barriers for optimal pain care on a patient's, healthcare provider's and societal level can be identified, and necessary content for pain neuroscience education for women with pain in the pelvis can be defined.

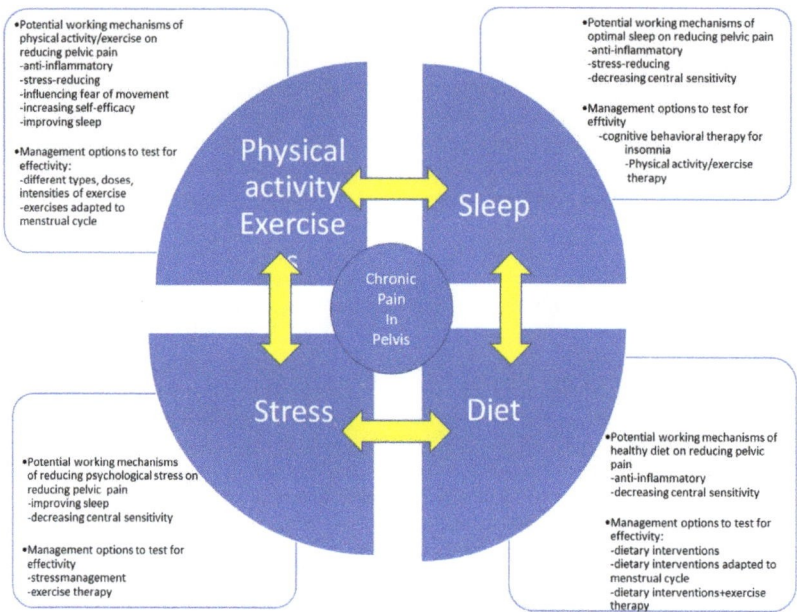

Figure 2. Research agenda of the potential working mechanisms of lifestyle factors on pain reduction in chronic pain in the pelvis, in parallel with potential management options.

6.2. A Broad View on Pain in Women with Pain in the Pelvis

Young menstruating women's pain experiences need to be better understood in the development of disability and chronic pain in the pelvis. A better understanding of the role of multiple factors, such as lifestyle, genetic, psychosocial and patho-anatomical factors as predictors for severe pain in the pelvis would create opportunities for developing early preventive and curative strategies. The underlying effects related to lifestyle interventions in endometriosis-related pelvic pain, such as an estrogen-dependent and an anti-inflammatory effect, need to be further explored. Such information is necessary to develop the specific content for pain neuroscience education programs in women with pain in the pelvis.

In the context of pregnancy-related pain, the pregnancy period is a period characterized by sleep deprivation, hormonal and psychological emotional changes, and less physical activity. For women after childbirth, pelvic floor trauma is an additional challenge in relation to lifestyle, besides those factors mentioned during pregnancy that all may prevail after pregnancy. Through shared neurophysiological mechanisms, these factors may contribute to the development of PGP in pregnancy and chronic PGP which lasts at postpartum. In this, the dominant pain mechanism in pregnancy-related PGP needs to be better understood. Since widespread pain, a characteristic feature of central sensitization [106], has been identified as the strongest predictor of poor long-term outcome in women with PGP [107], more studies on the role of central sensitization in the development of chronic PGP are needed to develop preventive strategies and individually tailored interventions (e.g., personalized pain education and behavior treatment).

Furthermore, the potential of lifestyle adaptations, adapted to pregnancy, as an opportunity for preventing and decreasing the impact of PGP after pregnancy must be explored. Research on how current treatments for lifestyle interventions such as cognitive behavioral therapy as a sleep intervention [121], can be adapted specifically for women with pain in the early time periods following childbirth, is of high priority. Indeed, women ask for more knowledge and support on strategies to (self-)manage pain in relation to pregnancy [10,115]. Therefore, studies on the content and delivery method of pain management programs in women with pregnancy-related pain in the pelvis are needed, i.e., how can treatment be implemented with potential barriers to approaching a healthy lifestyle (e.g., common sleep deprivation due to pregnancy or young children)? In terms of delivery form, management by means of mobile-and-internet-delivered programs for prevention, as well as pain management programs, must be further explored.

It is of interest to explore which barriers towards a healthy lifestyle exist in women with pain in the pelvis. It is, for example, of interest to explore whether transcutaneous electric nerve stimulation can be used as a nonpharmacological treatment to influence central sensitization in women with cyclic or periodic pain [122], and be an effective treatment for staying active and exercising during painful periods. Pelvic floor disorders as a consequence of childbirth need to be identified and managed, not only for the problems themselves but also as barriers to exercise. It is known that pregnancy and vaginal delivery are among the main risk factors for urinary and faecal incontinence [104], and that urinary incontinence affects exercise participation in one in two symptomatic women. Pelvic floor disorders including urinary and faecal incontinence, and pelvic floor prolapse are reported barriers to exercise with a moderate or great effect in 39% of women (95% CI: 22%, 57%) [123]. Therefore, it is clear that women with pelvic pain should always be approached in a multidimensional way, by a multidisciplinary team. Indeed, chronic pain in the pelvis requires competences from multiple disciplines that involve physiotherapists, midwives, gynecologists, psychologists, occupational therapists, and pain specialized medical doctors.

Finally future research on PGP should consider the recent published core outcome set of PGP to enable future compilation of results in systematic reviews [110]. To strengthen the quality of the evidence, future studies would benefit from designing and presenting results in accordance with accepted reporting standards (e.g., CONSORT and PRISMA).

7. Conclusions

During their lifespans, many women are exposed to pain in the pelvis in relation to menstruation and pregnancy, which is often considered normal and inherently linked to being a woman. This leads to insufficient treatment. Severe dysmenorrhea, as seen in endometriosis and pregnancy-related PGP, has a great impact on daily activities, school attendance and work ability. Lifestyle factors such as a low physical activity level, poor sleep, or periods of (di)stress are all common in these challenging periods of women's life.

Based on this state-of-the-art review, encouraging women with pain in the pelvis to be physically active and to exercise is supported to some extent. Clinicians are suggested to use a window of opportunity to prevent a potential transition from localized or periodic pain in the pelvis (e.g., pain during pregnancy and after delivery or severe dysmenorrhea) towards persistent chronic pain, by encouraging a healthy physical activity level and applying appropriate pain management. The available evidence on lifestyle factors such as sleep, (di)stress, diet, and tobacco/alcohol use is, however, inconclusive; very few studies are available, and the studies which are available are of general low quality.

Research to disentangle the relationship between lifestyle factors, such as physical activity level, sleep, diet, smoking, and psychological distress, and the experience of pain in the pelvis is highly needed. Studies which address the development of management strategies for adapting lifestyle, which are specifically tailored to women with pain in the pelvis, and take hormonal status, life events and context into account, are required.

Author Contributions: Conceptualization, A.G. and L.D.B.; methodology, A.G. and L.D.B.; validation, A.G., K.S. and L.D.B.; writing—A.G. and L.D.B.; writing—review and editing, A.G., K.S. and L.D.B. All authors have read and agreed to the published version of the manuscript.

Funding: Swedish state under the agreement between the Swedish government and the county council, the ALF-agreement (KS).

Institutional Review Board Statement: Not applicable.

Informed Consent Statement: Not applicable.

Conflicts of Interest: The authors declare no conflict of interest.

References

1. Armour, M.; Parry, K.; Al-Dabbas, M.A.; Curry, C.; Holmes, K.; MacMillan, F.; Ferfolja, T.; Smith, C.A. Self-care strategies and sources of knowledge on menstruation in 12,526 young women with dysmenorrhea: A systematic review and meta-analysis. *PLoS ONE* **2019**, *14*, e0220103. [CrossRef] [PubMed]
2. As-Sanie, S.; Kim, J.; Schmidt-Wilcke, T.; Sundgren, P.C.; Clauw, D.J.; Napadow, V.; Harris, R.E. Functional Connectivity is Associated with Altered Brain Chemistry in Women with Endometriosis-Associated Chronic Pelvic Pain. *J. Pain* **2016**, *17*, 1–13. [CrossRef] [PubMed]
3. Taylor, H.S.; Kotlyar, A.M.; Flores, V.A. Endometriosis is a chronic systemic disease: Clinical challenges and novel innovations. *Lancet* **2021**, *397*, 839–852. [CrossRef]
4. Liddle, S.D.; Pennick, V. Interventions for preventing and treating low-back and pelvic pain during pregnancy. *Cochrane Database Syst. Rev.* **2015**, *9*, CD001139. [CrossRef]
5. Vleeming, A.; Albert, H.B.; Ostgaard, H.C.; Sturesson, B.; Stuge, B. European guidelines for the diagnosis and treatment of pelvic girdle pain. *Eur. Spine J.* **2008**, *17*, 794–819. [CrossRef]
6. Wuytack, F.; Curtis, E.; Begley, C. Experiences of First-Time Mothers with Persistent Pelvic Girdle Pain after Childbirth: Descriptive Qualitative Study. *Phys. Ther.* **2015**, *95*, 1354–1364. [CrossRef]
7. Engeset, J.; Stuge, B.; Fegran, L. Pelvic girdle pain affects the whole life-a qualitative interview study in Norway on women's experiences with pelvic girdle pain after delivery. *BMC Res. Notes* **2014**, *7*, 686. [CrossRef]
8. Elden, H.; Gutke, A.; Kjellby-Wendt, G.; Fagevik-Olsen, M.; Ostgaard, H.C. Predictors and consequences of long-term pregnancy-related pelvic girdle pain: A longitudinal follow-up study. *BMC Musculoskelet. Disord.* **2016**, *17*, 276. [CrossRef]
9. Gutke, A.; Betten, C.; Degerskar, K.; Pousette, S.; Olsen, M.F. Treatments for pregnancy-related lumbopelvic pain: A systematic review of physiotherapy modalities. *Acta Obstet. Gynecol. Scand.* **2015**, *94*, 1156–1167. [CrossRef]
10. Gutke, A.; Boissonnault, J.; Brook, G.; Stuge, B. The Severity and Impact of Pelvic Girdle Pain and Low-Back Pain in Pregnancy: A Multinational Study. *J. Womens Health* **2018**, *27*, 510–517. [CrossRef]
11. Vermani, E.; Mittal, R.; Weeks, A. Pelvic girdle pain and low back pain in pregnancy: A review. *Pain Pract.* **2010**, *10*, 60–71. [CrossRef] [PubMed]
12. Shafrir, A.L.; Farland, L.V.; Shah, D.K.; Harris, H.R.; Kvaskoff, M.; Zondervan, K.; Missmer, S.A. Risk for and consequences of endometriosis: A critical epidemiologic review. *Best Pract. Res. Clin. Obstet. Gynaecol.* **2018**, *51*, 1–15. [CrossRef]
13. Zondervan, K.T.; Becker, C.M.; Missmer, S.A. Endometriosis. *N. Engl. J. Med.* **2020**, *382*, 1244–1256. [CrossRef] [PubMed]
14. As-Sanie, S.; Harris, R.E.; Napadow, V.; Kim, J.; Neshewat, G.; Kairys, A.; Williams, D.; Clauw, D.J.; Schmidt-Wilcke, T. Changes in regional gray matter volume in women with chronic pelvic pain: A voxel-based morphometry study. *Pain* **2012**, *153*, 1006–1014. [CrossRef] [PubMed]
15. Zondervan, K.T.; Becker, C.M.; Koga, K.; Missmer, S.A.; Taylor, R.N.; Vigano, P. Endometriosis. *Nat. Rev. Dis. Primers* **2018**, *4*, 9. [CrossRef]
16. Chiaffarino, F.; Cipriani, S.; Ricci, E.; Mauri, P.A.; Esposito, G.; Barretta, M.; Vercellini, P.; Parazzini, F. Endometriosis and irritable bowel syndrome: A systematic review and meta-analysis. *Arch. Gynecol. Obstet.* **2021**, *303*, 17–25. [CrossRef]
17. Prescott, J.; Farland, L.V.; Tobias, D.K.; Gaskins, A.J.; Spiegelman, D.; Chavarro, J.E.; Rich-Edwards, J.W.; Barbieri, R.L.; Missmer, S.A. A prospective cohort study of endometriosis and subsequent risk of infertility. *Hum. Reprod.* **2016**, *31*, 1475–1482. [CrossRef] [PubMed]
18. Rossi, H.R.; Uimari, O.; Arffman, R.; Vaaramo, E.; Kujanpaa, L.; Ala-Mursula, L.; Piltonen, T.T. The association of endometriosis with work ability and work life participation in late forties and lifelong disability retirement up till age 52: A Northern Finland Birth Cohort 1966 study. *Acta Obstet. Gynecol. Scand.* **2021**, *100*, 1822–1829. [CrossRef]
19. Alvarez-Salvago, F.; Lara-Ramos, A.; Cantarero-Villanueva, I.; Mazheika, M.; Mundo-Lopez, A.; Galiano-Castillo, N.; Fernández-Lao, C.; Arroyo-Morales, M.; Ocón-Hernández, O.; Artacho-Cordón, F. Chronic Fatigue, Physical Impairments and Quality of Life in Women with Endometriosis: A Case-Control Study. *Int. J. Environ. Res. Public Health* **2020**, *17*, 3610. [CrossRef]

20. Machairiotis, N.; Vasilakaki, S.; Thomakos, N. Inflammatory Mediators and Pain in Endometriosis: A Systematic Review. *Biomedicines* **2021**, *9*, 54. [CrossRef]
21. Rost, C.C.; Jacqueline, J.; Kaiser, A.; Verhagen, A.P.; Koes, B.W. Pelvic pain during pregnancy: A descriptive study of signs and symptoms of 870 patients in primary care. *Spine* **2004**, *29*, 2567–2572. [CrossRef]
22. Gutke, A.; Olsson, C.B.; Vollestad, N.; Oberg, B.; Wikmar, L.N.; Robinson, H.S. Association between lumbopelvic pain, disability and sick leave during pregnancy—A comparison of three Scandinavian cohorts. *J. Rehabil. Med.* **2014**, *46*, 468–474. [CrossRef] [PubMed]
23. Elden, H.; Hagberg, H.; Olsen, M.F.; Ladfors, L.; Ostgaard, H.C. Regression of pelvic girdle pain after delivery: Follow-up of a randomised single blind controlled trial with different treatment modalities. *Acta Obstet. Gynecol. Scand.* **2008**, *87*, 201–208. [CrossRef] [PubMed]
24. Aldabe, D.; Ribeiro, D.C.; Milosavljevic, S.; Dawn Bussey, M. Pregnancy-related pelvic girdle pain and its relationship with relaxin levels during pregnancy: A systematic review. *Eur. Spine J.* **2012**, *21*, 1769–1776. [CrossRef]
25. Gutke, A.; Josefsson, A.; Oberg, B. Pelvic girdle pain and lumbar pain in relation to postpartum depressive symptoms. *Spine* **2007**, *32*, 1430–1436. [CrossRef] [PubMed]
26. Virgara, R.; Maher, C.; Van Kessel, G. The comorbidity of low back pelvic pain and risk of depression and anxiety in pregnancy in primiparous women. *BMC Pregnancy Childbirth* **2018**, *18*, 288. [CrossRef]
27. Bryndal, A.; Majchrzycki, M.; Grochulska, A.; Glowinski, S.; Seremak-Mrozikiewicz, A. Risk Factors Associated with Low Back Pain among A Group of 1510 Pregnant Women. *J. Pers. Med.* **2020**, *10*, 51. [CrossRef]
28. Meijer, O.G.; Hu, H.; Wu, W.H.; Prins, M.R. The pelvic girdle pain deadlock: 1. Would 'deconstruction' help? *Musculoskelet. Sci. Pract.* **2020**, *48*, 102169. [CrossRef]
29. O'Sullivan, P.B.; Beales, D.J. Diagnosis and classification of pelvic girdle pain disorders—Part 1: A mechanism based approach within a biopsychosocial framework. *Man. Ther.* **2007**, *12*, 86–97. [CrossRef]
30. Willaert, W.; Leysen, L.; Lenoir, D.; Meeus, M.; Cagnie, B.; Nijs, J.; Sterling, M.; Coppieters, I. Combining Stress Management with Pain Neuroscience Education and Exercise Therapy in People with Whiplash-Associated Disorders: A Clinical Perspective. *Phys. Ther.* **2021**, *101*, pzab105. [CrossRef]
31. Malfliet, A.; Marnef, A.Q.; Nijs, J.; Clarys, P.; Huybrechts, I.; Elma, O.; Yilmaz, S.T.; Deliens, T. Obesity Hurts: The why and how of Integrating Weight Reduction with Chronic Pain Management. *Phys. Ther.* **2021**, *101*, pzab198. [CrossRef] [PubMed]
32. Nijs, J.; Mairesse, O.; Neu, D.; Leysen, L.; Danneels, L.; Cagnie, B.; Meeus, M.; Moens, M.; Ickmans, K.; Goubert, D. Sleep Disturbances in Chronic Pain: Neurobiology, Assessment, and Treatment in Physical Therapist Practice. *Phys. Ther.* **2018**, *98*, 325–335. [CrossRef] [PubMed]
33. Palagini, L.; Gemignani, A.; Banti, S.; Manconi, M.; Mauri, M.; Riemann, D. Chronic sleep loss during pregnancy as a determinant of stress: Impact on pregnancy outcome. *Sleep Med.* **2014**, *15*, 853–859. [CrossRef] [PubMed]
34. Okun, M.L.; Coussons-Read, M.E. Sleep disruption during pregnancy: How does it influence serum cytokines? *J. Reprod. Immunol.* **2007**, *73*, 158–165. [CrossRef]
35. Taveras, E.M.; Rifas-Shiman, S.L.; Rich-Edwards, J.W.; Mantzoros, C.S. Maternal short sleep duration is associated with increased levels of inflammatory markers at 3 years postpartum. *Metabolism* **2011**, *60*, 982–986. [CrossRef]
36. Wuytack, F.; Daly, D.; Curtis, E.; Begley, C. Prognostic factors for pregnancy-related pelvic girdle pain, a systematic review. *Midwifery* **2018**, *66*, 70–78. [CrossRef]
37. Youseflu, S.; Jahanian Sadatmahalleh, S.; Roshanzadeh, G.; Mottaghi, A.; Kazemnejad, A.; Moini, A. Effects of endometriosis on sleep quality of women: Does life style factor make a difference? *BMC Womens Health* **2020**, *20*, 168. [CrossRef]
38. Andrews, P.; Steultjens, M.; Riskowski, J. Chronic widespread pain prevalence in the general population: A systematic review. *Eur. J. Pain* **2018**, *22*, 5–18. [CrossRef]
39. World Health Organization. Prevalence of Insufficient Physical Activity among Adults. Available online: https://apps.who.int/gho/data/view.main.2463 (accessed on 19 September 2021).
40. Caspersen, C.J.; Powell, K.E.; Christenson, G.M. Physical activity, exercise, and physical fitness: Definitions and distinctions for health-related research. *Public Health Rep.* **1985**, *100*, 126–131.
41. Wu, W.H.; Meijer, O.G.; Uegaki, K.; Mens, J.M.; van Dieen, J.H.; Wuisman, P.I.; Östgaard, H.C. Pregnancy-related pelvic girdle pain (PPP), I: Terminology, clinical presentation, and prevalence. *Eur. Spine J.* **2004**, *13*, 575–589. [CrossRef]
42. Weis, C.A.; Pohlman, K.; Draper, C.; da Silva-Oolup, S.; Stuber, K.; Hawk, C. Chiropractic Care of Adults with Postpartum-Related Low Back, Pelvic Girdle, or Combination Pain: A Systematic Review. *J. Manip. Physiol. Ther.* **2020**, *43*, 732–743. [CrossRef]
43. Hansen, S.; Sverrisdottir, U.A.; Rudnicki, M. Impact of exercise on pain perception in women with endometriosis: A systematic review. *Acta Obstet. Gynecol. Scand.* **2021**, *100*, 1595–1601. [CrossRef] [PubMed]
44. Ricci, E.; Vigano, P.; Cipriani, S.; Chiaffarino, F.; Bianchi, S.; Rebonato, G.; Parazzini, F. Physical activity and endometriosis risk in women with infertility or pain: Systematic review and meta-analysis. *Medicine* **2016**, *95*, e4957. [CrossRef] [PubMed]
45. Huijs, E.; Nap, A. The effects of nutrients on symptoms in women with endometriosis: A systematic review. *Reprod. Biomed. Online* **2020**, *41*, 317–328. [CrossRef]
46. Nirgianakis, K.; Egger, K.; Kalaitzopoulos, D.R.; Lanz, S.; Bally, L.; Mueller, M.D. Effectiveness of Dietary Interventions in the Treatment of Endometriosis: A Systematic Review. *Reprod. Sci.* **2021**. [CrossRef] [PubMed]

47. Qi, X.; Zhang, W.; Ge, M.; Sun, Q.; Peng, L.; Cheng, W.; Li, X. Relationship Between Dairy Products Intake and Risk of Endometriosis: A Systematic Review and Dose-Response Meta-Analysis. *Front. Nutr.* **2021**, *8*, 701860. [CrossRef] [PubMed]
48. Evans, S.; Fernandez, S.; Olive, L.; Payne, L.A.; Mikocka-Walus, A. Psychological and mind-body interventions for endometriosis: A systematic review. *J. Psychosom. Res.* **2019**, *124*, 109756. [CrossRef]
49. Bravi, F.; Parazzini, F.; Cipriani, S.; Chiaffarino, F.; Ricci, E.; Chiantera, V.; Viganò, P.; Vecchia, C.L. Tobacco smoking and risk of endometriosis: A systematic review and meta-analysis. *BMJ Open* **2014**, *4*, e006325. [CrossRef]
50. Bonocher, C.M.; Montenegro, M.L.; Rosa, E.S.J.C.; Ferriani, R.A.; Meola, J. Endometriosis and physical exercises: A systematic review. *Reprod. Biol. Endocrinol.* **2014**, *12*, 4. [CrossRef]
51. Arion, K.; Orr, N.L.; Noga, H.; Allaire, C.; Williams, C.; Bedaiwy, M.A.; Yong, P.J. A Quantitative Analysis of Sleep Quality in Women with Endometriosis. *J. Womens Health* **2020**, *29*, 1209–1215. [CrossRef]
52. Nunes, F.R.; Ferreira, J.M.; Bahamondes, L. Pain threshold and sleep quality in women with endometriosis. *Eur. J. Pain* **2015**, *19*, 15–20. [CrossRef] [PubMed]
53. Stang, A. Critical evaluation of the Newcastle-Ottawa scale for the assessment of the quality of nonrandomized studies in meta-analyses. *Eur. J. Epidemiol.* **2010**, *25*, 603–605. [CrossRef]
54. Helbig, M.; Vesper, A.S.; Beyer, I.; Fehm, T. Does Nutrition Affect Endometriosis? *Geburtshilfe Frauenheilkd* **2021**, *81*, 191–199. [CrossRef] [PubMed]
55. Weis, C.A.; Pohlman, K.; Draper, C.; daSilva-Oolup, S.; Stuber, K.; Hawk, C. Chiropractic Care for Adults with Pregnancy-Related Low Back, Pelvic Girdle Pain, or Combination Pain: A Systematic Review. *J. Manip. Physiol. Ther.* **2020**, *43*, 714–731. [CrossRef] [PubMed]
56. Davenport, M.H.; Marchand, A.A.; Mottola, M.F.; Poitras, V.J.; Gray, C.E.; Jaramillo Garcia, A.; Barrowman, N.; Sobierajski, F.; James, M.; Meah, V.L.; et al. Exercise for the prevention and treatment of low back, pelvic girdle and lumbopelvic pain during pregnancy: A systematic review and meta-analysis. *Br. J. Sports Med.* **2019**, *53*, 90–98. [CrossRef]
57. Almousa, S.; Lamprianidou, E.; Kitsoulis, G. The effectiveness of stabilising exercises in pelvic girdle pain during pregnancy and after delivery: A systematic review. *Physiother. Res. Int.* **2018**, *23*, e1699. [CrossRef] [PubMed]
58. Shiri, R.; Coggon, D.; Falah-Hassani, K. Exercise for the prevention of low back and pelvic girdle pain in pregnancy: A meta-analysis of randomized controlled trials. *Eur. J. Pain* **2018**, *22*, 19–27. [CrossRef]
59. Tseng, P.C.; Puthussery, S.; Pappas, Y.; Gau, M.L. A systematic review of randomised controlled trials on the effectiveness of exercise programs on Lumbo Pelvic Pain among postnatal women. *BMC Pregnancy Childbirth* **2015**, *15*, 316. [CrossRef]
60. Stuge, B. Current knowledge on low back pain and pelvic girdle pain during pregnancy and after childbirth: A narrative review. *Curr. Women's Health Rev.* **2015**, *11*, 68–74. [CrossRef]
61. Fisseha, B.; Mishra, P.K. The effect of group training on pregnancy-induced lumbopelvic pain: Systematic review and meta-analysis of randomized control trials. *J. Exerc. Rehabil.* **2016**, *12*, 15–20. [CrossRef]
62. Caputo, E.L.; Ferreira, P.H.; Ferreira, M.L.; Bertoldi, A.D.; Domingues, M.R.; Shirley, D.; Silva, M.C. Physical Activity Before or During Pregnancy and Low Back Pain: Data From the 2015 Pelotas (Brazil) Birth Cohort Study. *J. Phys. Act. Health* **2019**, *16*, 886–893. [CrossRef] [PubMed]
63. Bellows-Riecken, K.H.; Rhodes, R.E. A birth of inactivity? A review of physical activity and parenthood. *Prev. Med.* **2008**, *46*, 99–110. [CrossRef] [PubMed]
64. Aota, E.; Kitagaki, K.; Tanaka, K.; Tsuboi, Y.; Matsuda, N.; Horibe, K.; Perrein, E.; Ono, R. The Impact of Sedentary Behavior after Childbirth on Postpartum Lumbopelvic Pain Prolongation: A Follow-Up Cohort Study. *J. Womens Health* **2021**. [CrossRef]
65. Bjelland, E.K.; Stuge, B.; Engdahl, B.; Eberhard-Gran, M. The effect of emotional distress on persistent pelvic girdle pain after delivery: A longitudinal population study. *BJOG* **2013**, *120*, 32–40. [CrossRef]
66. Palsson, T.S.; Beales, D.; Slater, H.; O'Sullivan, P.; Graven-Nielsen, T. Pregnancy is characterized by widespread deep-tissue hypersensitivity independent of lumbopelvic pain intensity, a facilitated response to manual orthopedic tests, and poorer self-reported health. *J. Pain* **2015**, *16*, 270–282. [CrossRef] [PubMed]
67. Horibe, K.; Isa, T.; Matsuda, N.; Murata, S.; Tsuboi, Y.; Okumura, M.; Kawaharada, R.; Kogaki, M.; Uchida, K.; Nakatsuka, K.; et al. Association between sleep disturbance and low back and pelvic pain in 4-month postpartum women: A cross-sectional study. *Eur. Spine J.* **2021**, *30*, 2983–2988. [CrossRef]
68. Beales, D.; Lutz, A.; Thompson, J.; Wand, B.M.; O'Sullivan, P. Disturbed body perception, reduced sleep, and kinesiophobia in subjects with pregnancy-related persistent lumbopelvic pain and moderate levels of disability: An exploratory study. *Man. Ther.* **2016**, *21*, 69–75. [CrossRef]
69. Ertmann, R.K.; Nicolaisdottir, D.R.; Kragstrup, J.; Siersma, V.; Lutterodt, M.C. Sleep complaints in early pregnancy. A cross-sectional study among women attending prenatal care in general practice. *BMC Pregnancy Childbirth* **2020**, *20*, 123. [CrossRef]
70. Hysing, M.; Harvey, A.G.; Torgersen, L.; Ystrom, E.; Reichborn-Kjennerud, T.; Sivertsen, B. Trajectories and predictors of nocturnal awakenings and sleep duration in infants. *J. Dev. Behav. Pediatr.* **2014**, *35*, 309–316. [CrossRef]
71. Sivertsen, B.; Hysing, M.; Dorheim, S.K.; Eberhard-Gran, M. Trajectories of maternal sleep problems before and after childbirth: A longitudinal population-based study. *BMC Pregnancy Childbirth* **2015**, *15*, 129. [CrossRef]
72. Wiezer, M.; Hage-Fransen, M.A.H.; Otto, A.; Wieffer-Platvoet, M.S.; Slotman, M.H.; Nijhuis-van der Sanden, M.W.G.; Pool-Goudzwaard, A.L. Risk factors for pelvic girdle pain postpartum and pregnancy related low back pain postpartum; a systematic review and meta-analysis. *Musculoskelet. Sci. Pract.* **2020**, *48*, 102154. [CrossRef]

73. Lim, S.; Hill, B.; Teede, H.J.; Moran, L.J.; O'Reilly, S. An evaluation of the impact of lifestyle interventions on body weight in postpartum women: A systematic review and meta-analysis. *Obes. Rev.* **2020**, *21*, e12990. [CrossRef]
74. Makama, M.; Awoke, M.A.; Skouteris, H.; Moran, L.J.; Lim, S. Barriers and facilitators to a healthy lifestyle in postpartum women: A systematic review of qualitative and quantitative studies in postpartum women and healthcare providers. *Obes. Rev.* **2021**, *22*, e13167. [CrossRef]
75. Hayes, L.; McParlin, C.; Azevedo, L.B.; Jones, D.; Newham, J.; Olajide, J.; McCleman, L.; Heslehurst, N. The Effectiveness of Smoking Cessation, Alcohol Reduction, Diet and Physical Activity Interventions in Improving Maternal and Infant Health Outcomes: A Systematic Review of Meta-Analyses. *Nutrients* **2021**, *13*, 1036. [CrossRef] [PubMed]
76. van der Pligt, P.; Olander, E.K.; Ball, K.; Crawford, D.; Hesketh, K.D.; Teychenne, M.; Campbell, K. Maternal dietary intake and physical activity habits during the postpartum period: Associations with clinician advice in a sample of Australian first time mothers. *BMC Pregnancy Childbirth* **2016**, *16*, 27. [CrossRef] [PubMed]
77. Downs, D.S.; Chasan-Taber, L.; Evenson, K.R.; Leiferman, J.; Yeo, S. Physical activity and pregnancy: Past and present evidence and future recommendations. *Res. Q. Exerc. Sport* **2012**, *83*, 485–502. [CrossRef]
78. World Health Organization. Physical Activity. Available online: https://www.who.int/news-room/fact-sheets/detail/physical-activity (accessed on 27 September 2021).
79. Buchbinder, R.; van Tulder, M.; Oberg, B.; Costa, L.M.; Woolf, A.; Schoene, M.; Croft, P.; Lancet Low Back Pain Series Working Group. Low back pain: A call for action. *Lancet* **2018**, *391*, 2384–2388. [CrossRef]
80. Nijs, J.; D'Hondt, E.; Clarys, P.; Deliens, T.; Polli, A.; Malfliet, A.; Coppieters, I.; Willaert, W.; Tumkaya Yilmaz, S.; Elma, O.; et al. Lifestyle and Chronic Pain across the Lifespan: An Inconvenient Truth? *PM R.* **2020**, *12*, 410–419. [CrossRef]
81. Malfliet, A.; Kregel, J.; Coppieters, I.; De Pauw, R.; Meeus, M.; Roussel, N.; Cagnie, B.; Danneels, L.; Nijs, J. Effect of Pain Neuroscience Education Combined with Cognition-Targeted Motor Control Training on Chronic Spinal Pain: A Randomized Clinical Trial. *JAMA Neurol.* **2018**, *75*, 808–817. [CrossRef] [PubMed]
82. Nijs, J.; Wijma, A.J.; Willaert, W.; Huysmans, E.; Mintken, P.; Smeets, R.; Goossens, M.; van Wilgen, C.P.; Van Bogaert, W.; Louw, A.; et al. Integrating Motivational Interviewing in Pain Neuroscience Education for People with Chronic Pain: A Practical Guide for Clinicians. *Phys. Ther.* **2020**, *100*, 846–859. [CrossRef] [PubMed]
83. Malfliet, A.; Bilterys, T.; Van Looveren, E.; Meeus, M.; Danneels, L.; Ickmans, K.; Cagnie, B.; Mairesse, O.; Neu, D.; Moens, M.; et al. The added value of cognitive behavioral therapy for insomnia to current best evidence physical therapy for chronic spinal pain: Protocol of a randomized controlled clinical trial. *Braz. J. Phys. Ther.* **2019**, *23*, 62–70. [CrossRef]
84. Lee, H.; Hubscher, M.; Moseley, G.L.; Kamper, S.J.; Traeger, A.C.; Mansell, G.; McAuley, J.H. How does pain lead to disability? A systematic review and meta-analysis of mediation studies in people with back and neck pain. *Pain* **2015**, *156*, 988–997. [CrossRef]
85. Armour, M.; Smith, C.A.; Steel, K.A.; Macmillan, F. The effectiveness of self-care and lifestyle interventions in primary dysmenorrhea: A systematic review and meta-analysis. *BMC Complement Altern. Med.* **2019**, *19*, 22. [CrossRef]
86. Stuge, B. Evidence of stabilizing exercises for low back- and pelvic girdle pain—A critical review. *Braz. J. Phys. Ther.* **2019**, *23*, 181–186. [CrossRef]
87. ACOG. Physical Activity and Exercise during Pregnancy and the Postpartum Period: ACOG Committee Opinion Summary, Number 804. *Obstet. Gynecol.* **2020**, *135*, 991–993.
88. O'Sullivan, P.B.; Beales, D.J. Diagnosis and classification of pelvic girdle pain disorders, Part 2: Illustration of the utility of a classification system via case studies. *Man. Ther.* **2007**, *12*, e1–e12. [CrossRef] [PubMed]
89. Beales, D.; Slater, H.; Palsson, T.; O'Sullivan, P. Understanding and managing pelvic girdle pain from a person-centred biopsychosocial perspective. *Musculoskelet. Sci. Pract.* **2020**, *48*, 102152. [CrossRef] [PubMed]
90. Meijer, O.G.; Barbe, M.F.; Prins, M.R.; Schipholt, I.J.L.; Hu, H.; Daffertshofer, A. The Pelvic Girdle Pain deadlock: 2. Topics that, so far, have remained out of focus. *Musculoskelet. Sci. Pract.* **2020**, *48*, 102166. [CrossRef]
91. Daenen, L.; Nijs, J.; Cras, P.; Wouters, K.; Roussel, N. Changes in Pain Modulation Occur Soon after Whiplash Trauma but are not Related to Altered Perception of Distorted Visual Feedback. *Pain Pract.* **2014**, *14*, 588–598. [CrossRef]
92. Parschau, L.; Fleig, L.; Warner, L.M.; Pomp, S.; Barz, M.; Knoll, N.; Schwarzer, R.; Lippke, S. Positive Exercise Experience Facilitates Behavior Change via Self-Efficacy. *Health Educ. Behav.* **2014**, *41*, 414–422. [CrossRef]
93. Estevez-Lopez, F.; Maestre-Cascales, C.; Russell, D.; Alvarez-Gallardo, I.C.; Rodriguez-Ayllon, M.; Hughes, C.M.; Davison, G.W.; Sanudo, B.; McVeigh, J.G. Effectiveness of Exercise on Fatigue and Sleep Quality in Fibromyalgia: A Systematic Review and Meta-analysis of Randomized Trials. *Arch. Phys. Med. Rehabil.* **2021**, *102*, 752–761. [CrossRef]
94. Belavy, D.L.; Van Oosterwijck, J.; Clarkson, M.; Dhondt, E.; Mundell, N.L.; Miller, C.T.; Owen, P.j. Pain sensitivity is reduced by exercise training: Evidence from a systematic review and meta-analysis. *Neurosci. Biobehav. Rev.* **2021**, *120*, 100–108. [CrossRef]
95. Gleeson, M.; Bishop, N.C.; Stensel, D.J.; Lindley, M.R.; Mastana, S.S.; Nimmo, M.A. The anti-inflammatory effects of exercise: Mechanisms and implications for the prevention and treatment of disease. *Nat. Rev. Immunol.* **2011**, *11*, 607–615. [CrossRef] [PubMed]
96. Nijs, J.; Leysen, L.; Vanlauwe, J.; Logghe, T.; Ickmans, K.; Polli, A.; Malfliet, A.; Coppieters, I.; Huysmans, E. Treatment of central sensitization in patients with chronic pain: Time for change? *Expert Opin. Pharmacother.* **2019**, *20*, 1961–1970. [CrossRef] [PubMed]
97. Nijs, J.; Kosek, E.; Van Oosterwijck, J.; Meeus, M. Dysfunctional endogenous analgesia during exercise in patients with chronic pain: To exercise or not to exercise? *Pain Physician* **2012**, *15* (Suppl. 3), ES205–ES213. [CrossRef] [PubMed]

98. Coll, C.V.; Domingues, M.R.; Goncalves, H.; Bertoldi, A.D. Perceived barriers to leisure-time physical activity during pregnancy: A literature review of quantitative and qualitative evidence. *J. Sci. Med. Sport* **2017**, *20*, 17–25. [CrossRef]
99. Haakstad, L.A.H.; Voldner, N.; Bo, K. Pregnancy and advanced maternal age—The associations between regular exercise and maternal and newborn health variables. *Acta Obstet. Gynecol. Scand.* **2020**, *99*, 240–248. [CrossRef]
100. Ekman, I.; Swedberg, K.; Taft, C.; Lindseth, A.; Norberg, A.; Brink, E.; Carlsson, J.; Dahlin-Ivanoff, S.; Johansson, I.L.; Kjellgren, K.; et al. Person-centered care—Ready for prime time. *Eur. J. Cardiovasc. Nurs.* **2011**, *10*, 248–251. [CrossRef]
101. Watson, J.A.; Ryan, C.G.; Cooper, L.; Ellington, D.; Whittle, R.; Lavender, M.; Dixon, J.; Atkinson, G.; Cooper, K.; Martin, D.J. Pain Neuroscience Education for Adults with Chronic Musculoskeletal Pain: A Mixed-Methods Systematic Review and Meta-Analysis. *J. Pain* **2019**, *20*, 1140.e1–1140.e22. [CrossRef]
102. Von Korff, M.; Crane, P.; Lane, M.; Miglioretti, D.L.; Simon, G.; Saunders, K.; Stang, P.; Brandenburg, N.; Kessler, R. Chronic spinal pain and physical-mental comorbidity in the United States: Results from the national comorbidity survey replication. *Pain* **2005**, *113*, 331–339. [CrossRef]
103. Armour, M.; Parry, K.; Manohar, N.; Holmes, K.; Ferfolja, T.; Curry, C.; MacMillan, F.; Smith, C.A. The Prevalence and Academic Impact of Dysmenorrhea in 21,573 Young Women: A Systematic Review and Meta-Analysis. *J. Womens Health* **2019**, *28*, 1161–1171. [CrossRef] [PubMed]
104. Woodley, S.J.; Lawrenson, P.; Boyle, R.; Cody, J.D.; Morkved, S.; Kernohan, A.; Hay-Smith, E.J.C. Pelvic floor muscle training for preventing and treating urinary and faecal incontinence in antenatal and postnatal women. *Cochrane Database Syst. Rev.* **2020**, *5*, CD007471. [PubMed]
105. Robinson, H.S.; Veierod, M.B.; Mengshoel, A.M.; Vollestad, N.K. Pelvic girdle pain-associations between risk factors in early pregnancy and disability or pain intensity in late pregnancy: A prospective cohort study. *BMC Musculoskelet. Disord.* **2010**, *11*, 91. [CrossRef]
106. Arendt-Nielsen, L.; Morlion, B.; Perrot, S.; Dahan, A.; Dickenson, A.; Kress, H.G.; Wells, C.; Bouhassira, D.; Mohr Drewes, A. Assessment and manifestation of central sensitisation across different chronic pain conditions. *Eur. J. Pain* **2018**, *22*, 216–241. [CrossRef]
107. Bergstrom, C.; Persson, M.; Nergard, K.A.; Mogren, I. Prevalence and predictors of persistent pelvic girdle pain 12 years postpartum. *BMC Musculoskelet. Disord.* **2017**, *18*, 399. [CrossRef]
108. Brosschot, J.F. Cognitive-emotional sensitization and somatic health complaints. *Scand. J. Psychol.* **2002**, *43*, 113–121. [CrossRef]
109. Gutke, A.; Kjellby-Wendt, G.; Oberg, B. The inter-rater reliability of a standardised classification system for pregnancy-related lumbopelvic pain. *Man. Ther.* **2009**, *15*, 13–18. [CrossRef]
110. Remus, A.; Smith, V.; Gutke, A.; Mena, J.J.S.; Morkved, S.; Wikmar, L.N.; Oberg, B.; Olsson, C.; Robinson, H.S.; Stuge, B.; et al. A core outcome set for research and clinical practice in women with pelvic girdle pain: PGP-COS. *PLoS ONE* **2021**, *16*, e0247466. [CrossRef] [PubMed]
111. Linton, S.J.; Hellsing, A.L.; Andersson, D. A controlled study of the effects of an early intervention on acute musculoskeletal pain problems. *Pain* **1993**, *54*, 353–359. [CrossRef]
112. Olson, C.M. Tracking of food choices across the transition to motherhood. *J. Nutr. Educ. Behav.* **2005**, *37*, 129–136. [CrossRef]
113. Bauman, A.E.; Reis, R.S.; Sallis, J.F.; Wells, J.C.; Loos, R.J.; Martin, B.W.; Lancet Physical Activity Series Working Group. Correlates of physical activity: Why are some people physically active and others not? *Lancet* **2012**, *380*, 258–271. [CrossRef]
114. Gutke, A.; Bullington, J.; Lund, M.; Lundberg, M. Adaptation to a changed body. Experiences of living with long-term pelvic girdle pain after childbirth. *Disabil. Rehabil.* **2018**, *40*, 3054–3060. [CrossRef] [PubMed]
115. Mackenzie, J.; Murray, E.; Lusher, J. Women's experiences of pregnancy related pelvic girdle pain: A systematic review. *Midwifery* **2018**, *56*, 102–111. [CrossRef] [PubMed]
116. van Benten, E.; Pool, J.; Mens, J.; Pool-Goudzwaard, A. Recommendations for physical therapists on the treatment of lumbopelvic pain during pregnancy: A systematic review. *J. Orthop. Sports Phys. Ther.* **2014**, *44*, 464–473. [CrossRef] [PubMed]
117. Fredriksen, E.H.; Harris, J.; Moland, K.M. Web-based Discussion Forums on Pregnancy Complaints and Maternal Health Literacy in Norway: A Qualitative Study. *J. Med. Internet Res.* **2016**, *18*, e113. [CrossRef]
118. Filipec, M.; Matijevic, R. Expert advice about therapeutic exercise during pregnancy reduces the symptoms of sacroiliac dysfunction. *J. Perinat. Med.* **2020**, *48*, 559–565. [CrossRef] [PubMed]
119. Gutke, A.; Ostgaard, H.C.; Oberg, B. Pelvic girdle pain and lumbar pain in pregnancy: A cohort study of the consequences in terms of health and functioning. *Spine* **2006**, *31*, E149–E155. [CrossRef]
120. Olsson, C.; Nilsson-Wikmar, L. Health-related quality of life and physical ability among pregnant women with and without back pain in late pregnancy. *Acta Obstet. Gynecol. Scand.* **2004**, *83*, 351–357. [CrossRef]
121. Nijs, J.; Meeus, M.; Cagnie, B.; Roussel, N.A.; Dolphens, M.; Van Oosterwijck, J.; Danneels, L. A modern neuroscience approach to chronic spinal pain: Combining pain neuroscience education with cognition-targeted motor control training. *Phys. Ther.* **2014**, *94*, 730–738. [CrossRef]
122. Nijs, J.; Meeus, M.; Van Oosterwijck, J.; Roussel, N.; De Kooning, M.; Ickmans, K.; Matic, M. Treatment of central sensitization in patients with 'unexplained' chronic pain: What options do we have? *Expert Opin. Pharmacother.* **2011**, *12*, 1087–1098. [CrossRef]
123. Dakic, J.G.; Hay-Smith, J.; Cook, J.; Lin, K.Y.; Calo, M.; Frawley, H. Effect of Pelvic Floor Symptoms on Women's Participation in Exercise: A Mixed-Methods Systematic Review With Meta-analysis. *J. Orthop. Sports Phys. Ther.* **2021**, *51*, 345–361. [CrossRef] [PubMed]

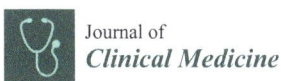

Journal of
Clinical Medicine

Review

Sleep Health Assessment and Treatment in Children and Adolescents with Chronic Pain: State of the Art and Future Directions

Emily F. Law [1,2,*], Agnes Kim [2,3], Kelly Ickmans [4,5,6] and Tonya M. Palermo [1,2]

1. Department of Anesthesiology & Pain Medicine, University of Washington School of Medicine, Seattle, WA 98195, USA; tonya.palermo@seattlechildrens.org
2. Center for Child Health, Behavior & Development, Seattle Children's Research Institute, Seattle, WA 98121, USA; agnkim@augusta.edu
3. Medical College of Georgia, Augusta University & University of Georgia Medical Partnership Campus, Augusta, GA 30912, USA
4. Pain in Motion Research Group (PAIN), Department of Physiotherapy, Human Physiology and Anatomy, Faculty of Physical Education & Physiotherapy, Vrije Universiteit Brussel, Laarbeeklaan 103, 1090 Brussels, Belgium; kelly.ickmans@vub.be
5. Movement & Nutrition for Health & Performance Research Group (MOVE), Department of Movement and Sport Sciences, Faculty of Physical Education and Physiotherapy, Vrije Universiteit Brussel, Pleinlaan 2, 1050 Brussels, Belgium
6. Department of Physical Medicine and Physiotherapy, Universitair Ziekenhuis Brussel, Laarbeeklaan 101, 1090 Brussels, Belgium
* Correspondence: emily.law@seattlechildrens.org

Citation: Law, E.F.; Kim, A.; Ickmans, K.; Palermo, T.M. Sleep Health Assessment and Treatment in Children and Adolescents with Chronic Pain: State of the Art and Future Directions. *J. Clin. Med.* **2022**, *11*, 1491. https://doi.org/10.3390/jcm11061491

Academic Editors: Jo Nijs and Felipe J. J. Reis

Received: 22 December 2021
Accepted: 4 March 2022
Published: 9 March 2022

Publisher's Note: MDPI stays neutral with regard to jurisdictional claims in published maps and institutional affiliations.

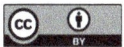

Copyright: © 2022 by the authors. Licensee MDPI, Basel, Switzerland. This article is an open access article distributed under the terms and conditions of the Creative Commons Attribution (CC BY) license (https://creativecommons.org/licenses/by/4.0/).

Abstract: Sleep is interrelated with the experience of chronic pain and represents a modifiable lifestyle factor that may play an important role in the treatment of children and adolescents with chronic pain. This is a topical review of assessment and treatment approaches to promote sleep health in children and adolescents with chronic pain, which summarizes: relevant and recent systematic reviews, meta-analyses, and methodologically sound prospective studies and clinical trials. Recommendations are provided for best practices in the clinical assessment and treatment of sleep health in youth with chronic pain. This overview can also provide researchers with foundational knowledge to build upon the best evidence for future prospective studies, assessment and intervention development, and novel clinical trials.

Keywords: child; adolescent; pediatric; chronic pain; sleep; insomnia

1. Introduction

Chronic pain is a major public health concern in children and adolescents, affecting up to 40% of youth [1,2]. Chronic pain in childhood can be nociplastic (i.e., arising from altered nociception in the central nervous system, such as fibromyalgia or central sensitization), as well as disease-related (i.e., arthritis, sickle cell disease) [1,2]. Headache, abdominal pain, and musculoskeletal pain are among the most common pain conditions in youth [1,2]. Across conditions, chronic pain in childhood is associated with decrements in children's physical, social, and psychological functioning (i.e., increased anxiety and depressive symptoms), and low health-related quality of life [3–10]. Longitudinal studies demonstrate that having childhood chronic pain increases the risk for continuing chronic pain in adulthood, as well as limitations in educational and vocational attainment in adulthood [11–16]. Therefore, identifying factors that predict the development and maintenance of chronic pain in children is an urgent priority.

Physical health conditions and lifestyle factors (e.g., sleep, physical activity, obesity) are one set of vulnerability factors identified as important in chronic pain development and persistence [17]. In particular, sleep disorders and poor quality of sleep commonly co-occur with chronic pain in youth. In a systematic review, Valrie and colleagues [18] found strong evidence for increased sleep problems across samples of youth with both nociplastic and diseases-related chronic pain conditions in comparison with healthy controls. For example, over 50% of adolescents with chronic pain vs. 10% same-age adolescents without pain endorse having significant insomnia symptoms [19]. Further, children with chronic pain report poor sleep quality, have higher sleep anxiety, more bedtime resistance, more frequent awakenings during the night, and more daytime fatigue than the controls [18]. Many cross-sectional studies in adolescents and adults with a variety of chronic pain conditions indicate that sleep disturbances are associated with greater pain sensitivity, as well as greater disability, poorer quality of life, and greater healthcare use and costs [19–22]. There is not only substantial evidence that chronic pain can disrupt sleep, but also that sleep disturbances contribute to pain—a bidirectional association between sleep and pain has been described.

Finan and colleagues [23] synthesized the evidence for the bidirectional effects of sleep and pain in a systematic review. In the included studies that assessed unidirectional effects of sleep on subsequent pain, there was a general consensus that sleep disturbance could: (1) increase the risk for new incidences of chronic pain in pain free individuals, (2) worsen long-term prognosis of existing headache and chronic musculoskeletal pain, and (3) influence daily fluctuations in clinical pain. There was also complementing evidence that good sleep improves long-term prognosis of individuals with tension-type headaches, migraine, and chronic musculoskeletal pain. In the studies that assessed bidirectional effects of sleep and pain, findings suggested that the direction of sleep to chronic pain were more strongly supported than vice versa. For example, in one of the included studies by Lewandowski and colleagues [24], adolescents with disrupted sleep on a given day had increased pain on the subsequent day, yet the reverse direction of this relationship was not significant. Overall, the direction of sleep disturbances influencing subsequent pain was more consistently supported such as in Figure 1.

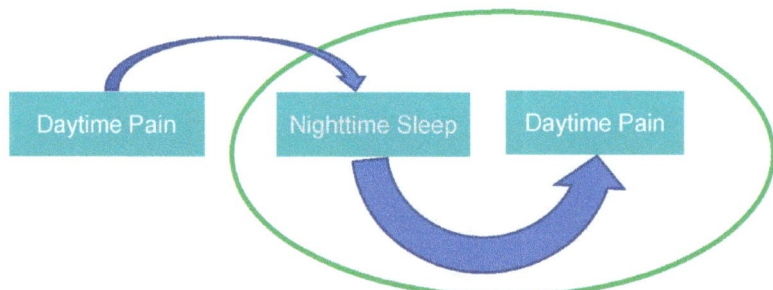

Figure 1. Direction of sleep–pain effects.

In this topical review, we use the term "sleep health" intentionally to highlight that sleep occurs along a continuum and is an important broad contributor to health and well-being. Sleep health is defined as "a multidimensional pattern of sleep-wakefulness, adapted to individual, social, and environmental demands, that promotes physical and mental well-being. Good sleep health is characterized by subjective satisfaction, appropriate timing, adequate duration, high efficiency, and sustained alertness during waking hours" [25].

This state of the art review aims to provide an overview of the role of sleep health in pediatric chronic pain, to present recommendations for clinical practice, and to provide a research agenda for designing future trials and prospective studies. Because studies consistently demonstrate that sleep disturbances are related to poor outcomes in children with chronic pain, including high pain-related disability and low health-related quality of life, sleep health has been proposed as a possible modifiable factor that may improve pain management for youth. We conducted a topical review to summarize the evidence for sleep health interventions in youth with chronic pain and also to highlight evidence in adult chronic pain, where gaps exist in the pediatric literature based on relevant and recent systematic reviews, meta-analyses, and methodologically sound prospective studies and clinical trials. We discuss future research needed to test the modulation of sleep as a potential therapeutic strategy for pain relief and prevention in children and adolescents.

2. Approaches for Sleep Health Assessment in Pediatric Pain Populations

Sleep health is a multi-dimensional construct, therefore a variety of approaches can be used in sleep assessment, including clinical interview, objective assessments, and self-report measures. In general, multi-method assessments of sleep health are recommended where possible in order to understand sleep patterns, sleep behaviors, perceptions of sleep quality, and experiences of daytime sleepiness. In a systematic review, de la Vega & Miro [26] identified three assessment procedures that have been used to assess sleep health specifically in adolescents with chronic pain: polysomnography, actigraphy, and questionnaires.

Polysomnography (PSG) is an objective measurement tool, and should be considered when evaluation of sleep stages and/or sleep-related breathing is indicated [26]. Polysomnography is the gold standard for diagnostic assessment of physiological causes of sleep disturbance (e.g., obstructive sleep apnea, restless leg syndrome). PSG is usually conducted in a specialized hospital sleep laboratory and is typically limited to a single overnight assessment. There are some limited data on PSG to assess sleep in youth with [27] chronic pain, mostly in small samples with rheumatological conditions [28,29], and it is not yet clear how PSG may help with the evaluation or management of sleep complaints in youth with chronic pain.

Daily sleep patterns in the adolescent's home environment can be assessed using actigraphy, which is a watch-like device worn on the wrist to record motor movements using a continuous actimetry sensor [30–32]. Actigraphy has been used to describe habitual sleep–wake patterns (e.g., sleep duration, sleep efficiency, time awake after sleep onset) and to identify associations with other pain outcomes in youth with chronic pain [24,33–35]. In other pediatric populations, actigraphy has been used to identify sleep disturbances such as insomnia and hypersomnolence [32]. The most commonly used devices across studies include the Actiwatch 2 (Philips Respironics, Murrysville, PA, USA) and the MicroMini-Motionlogger (Ambulatory Monitoring, Inc., Ardsley, NY, USA). Unlike PSG, actigraphy does not evaluate sleep stages or sleep-related breathing. Limitations of actigraphy include possible misclassification of sleep–wake periods, where periods of high activity during sleep are erroneously classified as time awake and periods of low activity during wakefulness are erroneously classified as sleep. To address this challenge, a daily sleep diary should be used to validate periods of wake versus sleep on actigraphy [27,32,36]. There can also be variability between different devices, placements, and scoring algorithms [27,36,37]. A multi-modal assessment of sleep (e.g., combining actigraphy with self-report questionnaires) can also help to address these limitations. Another potential limitation is the cost to purchase and score actigraphy devices. While there are lower costs such as commercially available wearable devices (e.g., Fitbit), the reliability and the validity for the measurement of sleep patterns in pediatric populations are unknown.

Self-report measures are useful for identifying behavioral factors that are contributing to sleep disturbances and can be used alone or in combination with objective measurements. Three self-report questionnaire measures have been identified as "well-established" for children and adolescents with chronic pain [26]: the Adolescent Sleep Wake Scale (ASWS) [38], the Adolescent Sleep Hygiene Scale (ASHS) [38], and the Children's Sleep Habits Questionnaire (CSHQ) [39] (see Table 1). The ASWS and the ASHS are adolescent self-report questionnaires that assess more targeted areas of behavioral sleep disturbances, including perceived sleep quality (ASWS) and sleep habits (ASHS). One limitation of these tools is the number of items and the length of administration, which are burdensome. To address this barrier, Essner and colleagues [40] proposed a 10-item short-form version of the ASWS (ASWS-SF) based upon exploratory factor analyses with a broad sample of youth with chronic health conditions, including youth with chronic pain, which has demonstrated adequate reliability and validity in subsequent studies of youth with chronic pain and co-occurring sleep disturbances [41,42]. The CSHQ is a multidimensional parent-report measure that can be useful for screening for a wide range of medical and behavioral sleep disorders in younger children.

Historically, a major gap in sleep assessment for youth has been the lack of brief developmentally informed self-report tools to screen for insomnia symptoms. Insomnia is characterized by persistent dissatisfaction with sleep quantity or quality that is associated with difficulty falling asleep, maintaining sleep, and/or early morning waking which results in daytime impairment [43]. Screening for insomnia is particularly important for youth with chronic pain, given the high prevalence of insomnia symptoms in this population [19]. To address this gap in insomnia measurement, Bromberg et al., [44] developed the 13-item Adolescent Insomnia Questionnaire (AIQ) and demonstrated acceptable psychometric properties in a heterogeneous sample of adolescents with chronic pain and other chronic health conditions. The ASWS-SF and AIQ are well-suited for use in clinical and research settings due to their brevity, ease of scoring, and established reliability and validity in pediatric chronic pain populations (see Table 1).

Table 1. Recommended self-report questionnaire assessments of sleep health for children and adolescents with chronic pain.

Measure Name	Domain	Age Range	Reporter	Items/Subscales	Primary Citation
Adolescent Sleep Wake Scale (ASWS)	Sleep quality	12–18 years	Youth	28 items, yields a total score and 5 subscale scores (Going to Bed, Falling Asleep, Maintaining Sleep, Reinitiating Sleep, Returning to Wakefulness)	LeBourgeois et al., [38]
Adolescent Sleep Wake Scale Short Form (ASWS-SF)	Sleep quality	12–18 years	Youth	10 items, yields a total score and 3 subscale scores (Falling Asleep and Reinitiating Sleep, Returning to Wakefulness, Going to Bed)	Essner et al., [40]
Adolescent Sleep Hygiene Scale (ASHS)	Sleep habits	12–18 years	Youth	28 items, yields a total score and 9 subscale scores (Physiological, Cognitive, Emotional, Sleep Environment, Daytime Sleep, Substances, Bedtime Routine, Sleep Stability, Bed/Bedroom Sharing)	LeBourgeois et al., [38]
Children's Sleep Habits Questionnaire (CSHQ)	Sleep disorders screen	4–10 years	Parent	45 items, yields a total score and 8 subscale scores (Bedtime Resistance, Parasomnia, Sleep Onset Delay, Sleep Duration, Sleep Anxiety, Night Wakings, Sleep-Disordered Breathing, Daytime Sleepiness)	Owens et al., [39]
Adolescent Insomnia Questionnaire (AIQ)	Insomnia screen	11–18 years	Youth	13 items, yields a total score and 3 subscale scores (Sleep Onset, Sleep Maintenance, Sleep Dissatisfaction and Impairments)	Bromberg et al., [44]

3. Interventions to Improve Sleep Health in Pediatric Pain Populations: Cognitive-Behavioral Therapy for Pain Management, Cognitive-Behavioral Therapy for Insomnia, and Sleep Hygiene Education

In general, psychological and behavioral treatments have been used to improve sleep health in children and adolescents [45–47]. There is limited rationale or evidence to use pharmacotherapy to address sleep health in youth, especially when the most common concerns center around behavioral insomnias [48,49].

Cognitive-behavioral therapy for pain management (CBT-Pain) is the gold standard psychological intervention for youth with chronic pain [50,51]. CBT-Pain incorporates training in cognitive skills, relaxation and distraction methods, and parent operant strategies in order to support adaptive coping with pain and participation in normal daily activities [51]. Although sleep health is recognized as an important outcome for pediatric chronic pain treatment [52], sleep has been rarely assessed or specifically targeted in psychosocial interventions. When sleep intervention is included, it is typically brief (one session or less) and focused on sleep hygiene education [53]. Sleep assessment in trials of CBT-Pain has also been limited, typically to a single modality (i.e., self-reported sleep quality or actigraphy).

A recent systematic review by Klausen et al., [54] found that sleep was reported as a treatment outcome in only two published RCTs of CBT-Pain in pediatric samples [55,56]. Sleep assessments included a self-report measure of sleep quality [56] and seven days of actigraphy monitoring [55]. Results were mixed. Findings from one trial indicated a small but significant benefit from CBT-Pain on sleep quality relative to pain education control [56], while the second trial found no difference in sleep duration or sleep efficiency on actigraphy between CBT-Pain and usual care [55]. The different pattern of findings between these two trials may reflect methodological differences in sleep assessment, as each was limited to a single assessment modality (i.e., self-reported sleep quality [56] and actigraphy [55]). In both trials, intervention specifically targeting sleep was limited to a brief education about sleep hygiene.

Cognitive-behavioral therapy for insomnia (CBT-I) is recommended by the American Academy of Sleep Medicine as a first line treatment for adults with sleep disturbances [57]. Core treatment strategies include education about sleep and sleep hygiene, stimulus control, and sleep restriction [57]. The overarching goal of treatment is to develop a consistent sleep–wake schedule and strengthen the association between bed and sleep by limiting time awake in bed. A recent systematic review identified 10 RCTs of CBT-I for adults with chronic pain and comorbid insomnia, some of which only delivered CBT-I while others delivered CBT-I followed by CBT-Pain [58]. Results of meta-analyses demonstrated large positive benefits of CBT-I on global measures of sleep at post-treatment (SMD = 0.89) and follow-up (SMD = 0.56) [58]. Small improvements in pain at post-treatment (SMD = 0.20) were also identified, but this was not maintained at follow-up [58]. Importantly, many of these prior trials have significant limitations, including small sample sizes, short follow-up periods and inadequate assessment of pain outcomes. Findings from two large rigorous trials with older adults with insomnia and comorbid osteoarthritis pain suggest that improvements in sleep in response to CBT-I may lead to both short- and long-term improvements in pain [59,60]. However, neither trial was designed to empirically test temporal associations between the sleep–pain relationship and more research is needed.

We are not aware of any published RCTs that evaluated the safety or efficacy of CBT-I in youth with chronic pain conditions. There is one published RCT which compared the efficacy of sleep hygiene guidelines to usual care in adolescents with migraine and co-occurring poor sleep health [61]. Results indicated that compared with usual care control youth who received the sleep hygiene guidelines had a greater reduction in migraine frequency from pre-treatment to 3-month and 6-month follow-ups [61]. However, this study was limited by the relatively small sample size (total n = 70) and lack of validated assessment tools measuring headache and sleep outcomes.

While controlled trials evaluating efficacy of CBT-I in pediatric pain populations are lacking, there are a few single arm pilot trials in mixed samples of adolescents with chronic pain and other medical and mental health comorbidities [41,62]. These studies used brief 4–6 session CBT-I protocols delivered to youth and their parents following standard core treatment elements, including education about sleep and sleep hygiene, stimulus control, and sleep restriction. Results of this pilot work demonstrated feasibility for in-person treatment delivery and preliminary efficacy, where youth showed improvements in sleep quality, sleep hygiene, sleep duration, sleep efficiency, and mood and anxiety symptoms [41,62].

Hybrid CBT programs have also been developed for adults and youth with co-occurring chronic pain and insomnia, which combine CBT-I with CBT-Pain. By providing treatment for two problems simultaneously, hybrid CBT may offer some practical advantages for both patients and healthcare systems. A recent topical review found emerging evidence for the feasibility, acceptability, and preliminary efficacy of hybrid CBT programs for improving pain and sleep outcomes in adults with coexisting chronic pain and insomnia [63]. However, these studies are limited to a handful of relatively small single-arm pilot trials [64–66]. We are not aware of any published randomized controlled trials evaluating hybrid CBT protocols for youth with comorbid insomnia and chronic pain, although related work is underway in adult chronic pain populations (e.g., [67]).

To address this gap, Law and colleagues [42] developed a six-session hybrid CBT program delivered in person to youth with chronic migraine and comorbid insomnia symptoms (see Table 2). The treatment protocol integrates core components of CBT-I (sleep restriction, stimulus control, sleep hygiene) with core components of CBT-Pain (relaxation and distraction methods, cognitive skills, and parent operant training). In a single-arm pilot trial, preliminary evidence for efficacy was demonstrated on improvements in sleep quality, sleep hygiene, sleep duration, and sleep efficiency. Notably, youth also experienced reductions in headache-related disability and headache frequency from pre- to post-hybrid CBT treatment [42].

Table 2. Best evidence psychological interventions for addressing sleep health in youth with chronic pain.

Intervention	Target Population	Level of Evidence	Setting of Care Delivery	Provider Discipline
Sleep hygiene education	Youth with chronic pain	Promising	Tertiary care clinic (e.g., Pain Medicine Clinic, Sleep Clinic), Digital health technology	Psychologist, Behavioral Sleep Specialist, Pain medicine specialist
Cognitive-Behavioral Therapy for Insomnia (CBT-I)	Youth with comorbid chronic pain, insomnia, and mental health conditions	Promising	Tertiary care clinic (e.g., Pain Medicine Clinic, Sleep Clinic), Self-guided digital health technology	Psychologist, Behavioral sleep specialist

Given the lack of behavioral sleep medicine specialists in many communities, there is also interest in digital health interventions (e.g., mobile apps, internet interventions) to improve sleep health. There is robust evidence indicating that self-guided web-based CBT-I produces similar effect sizes for improving insomnia symptoms in adults compared to face-to-face CBT-I [68], although similar data in youth are lacking. Recently, Carmona and colleagues [69] demonstrated feasibility and acceptability of a transdiagnostic web-based app for adolescents and young adults (AYAs), which provides self-guided training in sleep education, personalized feedback comparing the user's sleep patterns to age-based norms, and tailored goal setting to improve sleep habits. We are not aware of any published randomized controlled trials testing technology delivered sleep health interventions for youth, although studies are currently underway (e.g., [70]).

4. Future Directions for Clinical Practice

Our review uncovers a number of areas important to consider in clinical practice (see Table 3). Given evidence of the high prevalence of sleep disturbances among youth with chronic pain and the importance of overall sleep health on pain and well-being, routine screening should be implemented. In addition to the clinical interview, there are brief validated self-report screening measures to assess insomnia, sleep quality, and sleep impairment in youth, which should be used. The assessment of sleep health in all children and adolescents presenting with chronic pain is recommended. Interventions targeting sleep hygiene and insomnia symptoms can be offered to youth; this may include education about sleep needs, importance of consistency in sleep–wake schedules, and tips for healthy sleep (e.g., establish a positive bedtime and waking routine, limit electronics in the bedroom). Additional consideration may be needed to tailor education to the unique challenges that impact sleep health in youth with chronic pain such as a lack of scheduled activities and routines, low levels of physical activity, and the use of napping as a coping strategy for pain management. Youth with clinically significant insomnia symptoms should be referred to a sleep specialist. Once the efficacy and the safety of insomnia interventions are established in youth with chronic pain, considerations for implementation would include the use of telehealth and digital health technologies to improve access and potentially reduce costs.

Table 3. Future Directions for Clinical Practice.

1.	Integrate screening for sleep disturbances into the assessment of all children and adolescents presenting with chronic pain.
2.	Provide sleep health interventions to target sleep hygiene and insomnia in youth presenting with sleep disturbances.
3.	Where available, use technology to deliver sleep health treatments, e.g., via telehealth and digital health technologies.
4.	Disseminate evidence-based sleep interventions.
5.	Before considering approaches to dissemination and implementation, further work is needed to understand safety and efficacy of CBT-I and Hybrid CBT-I/CBT-Pain interventions for youth with chronic pain via controlled trials.

5. Future Directions for Research

Our review also highlights the need for research in multiple areas of sleep health in adolescents with chronic pain (see Table 4). First, there is an incomplete understanding of the impact of pain treatments on sleep outcomes in youth with chronic pain as sleep is not often measured in pain clinical trials. Knowledge of the safety and efficacy of sleep treatments such as CBT-I and Hybrid CBT-I/CBT Pain has not yet been fully established in youth with chronic pain. In particular, future research of sleep treatments using randomized controlled trial designs with long-term follow-up is needed. Sleep has been shown to influence subsequent pain, therefore research to understand the optimal sequence of pain and sleep interventions is needed. In particular, it will be important to evaluate whether intervening to improve sleep first may boost the effects of subsequent pain interventions. There are also gaps in the understanding of the longitudinal and causal relationships between sleep health and chronic pain, including whether there are key vulnerability periods (e.g., puberty) that may influence the linkage between sleep and pain. Few studies have focused on how positive aspects of sleep health may influence pain and pain management in youth. Furthermore, there is limited understanding of how sleep health influences motivation and self-efficacy among youth with chronic pain and how this may influence their ability to engage in pain self-management behaviors. Another future direction for research is to understand sociodemographic influences on sleep health, including possible disparities in the impact of sleep health on youth. Last, it will be important to identify shared biopsychosocial mechanisms that underlie the treatment benefits of pain and sleep interventions for youth to better inform optimization of these interventions in the context of comorbid pain and sleep problems.

Table 4. Future Directions for Research.

1.	Comprehensively characterize the impact of pain treatments on sleep health in youth with chronic pain.
2.	Evaluate the safety and efficacy of CBT-I and Hybrid CBT-I/CBT-Pain interventions for youth with chronic pain and co-occurring sleep disturbances.
3.	Conduct research to understand optimal sequencing of pain and sleep interventions, in particular to understand whether children and adolescents may benefit synergistically from improvements in sleep prior to beginning pain self-management interventions.
4.	Conduct longitudinal studies to identify the causal relationship between sleep health and chronic pain over time to uncover mechanisms and identify key vulnerability periods.
5.	Characterize resiliency in sleep health and how this can be enhanced among youth with chronic pain.
6.	Understand sociodemographic influences on sleep health among youth with chronic pain.
7.	Understand how sleep health influences motivation and self-efficacy among youth with chronic pain.
8.	Identify shared biopsychosocial mechanisms that underlie treatment benefits of pain and sleep interventions for individuals with co-occurring conditions.

6. Conclusions

There is growing consensus among experts that sleep health has a direct effect on pain perception, pain intensity, and pain-related disability among youth with chronic pain. Validated assessment tools that can be considered in clinical practice and research settings vary in terms of their cost and burden, and include polysomnography, actigraphy, and self-report questionnaire measures. Appropriate assessment tools have been developed and validated for pediatric populations with chronic pain, which can be used in clinical practice and research studies. Sleep health can be modified through psychological and behavioral interventions. Although randomized controlled trials of psychological interventions specifically targeting sleep health in youth with chronic pain are limited, a growing number of pilot studies supports the feasibility and preliminary efficacy of sleep hygiene education and cognitive-behavioral therapy for insomnia (CBT-I) for improving sleep patterns, improving perceived sleep quality, and reducing pain and pain-related disability in adolescents and young adults with chronic pain when delivered face-to-face and via digital health technologies. Clinicians are encouraged to routinely screen sleep health in all children and youth presenting with chronic pain. Research is still needed to characterize the sleep–pain relationship over time in youth with chronic pain to identify mechanisms that account for their interrelationship and to definitively evaluate the safety and the efficacy of psychological interventions targeting sleep health in pediatric chronic pain populations.

Author Contributions: Conceptualization, T.M.P., K.I. and E.F.L.; Methodology, T.M.P., A.K. and E.F.L., Writing—Original Draft Preparation, T.M.P., A.K. and E.F.L., Writing—Review & Editing, T.M.P., A.K., K.I. and E.F.L. All authors have read and agreed to the published version of the manuscript.

Funding: A.K. received funding from the Medical Scholars Program, Medical College of Georgia, Augusta University & University of Georgia Medical Partnership Campus.

Institutional Review Board Statement: Not applicable.

Informed Consent Statement: Not applicable.

Data Availability Statement: Not applicable.

Acknowledgments: We thank the patients and families who participated in the research studies summarized in this review.

Conflicts of Interest: The authors declare no conflict of interest. Funders had no role in the design of the study; in the collection, analyses, or interpretation of data; in the writing of the manuscript, or in the decision to publish the results.

References

1. Gobina, I.; Villberg, J.; Valimaa, R.; Tynjala, J.; Whitehead, R.; Cosma, A.; Brooks, F.; Cavallo, F.; Ng, K.; de Matos, M.G.; et al. Prevalence of self-reported chronic pain among adolescents: Evidence from 42 countries and regions. *Eur. J. Pain* **2019**, *23*, 316–326. [CrossRef] [PubMed]
2. Swain, M.S.; Henschke, N.; Kamper, S.J.; Gobina, I.; Ottova-Jordan, V.; Maher, C.G. An international survey of pain in adolescents. *BMC Public Health* **2014**, *14*, 447. [CrossRef] [PubMed]
3. Gold, J.I.; Mahrer, N.E.; Yee, J.; Palermo, T.M. Pain, fatigue, and health-related quality of life in children and adolescents with chronic pain. *Clin. J. Pain* **2009**, *25*, 407–412. [CrossRef] [PubMed]
4. Kashikar-Zuck, S.; Goldschneider, K.R.; Powers, S.W.; Vaught, M.H.; Hershey, A.D. Depression and functional disability in chronic pediatric pain. *Clin. J. Pain* **2001**, *17*, 341–349. [CrossRef]
5. Lewandowski, A.S.; Palermo, T.M.; Peterson, C.C. Age-dependent relationships among pain, depressive symptoms, and functional disability in youth with recurrent headaches. *Headache* **2006**, *46*, 656–662. [CrossRef]
6. Palermo, T.M.; Putnam, J.; Armstrong, G.; Daily, S. Adolescent autonomy and family functioning are associated with headache-related disability. *Clin. J. Pain* **2007**, *23*, 458–465. [CrossRef]
7. Hoff, A.L.; Palermo, T.M.; Schluchter, M.; Zebracki, K.; Drotar, D. Longitudinal relationships of depressive symptoms to pain intensity and functional disability among children with disease-related pain. *J. Pediatr. Psychol.* **2006**, *31*, 1046–1056. [CrossRef]
8. Fales, J.L.; Murphy, L.K.; Rights, J.D.; Palermo, T.M. Daily Peer Victimization Experiences of Adolescents With and Without Chronic Pain: Associations With Mood, Sleep, Pain, and Activity Limitations. *J. Pain* **2020**, *21*, 97–107. [CrossRef]

9. Arruda, M.A.; Arruda, R.; Guidetti, V.; Bigal, M.E. Psychosocial adjustment of children with migraine and tension-type headache—A nationwide study. *Headache* **2015**, *55* (Suppl. 1), 39–50. [CrossRef]
10. Logan, D.E.; Simons, L.E.; Kaczynski, K.J. School functioning in adolescents with chronic pain: The role of depressive symptoms in school impairment. *J. Pediatr. Psychol.* **2009**, *34*, 882–892. [CrossRef]
11. Murray, C.B.; Groenewald, C.B.; de la Vega, R.; Palermo, T.M. Long-term impact of adolescent chronic pain on young adult educational, vocational, and social outcomes. *Pain* **2020**, *161*, 439–445. [CrossRef] [PubMed]
12. Kashikar-Zuck, S.; Cunningham, N.; Peugh, J.; Black, W.R.; Nelson, S.; Lynch-Jordan, A.M.; Pfeiffer, M.; Tran, S.T.; Ting, T.V.; Arnold, L.M.; et al. Long-term outcomes of adolescents with juvenile-onset fibromyalgia into adulthood and impact of depressive symptoms on functioning over time. *Pain* **2019**, *160*, 433–441. [CrossRef] [PubMed]
13. Kashikar-Zuck, S.; Cunningham, N.; Sil, S.; Bromberg, M.H.; Lynch-Jordan, A.M.; Strotman, D.; Peugh, J.; Noll, J.; Ting, T.V.; Powers, S.W.; et al. Long-term outcomes of adolescents with juvenile-onset fibromyalgia in early adulthood. *Pediatrics* **2014**, *133*, e592–e600. [CrossRef] [PubMed]
14. Walker, L.S.; Dengler-Crish, C.M.; Rippel, S.; Bruehl, S. Functional abdominal pain in childhood and adolescence increases risk for chronic pain in adulthood. *Pain* **2010**, *150*, 568–572. [CrossRef]
15. Walker, L.S.; Sherman, A.L.; Bruehl, S.; Garber, J.; Smith, C.A. Functional abdominal pain patient subtypes in childhood predict functional gastrointestinal disorders with chronic pain and psychiatric comorbidities in adolescence and adulthood. *Pain* **2012**, *153*, 1798–1806. [CrossRef]
16. Horst, S.; Shelby, G.; Anderson, J.; Acra, S.; Polk, D.B.; Saville, B.R.; Garber, J.; Walker, L.S. Predicting persistence of functional abdominal pain from childhood into young adulthood. *Clin. Gastroenterol. Hepatol.* **2014**, *12*, 2026–2032. [CrossRef]
17. Palermo, T.M. Pain prevention and management must begin in childhood: The key role of psychological interventions. *Pain* **2020**, *161* (Suppl. 1), S114–S121. [CrossRef]
18. Valrie, C.R.; Bromberg, M.H.; Palermo, T.; Schanberg, L.E. A systematic review of sleep in pediatric pain populations. *J. Dev. Behav. Pediatr.* **2013**, *34*, 120–128. [CrossRef]
19. Palermo, T.M.; Wilson, A.C.; Lewandowski, A.S.; Toliver-Sokol, M.; Murray, C.B. Behavioral and psychosocial factors associated with insomnia in adolescents with chronic pain. *Pain* **2011**, *152*, 89–94. [CrossRef]
20. Butbul Aviel, Y.; Stremler, R.; Benseler, S.M.; Cameron, B.; Laxer, R.M.; Ota, S.; Schneider, R.; Spiegel, L.; Stinson, J.N.; Tse, S.M.; et al. Sleep and fatigue and the relationship to pain, disease activity and quality of life in juvenile idiopathic arthritis and juvenile dermatomyositis. *Rheumatology* **2011**, *50*, 2051–2060. [CrossRef]
21. LaPlant, M.M.; Adams, B.S.; Haftel, H.M.; Chervin, R.D. Insomnia and quality of life in children referred for limb pain. *J. Rheumatol.* **2007**, *34*, 2486–2490. [PubMed]
22. Meltzer, L.J.; Logan, D.E.; Mindell, J.A. Sleep patterns in female adolescents with chronic musculoskeletal pain. *Behav. Sleep. Med.* **2005**, *3*, 193–208. [CrossRef] [PubMed]
23. Finan, P.H.; Goodin, B.R.; Smith, M.T. The association of sleep and pain: An update and a path forward. *J. Pain* **2013**, *14*, 1539–1552. [CrossRef] [PubMed]
24. Lewandowski, A.S.; Palermo, T.M.; Motte, S.D.l.; Fu, R. Temporal daily associations between pain and sleep in adolescents with chronic pain versus healthy adolescents. *Pain* **2010**, *151*, 220–225. [CrossRef] [PubMed]
25. Buysse, D.J. Sleep health: Can we define it? Does it matter? *Sleep* **2014**, *37*, 9–17. [CrossRef] [PubMed]
26. de la Vega, R.; Miro, J. The assessment of sleep in pediatric chronic pain sufferers. *Sleep Med. Rev.* **2012**, *17*, 185–192. [CrossRef]
27. Galland, B.; Meredith-Jones, K.; Terrill, R.; Taylor, R. Challenges and Emerging Technologies within the Field of Pediatric Actigraphy. *Front. Psychiatry* **2014**, *5*, 99. [CrossRef]
28. Ward, T.M.; Brandt, P.; Archbold, K.; Lentz, M.; Ringold, S.; Wallace, C.A.; Landis, C.A. Polysomnography and self-reported sleep, pain, fatigue, and anxiety in children with active and inactive juvenile rheumatoid arthritis. *J. Pediatr. Psychol.* **2008**, *33*, 232–241. [CrossRef]
29. Ward, T.M.; Chen, M.L.; Landis, C.A.; Ringold, S.; Beebe, D.W.; Pike, K.C.; Wallace, C.A. Congruence between polysomnography obstructive sleep apnea and the pediatric sleep questionnaire: Fatigue and health-related quality of life in juvenile idiopathic arthritis. *Qual. Life Res.* **2017**, *26*, 779–788. [CrossRef]
30. Acebo, C. *Using and Scoring Actigraphy*; E.P. Bradley Hospital Sleep Research Lab, Brown Medical School: Providence, RI, USA, 2006.
31. Sadeh, A.; Acebo, C. The role of actigraphy in sleep medicine. *Sleep Med. Rev.* **2002**, *6*, 113–124. [CrossRef]
32. Meltzer, L.J.; Montgomery-Downs, H.E.; Insana, S.P.; Walsh, C.M. Use of actigraphy for assessment in pediatric sleep research. *Sleep Med. Rev.* **2012**, *16*, 463–475. [CrossRef] [PubMed]
33. Palermo, T.M.; Toliver-Sokol, M.; Fonareva, I.; Koh, J.L. Objective and subjective assessment of sleep in adolescents with chronic pain compared to healthy adolescents. *Clin. J. Pain* **2007**, *23*, 812–820. [CrossRef] [PubMed]
34. Pavlova, M.; Kopala-Sibley, D.C.; Nania, C.; Mychasiuk, R.; Christensen, J.; McPeak, A.; Tomfohr-Madsen, L.; Katz, J.; Palermo, T.M.; Noel, M. Sleep disturbance underlies the co-occurrence of trauma and pediatric chronic pain: A longitudinal examination. *Pain* **2020**, *161*, 821–830. [CrossRef] [PubMed]
35. Tsai, S.Y.; Labyak, S.E.; Richardson, L.P.; Lentz, M.J.; Brandt, P.A.; Ward, T.M.; Landis, C.A. Actigraphic sleep and daytime naps in adolescent girls with chronic musculoskeletal pain. *J. Pediatric. Psychol.* **2008**, *33*, 307–311. [CrossRef]

36. Meltzer, L.J.; Westin, A.M. A comparison of actigraphy scoring rules used in pediatric research. *Sleep Med.* **2011**, *12*, 793–796. [CrossRef]
37. Galland, B.C.; Short, M.A.; Terrill, P.; Rigney, G.; Haszard, J.J.; Coussens, S.; Foster-Owens, M.; Biggs, S.N. Establishing normal values for pediatric nighttime sleep measured by actigraphy: A systematic review and meta-analysis. *Sleep* **2018**, *41*, zsy017. [CrossRef]
38. LeBourgeois, M.K.; Giannotti, F.; Cortesi, F.; Wolfson, A.R.; Harsh, J. The relationship between reported sleep quality and sleep hygiene in Italian and American adolescents. *Pediatrics* **2005**, *115*, 257–265. [CrossRef]
39. Owens, J.A.; Spirito, A.; McGuinn, M. The Children's Sleep Habits Questionnaire (CSHQ): Psychometric properties of a survey instrument for school-aged children. *Sleep* **2000**, *23*, 1043–1051. [CrossRef]
40. Essner, B.; Noel, M.; Myrvik, M.; Palermo, T. Examination of the Factor Structure of the Adolescent Sleep-Wake Scale (ASWS). *Behav. Sleep Med.* **2015**, *13*, 296–307. [CrossRef]
41. Palermo, T.M.; Beals-Erickson, S.; Bromberg, M.; Law, E.; Chen, M. A Single Arm Pilot Trial of Brief Cognitive Behavioral Therapy for Insomnia in Adolescents with Physical and Psychiatric Comorbidities. *J. Clin. Sleep Med.* **2017**, *13*, 401–410. [CrossRef]
42. Law, E.F.; Tham, S.W.; Aaron, R.V.; Dudeney, J.; Palermo, T.M. Hybrid cognitive-behavioral therapy intervention for adolescents with co-occurring migraine and insomnia: A single-arm pilot trial. *Headache* **2018**, *58*, 1060–1073. [CrossRef] [PubMed]
43. Olufsen, I.S.; Sorensen, M.E.; Bjorvatn, B. New diagnostic criteria for insomnia and the association between insomnia, anxiety and depression. *Tidsskr. Nor. Laegeforen.* **2020**, *140*. [CrossRef]
44. Bromberg, M.H.; de la Vega, R.; Law, E.F.; Zhou, C.; Palermo, T.M. Development and Validation of the Adolescent Insomnia Questionnaire. *J. Pediatr. Psychol.* **2020**, *45*, 61–71. [CrossRef] [PubMed]
45. Meltzer, L.J.; Wainer, A.; Engstrom, E.; Pepa, L.; Mindell, J.A. Seeing the Whole Elephant: A scoping review of behavioral treatments for pediatric insomnia. *Sleep Med. Rev.* **2021**, *56*, 101410. [CrossRef]
46. Maski, K.; Owens, J. Pediatric Sleep Disorders. *Continuum* **2018**, *24*, 210–227. [CrossRef] [PubMed]
47. Meltzer, L.J.; Plaufcan, M.R.; Thomas, J.H.; Mindell, J.A. Sleep problems and sleep disorders in pediatric primary care: Treatment recommendations, persistence, and health care utilization. *J. Clin. Sleep Med.* **2014**, *10*, 421–426. [CrossRef]
48. Owens, J.A.; Rosen, C.L.; Mindell, J.A.; Kirchner, H.L. Use of pharmacotherapy for insomnia in child psychiatry practice: A national survey. *Sleep Med.* **2010**, *11*, 692–700. [CrossRef]
49. Meltzer, L.J.; Mindell, J.A. Systematic Review and Meta-Analysis of Behavioral Interventions for Pediatric Insomnia. *J. Pediatr. Psychol.* **2014**, *39*, 932–948. [CrossRef]
50. Fisher, E.; Law, E.; Dudeney, J.; Palermo, T.M.; Stewart, G.; Eccleston, C. Psychological therapies for the management of chronic and recurrent pain in children and adolescents. *Cochrane Database Syst. Rev.* **2018**, *9*, CD003968.
51. Palermo, T.M. *Cognitive-Behavioral Therapy for Chronic Pain in Children and Adolescents*; Oxford University Press: New York, NY, USA, 2012.
52. Palermo, T.M.; Walco, G.A.; Paladhi, U.R.; Birnie, K.A.; Crombez, G.; de la Vega, R.; Eccleston, C.; Kashikar-Zuck, S.; Stone, A.L. Core outcome set for pediatric chronic pain clinical trials: Results from a Delphi poll and consensus meeting. *Pain* **2021**, *162*, 2539–2547. [CrossRef]
53. Law, E.F.; Beals-Erickson, S.E.; Fisher, E.; Lang, E.A.; Palermo, T.M. Components of Effective Cognitive-Behavioral Therapy for Pediatric Headache: A Mixed Methods Approach. *Clin. Pract. Pediatric Psychol.* **2017**, *5*, 376–391. [CrossRef] [PubMed]
54. Klausen, S.H.; Ronde, G.; Tornoe, B.; Bjerregaard, L. Nonpharmacological Interventions Addressing Pain, Sleep, and Quality of Life in Children and Adolescents with Primary Headache: A Systematic Review. *J. Pain Res.* **2019**, *12*, 3437–3459. [CrossRef] [PubMed]
55. Law, E.F.; Beals-Erickson, S.E.; Noel, M.; Claar, R.; Palermo, T.M. Pilot randomized controlled trial of internet-delivered cognitive-behavioral treatment for pediatric headache. *Headache* **2015**, *55*, 1410–1425. [CrossRef] [PubMed]
56. Palermo, T.M.; Law, E.F.; Fales, J.; Bromberg, M.H.; Jessen-Fiddick, T.; Tai, G. Internet-delivered cognitive-behavioral treatment for adolescents with chronic pain and their parents: A randomized controlled multicenter trial. *Pain* **2016**, *157*, 174–185. [CrossRef] [PubMed]
57. Edinger, J.D.; Arnedt, J.T.; Bertisch, S.M.; Carney, C.E.; Harrington, J.J.; Lichstein, K.L.; Sateia, M.J.; Troxel, W.M.; Zhou, E.S.; Kazmi, U.; et al. Behavioral and psychological treatments for chronic insomnia disorder in adults: An American Academy of Sleep Medicine clinical practice guideline. *J. Clin. Sleep Med.* **2021**, *17*, 255–262. [CrossRef] [PubMed]
58. Selvanathan, J.; Pham, C.; Nagappa, M.; Peng, P.W.H.; Englesakis, M.; Espie, C.A.; Morin, C.M.; Chung, F. Cognitive behavioral therapy for insomnia in patients with chronic pain—A systematic review and meta-analysis of randomized controlled trials. *Sleep Med. Rev.* **2021**, *60*, 101460. [CrossRef]
59. McCurry, S.M.; Zhu, W.; Von Korff, M.; Wellman, R.; Morin, C.M.; Thakral, M.; Yeung, K.; Vitiello, M.V. Effect of Telephone Cognitive Behavioral Therapy for Insomnia in Older Adults With Osteoarthritis Pain: A Randomized Clinical Trial. *JAMA Intern. Med.* **2021**, *181*, 530–538. [CrossRef]
60. Vitiello, M.V.; McCurry, S.M.; Shortreed, S.M.; Baker, L.D.; Rybarczyk, B.D.; Keefe, F.J.; Von Korff, M. Short-term improvement in insomnia symptoms predicts long-term improvements in sleep, pain, and fatigue in older adults with comorbid osteoarthritis and insomnia. *Pain* **2014**, *155*, 1547–1554. [CrossRef]
61. Bruni, O.; Galli, F.; Guidetti, V. Sleep hygiene and migraine in children and adolescents. *Cephalalgia* **1999**, *19* (Suppl. 25), 57–59. [CrossRef]

62. Aslund, L.; Lekander, M.; Wicksell, R.K.; Henje, E.; Jernelov, S. Cognitive-behavioral therapy for insomnia in adolescents with comorbid psychiatric disorders: A clinical pilot study. *Clin. Child. Psychol. Psychiatry* **2020**, *25*, 958–971. [CrossRef]
63. Babiloni, A.H.; Beetz, G.; Tang, N.K.Y.; Heinzer, R.; Nijs, J.; Martel, M.O.; Lavigne, G.J. Towards the endotyping of the sleep-pain interaction: A topical review on multitarget strategies based on phenotypic vulnerabilities and putative pathways. *Pain* **2021**, *162*, 1281–1288. [CrossRef] [PubMed]
64. Finan, P.H.; Buenaver, L.F.; Coryell, V.T.; Smith, M.T. Cognitive-Behavioral Therapy for Comorbid Insomnia and Chronic Pain. *Sleep Med. Clin.* **2014**, *9*, 261–274. [CrossRef] [PubMed]
65. Tang, N.K.; Lereya, S.T.; Boulton, H.; Miller, M.A.; Wolke, D.; Cappuccio, F.P. Nonpharmacological Treatments of Insomnia for Long-Term Painful Conditions: A Systematic Review and Meta-analysis of Patient-Reported Outcomes in Randomized Controlled Trials. *Sleep* **2015**, *38*, 1751–1764. [CrossRef] [PubMed]
66. Tang, W.-X.; Zhang, L.-F.; Ai, Y.-Q.; Li, Z.-S. Efficacy of Internet-delivered cognitive-behavioral therapy for the management of chronic pain in children and adolescents: A systematic review and meta-analysis. *Medicine* **2018**, *97*, e12061. [CrossRef]
67. Malfliet, A.; Bilterys, T.; Van Looveren, E.; Meeus, M.; Danneels, L.; Ickmans, K.; Cagnie, B.; Mairesse, O.; Neu, D.; Moens, M.; et al. The added value of cognitive behavioral therapy for insomnia to current best evidence physical therapy for chronic spinal pain: Protocol of a randomized controlled clinical trial. *Braz. J. Phys. Ther.* **2019**, *23*, 62–70. [CrossRef]
68. Zachariae, R.; Lyby, M.S.; Ritterband, L.M.; O'Toole, M.S. Efficacy of internet-delivered cognitive-behavioral therapy for insomnia—A systematic review and meta-analysis of randomized controlled trials. *Sleep Med. Rev.* **2016**, *30*, 1–10. [CrossRef]
69. Carmona, N.E.; Usyatynsky, A.; Kutana, S.; Corkum, P.; Henderson, J.; McShane, K.; Shapiro, C.; Sidani, S.; Stinson, J.; Carney, C.E. A Transdiagnostic Self-management Web-Based App for Sleep Disturbance in Adolescents and Young Adults: Feasibility and Acceptability Study. *JMIR Form. Res.* **2021**, *5*, e25392. [CrossRef]
70. Peersmann, S.H.M.; van Straten, A.; Kaspers, G.J.L.; Thano, A.; van den Bergh, E.; Grootenhuis, M.A.; van Litsenburg, R.R.L. Does the guided online cognitive behavioral therapy for insomnia i-"Sleep youth" improve sleep of adolescents and young adults with insomnia after childhood cancer? (MICADO-study): Study protocol of a randomized controlled trial. *Trials* **2021**, *22*, 307. [CrossRef]

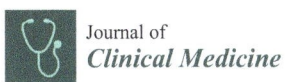

Review

Diet and Chronic Non-Cancer Pain: The State of the Art and Future Directions

Katherine Brain [1,2,3], Tracy L. Burrows [1,2], Laura Bruggink [3], Anneleen Malfliet [4,5,6,7], Chris Hayes [3], Fiona J. Hodson [3] and Clare E. Collins [1,2,*]

1. School of Health Science, College of Health, Medicine and Wellbeing, University of Newcastle, Callaghan, NSW 2308, Australia; katherine.brain@newcastle.edu.au (K.B.); tracy.burrows@newcastle.edu.au (T.L.B.)
2. Priority Research Centre for Physical Activity and Nutrition, University of Newcastle, Callaghan, NSW 2308, Australia
3. Hunter Integrated Pain Service, Newcastle, NSW 2300, Australia; laura.bruggink@health.nsw.gov.au (L.B.); chris.hayes@health.nsw.gov.au (C.H.); fiona.hodson@health.nsw.gov.au (F.J.H.)
4. Department of Physiotherapy, Human Physiology and Anatomy, Faculty of Physical Education & Physiotherapy, Vrije Universiteit Brussel, 1050 Brussels, Belgium; anneleen.malfliet@vub.be
5. Pain in Motion International Research Group, 1000 Brussels, Belgium
6. Research Foundation Flanders (FWO), 1000 Brussels, Belgium
7. Department of Physical Medicine and Physiotherapy, University Hospital Brussels, 1090 Brussels, Belgium
* Correspondence: clare.collins@newcastle.edu.au

Abstract: Nutrition plays an important role in pain management. Healthy eating patterns are associated with reduced systemic inflammation, as well as lower risk and severity of chronic non-cancer pain and associated comorbidities. The role of nutrition in chronic non-cancer pain management is an emerging field with increasing interest from clinicians and patients. Evidence from a number of recent systematic reviews shows that optimising diet quality and incorporating foods containing anti-inflammatory nutrients such as fruits, vegetables, long chain and monounsaturated fats, antioxidants, and fibre leads to reduction in pain severity and interference. This review describes the current state of the art and highlights why nutrition is critical within a person-centred approach to pain management. Recommendations are made to guide clinicians and highlight areas for future research.

Keywords: nutrition; diet quality; chronic non-cancer pain

1. Introduction

Chronic non-cancer pain (CNCP) is defined as pain that persists for more than three months, which exceeds the time it typically takes for tissues to heal [1]. Globally, the prevalence of CNCP is approximately 20%, with a higher prevalence among vulnerable populations such as the elderly and those from culturally and linguistically diverse backgrounds (≥40%) [2–4]. In 2010, the economic burden of CNCP in the United States was reported to be $635 billion, exceeding that of heart disease ($309 billion), diabetes ($188 billion), and cancer ($243 billion) [5]. In Australia, the cost of chronic pain in 2018 was $139.3 billion and expected to increase to $215.6 billion by 2050 [4]. CNCP is a major burden on both individuals and the community due to absenteeism and loss of productivity [4]. In Australia in 2018, $48.3 billion of the financial cost associated with CNCP was attributed to productivity losses and $66.1 billion was attributed to reductions in quality of life [4]. CNCP also causes increased stress on the health care system, as many people experiencing pain have exacerbations of other chronic health conditions requiring specialised treatment. In 2019, self-reported data from 72 adult CNCP services (30,000 patients) across Australia and New Zealand reported approximately 40% of patients had mental health issues, 23% had digestive diseases, 22% had high blood pressure and/or high cholesterol, and 10% had diabetes [6]. Individuals who live with pain can find it difficult to move about and

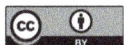

socialise. Pain also impacts their mood, ability to shop and cook, and the food and drinks they consume.

A whole-person approach to pain management is a patient-centred framework that encourages the adoption of active strategies to address biopsychosocial and lifestyle modulators of pain experiences [7]. In this broad context, there is recognition of the multidirectional relationships between diet, mental health, sleep, food preparation, and mobility [7]. Addressing these dimensions of pain experience in specialist multidisciplinary pain services reduces pain and improves quality of life [6,8]. There are, however, challenges in implementing multidisciplinary approaches in primary care [9]. Nutrition is a central component of the whole-person approach and emerging evidence, explored in this review, suggests that dietary interventions can be effective in improving quality of life and managing CNCP, as well as comorbid mental and physical health problems [10].

This state-of-the-art overview explores the role of diet in CNCP. The available evidence is reviewed with the aim of helping clinicians translate findings into practice and assisting researchers to optimise the design of future trials and implementation studies.

1.1. Diet, Pain, and Systemic Inflammation

Persisting low-grade systemic inflammation is associated with CNCP and multiple comorbid chronic health conditions. Diet plays a complex role in modulating systemic inflammation. Knowledge is expanding rapidly in this area and multiple links between diet and inflammation have been identified. Metabolic mechanisms associated with post prandial hyperglycaemia and frequent and prolonged rises in plasma insulin levels, influenced by dietary intake, can produce systemic inflammation [11,12]. This has been shown in insulin-resistant states where increasing adiposity is associated with the increased secretion of pro-inflammatory cytokines in adipose tissue, liver, and skeletal muscle [13].

There are several mechanisms associated with fat metabolism. An excess of omega-6 fatty acids relative to omega-3 fatty acids loads the arachidonic acid pathway and contributes to a pro-inflammatory state [14,15]. The body requires both omega-3 and omega-6 fatty acids, ideally in a ratio of approximately 1:1 [16]. Dominance of omega-6 polyunsaturated fats in Westernised diets over the last few decades has led to ratios of omega-3 to omega-6 in the range of 1 to 15–30, which has been shown to promote systemic inflammation [14]. Industrial trans fats, or hydrogenated oils, also promote inflammation and raise LDL cholesterol and lower HDL cholesterol [17,18].

In the context of CNCP, an aspect of systemic inflammation of particular interest manifests in the central nervous system. This neuroinflammation is mediated by neuroglia cells, which are found in the brain and central nervous system [19]. They are thought to be activated by overall poor dietary patterns (i.e., energy-dense, nutrient-poor diets) through a variety of mechanisms such as oxidative stress, peripheral inflammation, and changes in the gut microbiome [19]. This leads to central nervous system sensitisation, a dominant contributor to CNCP [19,20]. The corollary of this is that the adoption of a high-quality diet facilitates normalisation of glial activity and reduced central nervous system inflammation and sensitisation [19].

Alterations in the gut microbiome and associated auto-immune mechanisms also influence systemic inflammation. A range of mechanistic, animal, and observational human studies have found that changes in gut microbiota can influence immune function and may contribute to an increased risk or severity of auto-immune diseases [21]. Increased intestinal permeability potentially allows the translocation of bacterial fragments such as lipopolysaccharides, which can trigger inflammation and auto-immune responses [21].

While metabolic pathways can produce inflammation, they can also have anti-inflammatory activity and reduce oxidative stress [19]. Non-nutritive bioactive compounds such as polyphenols mitigate oxidative stress and inflammation, as well as modulating pain experiences [22]. One such mechanism operates through the inhibition of COX-2 in neuromodulating pathways [22]. Polyphenols are found in a range of foods such as fruits, vegetables, whole grains, cocoa, tea, coffee, and alcohol [23]. Food's rich in polyphenols, such as cherries, strawberries, blueberries, and plums, have been used in a variety of clinical studies showing anti-inflammatory benefits, as well as cardio-metabolic benefits and neuroprotective effects [24–28]. Dietary fibre intake and the consequent colonic production of short chain fatty acids also reduces inflammation through its beneficial role in the gut microbiome–brain axis and in immunomodulation [22].

As such, dietary factors mediate systemic inflammation and so therapeutic focus should be placed on reducing inflammation through optimising overall dietary quality, addressing the ratio of omega-3 to omega-6 PUFAs, and increasing the intake of polyphenols and fibre.

1.2. Diet, Pain, and Comorbidities

Systemic inflammation is linked with CNCP and multiple other comorbidities impacting both physical and mental health [6,29–31]. These varied conditions include type 2 diabetes, cardiovascular disease (CVD), respiratory and kidney disease, obesity, cancer, non-alcoholic fatty liver disease, autoimmune disorders, neurodegenerative disorders, and depression [32–34]. The specific mechanisms and predominant sites of inflammation, along with the genetic and epigenetic vulnerabilities of the person, influence disease expression. For example, oxidative stress may exacerbate neuropathy [35]. Changes in the vascular endothelium are correlated with cardiovascular disease and metabolic syndrome [36,37]. Neuroinflammation involving immune cells such as glia and cytokine cascades [38–40] plays a role in the central sensitisation that is strongly correlated with CNCP.

Systemic inflammation can contribute to CNCP at multiple levels impacting both structural tissues and the nervous system. In osteoarthritis, for example, inflammation is expressed within the affected joint [41] in addition to neuroinflammation in the central nervous system [42].

In a clinical audit in 2017 at a tertiary pain service in Australia, 64% of patients reported having two or more comorbidities [29]. This is supported by a Scottish primary care study which found that 46% of patients presenting with CNCP had three or more long-term conditions [43]. A cross sectional study conducted on a sample of 3000 individuals in Germany also found that those suffering from depression were three times more likely to experience non-neuropathic chronic pain (18%) and six times more likely to experience neuropathic pain (7%) [44]. People with obesity, diabetes, hypertension, and cerebrovascular disease were also at a higher risk of having non-neuropathic chronic pain [44]. A recent systematic review of 20 studies found that people experiencing chronic musculoskeletal pain were almost twice as likely to report having CVD than those people without chronic musculoskeletal pain [45]. Another meta-analysis found that people with diabetes were 1.4 times more likely to report lower back pain and 1.2 times more likely to report neck pain compared to those without diabetes [46]. There is also an association between CNCP and obesity. This is evidenced in two large studies conducted in the United States of America in which it was found that those with a higher Body Mass Index (BMI) were more likely to self-report moderate and severe pain intensity [47,48]. Participants who were classified as obese (Body Mass Index ≥ 30 kg/m^2) were approximately 1.3 to 2 times more likely to experience pain [47,48]. Obesity can contribute to pain via increased mechanical load in addition to pro-inflammatory mechanisms [49]. Pain can contribute to obesity by interfering with food preparation and healthy dietary choices.

Given the prevalence of nutrition-related comorbidities associated with CNCP and the overlap of the underlying mechanisms, it is important to consider the role of nutrition in simultaneously reducing the severity and risk of CNCP and other chronic health conditions. Many of these conditions and their associated risk factors can be modulated through changes in diet.

1.3. Dietary Intake of People Experiencing Pain

A limited amount of research has assessed dietary intake in people experiencing CNCP. The studies that do exist largely report on diet quality, total energy intake, and macronutrient distribution. A study by VanDenKerkhof et al. analysed data from the British Birth Cohort Study (n = 89,673, aged $\geq$45 years, 12% with CNCP) and found that fruit and vegetable consumption of women experiencing CNCP pain was more likely to decrease over time, compared to women with no pain [50]. Overall diet quality was lower in women with CNCP ($\leq$1 serve/week of fruit and vegetables and $\geq$1 serve/day of fatty foods and chips), compared to women without pain [50]. A study conducted by Collins et al. examined diet-related survey data from 10,000 Australian women aged 50–55 years [51]. Findings showed that poorer diet quality was associated with higher pain scores as reported using the pain subscale within SF-36 [51]. Conversely, higher diet quality was associated with lower pain levels [51]. Long term opioid use is associated with excessive energy intakes as shown in a study conducted by Meleger et al., where one third of male and half of female patients receiving long-term opioid therapy were exceeding recommended energy intake targets [52]. A pilot study conducted in 2019 found that at baseline, participants' mean percentage of energy derived from core foods (fruit, vegetables, breads, and cereals, meat and meat alternatives, and dairy and dairy alternatives) was 58% and their mean percentage of energy from energy-dense nutrient-poor foods (e.g., confectionary, sugar sweetened beverages, and takeaway foods) was 42% [53]. Ideally, at least 85–90% energy should come from nutrient-rich core foods and no more than 10–15% from energy-dense nutrient-poor foods [54,55]. The intervention in this pilot study consisted of 6 weeks of personalised dietary consultations and cherry juice high in antioxidants vs. a placebo fruit (apple) juice [53]. After 6 weeks, all groups had a statistically significant increase in percentage of energy from core foods (63%) and a reduction in percentage of energy from energy-dense, nutrient-poor foods (37%) [53]. The group that received the personalised dietary consultations had a significant reduction in percentage of energy from total fat (-3.36%) compared to the control group (+2%) [53]. Participants who received the cherry juice did no better than those who received the apple juice [53].

1.4. Diet and the Whole-Person Approach to Pain Management

The biopsychosocial and lifestyle factors that influence pain all interact, and these factors rarely stand alone in terms of contribution to pain experiences. Figure 1 depicts the relationship between nutrition and the whole-person approach to pain management.

1.4.1. Diet and Biomedical Aspects

There is a complex relationship between the biomedical and psychosocial aspects of pain and nutrition. From a biomedical perspective, as previously discussed, dietary intake can affect pain by modulating systemic inflammation and oxidative stress, as well as by its impact comorbid conditions.

The adverse effects of medications used for pain and other chronic health conditions can be substantial and add to nutritional challenges. Opioid medications commonly reduce motility, delay transit and gastric emptying, and suppress androgen and adrenal function [56]. This in turn can adversely impact metabolism and increase feelings of fullness, bloating, nausea, and constipation. Mechanism-based studies conducted in animals and humans have shown that non-steroidal anti-inflammatory drugs (NSAIDs) can increase gut permeability, inflammation, and the risk of gastrointestinal injury (e.g., ulcers) [57,58]. Antidepressants and anticonvulsants commonly used for pain management are also associated with gastrointestinal side effects such as nausea, constipation, diarrhoea, and changes in appetite [59,60]. Medications can also impact the gut microbiome. Antibiotics and proton pump inhibitors, for example, can have major adverse impacts on microbiome diversity [58].

Tapering and ceasing, or minimising the dose of pain related medications, will improve gastrointestinal and nutrition-related problems [61]. Adequate intake of soluble and insoluble fibre and water can assist in relieving the side effects of constipating medications [62]. More information about fibre and fluid can be found in Section 2.2.5 and Appendix A.

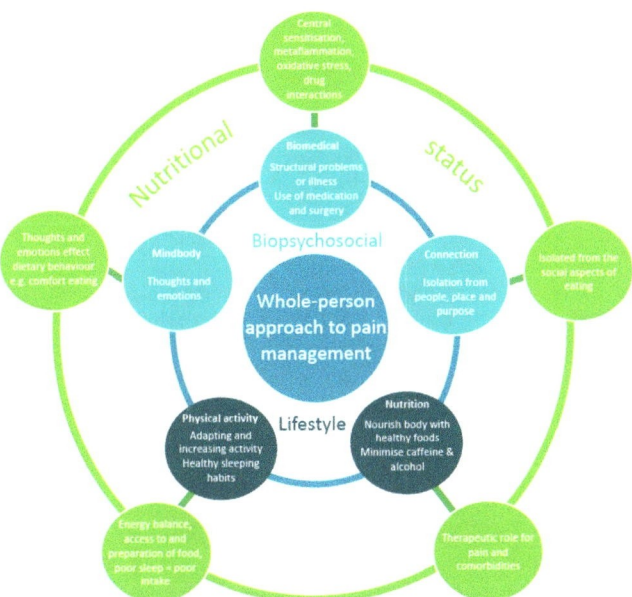

Figure 1. The relationship between nutrition and the whole-person approach to pain management (adapted and reprinted with permission).

1.4.2. Relationships between Diet, Mental Health, and Lifestyle

Mental health comorbidities such as anxiety and depression, as well as feelings of isolation and loss of connection to people, place, and purpose, are also common in people experiencing CNCP [6,63,64]. Self-reported data from 72 adult pain services (30,000 patients) in Australia and New Zealand shows that 40% of patients have depression, anxiety, and/or post-traumatic stress disorder [6]. A bivariate adjusted analysis of the Canadian Longitudinal Study of Ageing ($n = 28,000$) found that those who were socially isolated and/or lonely had an increased likelihood of psychological distress relative to those who were neither isolated nor lonely [65]. Subsequent studies have found that interventions targeting social isolation have led to significant improvements in self-reported pain intensity and emotional and physical functioning [63,64].

Mental health issues and isolation can lead to changes in dietary behaviours such as comfort eating, low motivation for meal preparation, loss of appetite, and lack of meaning around meal times. Qualitative data show that people experiencing CNCP report using emotional eating or binge eating behaviours as a response to their pain [66]. Participants reported that this often coincides with depression and guilt [66]. Depression and anxiety are associated with overall low diet quality [67,68]. Low diet quality is associated with lower intakes of key essential macro and micronutrients often found in foods such as fruits and vegetables [51,69].

Overeating is also associated with CNCP. Mechanisms for overeating in response to pain are likely highly varied due to the clustering of a range of comorbidities in this population group, which may include depression and anxiety. Overconsumption could be related to hedonic hunger triggered by physical pain, as well as emotional eating as a coping strategy [66]. Consuming food may elevate low mood or provide a distraction from anxious or traumatic thoughts via activation of brain reward pathways involving neurotransmitters such as dopamine [70]. Data from a survey of over 200 adults with CNCP reported that approximately 12% of respondents ate more to feel better when they experienced pain [70]. In another study of 126 veterans, the Yale Emotional Overeating Questionnaire (YEOQ) was used to examine overeating responses to physical pain [71]. Approximately 43% of participants had engaged in at least one overeating episode in response to pain in the past month and 14% engaged in this behaviour daily [71]. This study proposed that those with higher pain interference are more likely to have depression and may have maladaptive pain-related coping, including overeating [71]. This may be due in part to associations between higher pain catastrophizing, low distress tolerance, and higher levels of unhealthy eating [72].

Pain can lead to reduced mobility and functional strength, which in turn can make shopping, cooking, and preparing meals difficult and may exacerbate pain [73]. Given the range of living conditions of those with CNCP, there may be increased vulnerability of some population groups to these factors such as those living alone, in group homes, or in aged care. Decreased mobility due to pain often means regular employment is difficult, and there may be large periods of unemployment contributing to financial burden. Reliance on takeaway or convenience foods may be an appealing solution to some people experiencing pain. However, this can lead to low diet quality.

Pain can also significantly impact sleep. This may include quantity, quality, sleep hygiene, and how long it takes to get to sleep, which are all important elements that need to be considered. A lack of restorative sleep leads to increased tiredness, caffeine consumption, overall daily energy intake, and fat, protein, and carbohydrate intake, and can also lead to impaired hormone regulation [74,75]. For example, leptin may be reduced, with a consequent decrease in satiety signals to the brain. In addition, levels of ghrelin, a 'hunger hormone', may be increased by lack of sleep [74,76]. Poor sleep can also affect glucose tolerance and insulin levels, with an increased risk of type 2 diabetes, which is highly prevalent in people experiencing CNCP [6,46,74,76].

It is clear that nutrition does not stand alone in the management of pain, but there is equally a need to recognise that food has important direct and indirect influences on the whole-person pain management approach.

1.4.3. Diet and the Whole-Person Approach to Pain Management and Behaviour Change

It is important to consider tips and strategies to address dietary behaviours as well as dietary intake. Given the complexities surrounding the relationship between nutrition, pain, and the whole-person approach to pain management, behaviour change strategies are well placed to support people to change their habits. The Behaviour Change Model is an evidence-based approach that incorporates the overarching aspects of environment, policy, and regulation, combined with clinician-delivered interventions, and patient factors of capability, opportunity, and motivation [77]. At an individual patient level, it is vital that health professionals identify their patients' capabilities, opportunities, and motivations to help set specific nutrition goals and facilitate successful behaviour change [77]. Health professionals can use the sources of behaviours as a way to identify patient' barriers and/or facilitators. They can then assist patients to overcome barriers or harness facilitators to ensure successful behaviour change [77]. For example, your patient may not know the relationship between diet and CNCP (capability), they may not have time or access (opportunity), and they may not have the belief or confidence to change (motivation).

To ensure consistent and high-quality care, it is important to follow a process to comprehensively assess dietary intake, take challenges into consideration, implement strategies, and monitor progress. The first step of this process is to assess dietary intake. There are a variety of tools including brief dietary screeners, such as the Healthy Eating Quiz [78], that provide an indication of overall diet quality, and more comprehensive tools (e.g., food frequency questionnaires, food records, or 24-h recalls), that can be used to assess the adequacy of food and nutrient intakes relative to national recommendations. Which one should be used depends on the situation and purpose? Many variations on these tools are available to the public online or via apps, which makes it easier for patients to access them. Some online tools and apps can also provide instant analysis. The next step is comparing the dietary assessment to recommendations such as national guidelines or nutrient reference values. Comparison to recommendations allows the identification of areas for improvement and these are often the basis of goals. Exploring barriers to and motivators for change will assist making a SMART (Specific, Measurable, Achievable, Relevant, and Time-bound) goal that is realistic and achievable. There are a number of potential barriers that need to be taken into consideration such as socioeconomic and cultural preferences, food availability, mental health and mobility issues, and poor health literacy [79]. These barriers need to be addressed with appropriate and relevant strategies. Working with patients to identify relevant barriers and strategies will make it easier for patients to achieve their goals. This can be done using the COM-B model. For example, identifying culturally and linguistically diverse (CALD) services in your area can help assist CALD patients. Self-monitoring progress is helpful for patients to maintain their level of awareness and motivation towards change. Self-monitoring also gives clinicians an indication on how their patient is progressing and allows the revision of goals if needed.

2. State of the Art

2.1. Nutrition Interventions for People Experiencing Chronic Non-Cancer Pain

Research from a pilot study (evidence level 1c) (Table 1) conducted in 2019 found that a personalised dietary intervention that included a dietary assessment, dietary advice for pain management, and strategies to overcome barriers to assist with behaviour change that was delivered by a dietitian had a clinically meaningful effect on self-reported pain interference and pain self-efficacy [53]. Participants also had improvements in quality of life and dietary intake [53]. However, given that this was a pilot study, the intervention needs to be implemented and tested in fully powered trials. Another quasi-experimental study (evidence level 2d) in a cohort of people with chronic musculoskeletal pain found that an 8-week plant-based diet led to a statistically significant reduction in pain (mean change 3.14, $p = 0.0001$) measured on a numerical pain rating scale [80], although this study had a small sample size ($n = 14$).

Table 1. Best evidence table.

Experimental Study Designs	Level of Evidence [81]	Study Type	Target Population	Intervention(s)	Length of Intervention	Risk of Bias (ROB)/Methodological Quality	Results	Evidence Gaps
Field et al., 2021 [82]	1b	SR and MA (exp); $n = 43$	Chronic non-cancer MSK pain	Veg/vegan ($n = 11$), single food changes ($n = 11$), elimination (n-11), energy or macronutrient restriction ($n = 8$), omega-3 ($n = 5$), Mediterranean diet ($n = 2$)	Ave 18 weeks (2 weeks–2 years)	RCT's and pre-post studies: Good ($n = 7$), fair ($n = 19$), poor ($n = 11$)	N= 23/32 controlled studies included in MA. SMD −0.44; 95% CI: −0.63 to −0.24; $p < 0.0001$; $I^2 = 62\%$ (high heterogeneity)	Poor methodological quality, heterogeneity, most common pain measure unidimensional
Elma et al., 2020 [83]	1b	SR (exp and obs); $n = 12$	Chronic MSK pain	Exp studies: Veg/vegan ($n = 4$), weight loss ($n = 2$), peptide diet ($n = 1$), aspartame elimination ($n = 1$), low FODMAP ($n = 1$)	Exp studies: Ave 16 weeks (4 weeks–1 year)	RCT's: Good ($n = 1$), poor ($n = 3$)	7/9 exp studies reported pain relieving effect of dietary changes. Two studies reported no effect (aspartame elimination and vegetarian).	Poor methodological quality, heterogeneity, most common pain measure unidimensional
Genel et al., 2020 [84]	1b	SR and MA (exp); $n = 7$	Arthritis	Mediterranean diet ($n = 4$), anti-inflammatory food ($n = 2$), low inflammatory diet ($n = 1$)	Ave 17 weeks (12–24 weeks)	RCTs: low ROB ($n = 1$), high ROB ($n = 4$), non RCTs: moderate risk ($n = 1$), serious risk ($n = 1$)	Overall no significant change in pain. Subgroup analysis for RA had reduction, SMD −2.81 (95 % CI −3.60, −2.02), $p <0.00001$	Small sample size, poor methodological quality, heterogeneity
Brain et al., 2019 [85]	1b	SR and MA (exp); $n = 71$	CNCP	Altered overall diet ($n = 16$), altered specific nutrient ($n = 5$), supplement-based ($n = 46$), fasting ($n = 4$)	Ave 17 weeks (2 to 2 years)	Positive ($n = 31$), neutral ($n = 36$), negative ($n = 4$)	MA ($n = 23$): −0.905 (95% CI −0.537 to −1.272), $p < 0.001$ Qual synthesis: 12/16, 2/5, 11/46 and 1/4 studies from each respective group had significant reduction in pain	Poor methodological quality, small sample size, heterogeneity, most common pain measure unidimensional

Table 1. Cont.

Study	Level	Design (n)	Condition	Intervention	Duration	Evidence quality	Results	Limitations
Silva et al., 2019 [86]	1b	SR (exp); n = 7	Fibromyalgia	Weight loss (n = 2), vegetarian (n = 2), low FODMAP (n = 1), gluten free (n = 1), MSG and aspartame free diet (n = 1)	Ave 18 weeks (4 weeks to 6 months)	All very low or low uncertainty of evidence, except n = 1 moderate	All but 2 studies (gluten free and MSG/aspartame free diet) had significant reduction in pain	Poor methodological quality, small sample size
Brain et al., 2019 [53]	1c	Pilot RCT (n = 60)	CNCP	Personalised dietary assessment, education (i.e., F&V, good quality fats, antioxidants and micronutrients and fibre) and advice using the Behaviour Change Wheel and provided by a dietitian +/− antioxidant supplement	6 weeks	N/A	All groups had statastically signigicant improvement in pain interference, pain self-efficacy and pain catastrophizing. Personalised dietary support groups had clinically meaningful improvement in pain interference and pain self-efficacy	Small sample size, loss to follow up (30%), placebo effect
Dragan et al., 2020 [87]	2b	Literature Review (exp); n = 38	CNCP	Antioxidant, vitamin and minerals (n = 9), elimination diet (n = 7), energy restriction (n = 5), low-fat/plant based (n = 5), pre and probiotics (n = 5), fruit and fibre (n = 4), enriched PUFA (n = 2), high protein (n = 1)	Ave 15 weeks (4 weeks–1.5 years)	Not reported	Antioxidants, vitamins and minerals: 8 improvement in pain (IP), 1 no difference (ND) Elimination: 4 IP, 3 ND Energy restriction: 5 IP Low fat/plant based: 5 IP Pre/probiotics: 3 IP, 2 ND Fruit/fibre: 4 IP Enriched PUFA: 2 IP High protein: 1 IP (Note IP included a variety of measures e.g., severity or frequency and strength of improvements ranged from trends to significant improvements)	Small sample size, poor methodological quality

Table 1. Cont.

Study	Level	Design	Condition	Intervention	Duration	Results	Conclusion	Limitations
Kaushik et al., 2020 [35]	2b	Literature review ($n = 8$)	CNCP	Antioxidant ($n = 3$), Mediterranean diet ($n = 2$), low carbohydrate ($n = 2$), saturated fat ($n = 1$)	Ave 17 weeks (1 day–1 year)	Not reported	Summary of oxidative stress and inflammation provided. Low carbohydrate, 2/3 antioxidant and Mediterranean diet had reduction in oxidative stress and inflammation. 1 antioxidant study showed no change and saturated fat showed increase in oxidative stress and inflammation	Small number of clinical studies, only 2 studies were specifically measured pain, hard to compare dietary studies when variety of interventions
Fondanelli et al., 2018 [88]	2b	Narrative review ($n = 172$)	CNCP	Red wine ($n = 26$), olive oil ($n = 24$), zinc and selenium ($n = 18$), oil seeds ($n = 14$), yoghurt ($n = 11$), F&V ($n = 10$), spices ($n = 8$), vitamin D ($n = 7$), fibre in opioid induced constipation ($n = 7$), cheese ($n = 7$), legumes ($n = 6$), sweets ($n = 6$), omega-3 ($n = 6$), meat and fish ($n = 5$), eggs ($n = 4$), vitamin B12 ($n = 3$), water ($n = 3$), fibre ($n = 2$)	Not reported	Level of evidence: $n = 1$ SR, $n = 6$ RCT or obs study with dramatic effect, $n = 7$ non-RCT, cohort/follow-up studies, $n = 3$ case series, case-control or historically controlled studies, $n = 149$ mechanism based reasoning	A food pyramid was developed and presented as the results of the paper. This divided foods into those that should be consumed daily, consumed 1, 2, or 4 times per week and foods to be eaten occasionally.	Combination of human, in vitro and animal models included, reliance on lower levels of evidence, casual relationships unknown
Towery et al., 2018 [80]	2d	Quasi-exp cohort study ($n = 14$)	Chronic MSK pain	Education on plant based diet and sample menu cycle. Included grains, F&V, legumes, dairy products and eggs. Meat, poultry, seafood and fish not allowed and processed foods and drinks discouraged	8 weeks	N/A	Pain: mean change 3.14 on NPRS (95% CI 2.16–4.12), $p = 0.0001$. Quality of life: mean change 24.991 on SF-36 (95% CI 18.16–31.97), $p = 0.0001$	Small sample (although powered), unable to blind, accuracy of reported intake, convenience sample, self-reported food intake can increase motivation to change eating habits

Table 1. Cont.

Expert Consensus Papers	Level of Evidence	Study Type	Population	Summary	Evidence Gaps
Brain et al., 2020 [89]	5b	Expert opinion factsheet	CNCP	• Brief summary on how dietary intake effects CNCP (enhancing nervous system and reducing inflammation), reduces or maintains weight, and improves comorbidities • Acknowledges how diet can be impacted (and vice versa) by limited mobility and strength affecting shopping, cooking, and preparation of food, mental health issues, feelings of isolation, and lack of sleep • Provides tips for nutrition and pain management with a focus on F&V, good quality fats, micronutrient deficiencies, water, fibre, ultra-processed food and added sugar	N/A
Nijs J et al., 2020 [19]	5b	Expert opinion review	CNCP (animal and human studies)	• Focus on role of neuroinflammation and the possibility that the interaction between nutrition and central sensitisation is mediated via bidirectional gut-brain interactions • Low saturated fat, low added sugar and anti-inflammatory dietary patterns have the following potential therapeutic targets: reduce oxidative stress, preventing toll-like receptor activation, prevent afferent vagal nerve fibres sensing pro-inflammatory mediators, normalise microglial, optimise gut microbiota, reduce polyamine production, and enhance neurotransmitters • Beneficial dietary pattern includes polyphenols, fruits, vegetables, and cereals • Important focus on long term changes and improvements (pain interference) from dietary changes and does not rely on short term changes (i.e., pain severity)	Need to explore interactions in human studies
Philpot et al., 2019 [79]	5b	Expert opinion editorial	CNCP	• Focus on dietary modification to reduce inflammation and therefore alleviate pain. • Highlights the potential role of the Dietary Inflammatory Index. • Diets high in daily consumption of F&V, olive oil, nuts, and legumes (i.e., Mediterranean-style diet) with adequate micronutrients (omega-3, vitamin B12, and magnesium) in conjunction with a reduction of processed food is anti-inflammatory and potentially beneficial for CNCP • Acknowledges challenges faced by patients that impact dietary intake such as financial, physical, and psychological or practice difficulties. • Suggests CNCP services would substantially benefit from access to dietitians' skills in assessment, modification, and support of diets specific to pain patients	Lack of research on the efficacy of diet therapy for people with CNCP and on the barriers to implementing diet therapy into clinical practice.

Table 1. *Cont.*

Bjørklund. 2019 [22]	5b	Expert opinion review	CNCP	• Focus on anti-inflammatory compounds (i.e., antioxidants, vitamins, and minerals) and anti-nociceptive/analgesic compounds (e.g., flavonoids and omega-3) • Main themes: fruit and vegetables, antioxidants, deficiency of vitamin D, and the ratio of omega-3 to omega-6 • Acknowledges additional considerations such as cultural differences, socioeconomic burden, and food availability • Despite inconsistency in the literature, diet (in combination with physical activity and a good lifestyle) is still a promising strategy for reducing pain burden and should not be ignored	More research on the best dietary program for CNCP is needed

SR = systematic review, MA = meta-analysis, exp = experimental, obs = observational, MSK = musculoskeletal, RCT = randomised controlled trial, Veg = vegetarian, PUFA = polyunsaturated fats, ROB = risk of bias, MSG = monosodium glutamate, FODMAP = fermentable oligosaccharides, disaccharides, monosaccharides, and polyols, F&V = fruits and vegetables, CNCP = chronic non-cancer pain.

A recent systematic review (evidence level 1b) collated and summarised experimental studies exploring the effect of dietary interventions on chronic non-cancer musculoskeletal pain, arthritis, and fibromyalgia [82]. Through a synthesis of results from 43 studies overall, a positive effect was found for a number of whole food dietary interventions (i.e., foods commonly found in the diet, excluding nutraceuticals) with an average reduction in pain score, -0.44, $p < 0.0001$ [82]. Other systematic reviews in people with chronic musculoskeletal pain, arthritis, and fibromyalgia have found similar results. Elma et al. found that in 12 experimental and observational studies, vegetarian, vegan, weight loss, or peptide diets were associated with improved pain outcomes (evidence level 1b) [83]. Two other systematic reviews (evidence level 1b) in people with arthritis (n = 7 studies) and fibromyalgia (n = 7 studies) included studies with interventions focused on diets that are predominantly plant rich and/or contain anti-inflammatory aspects (e.g., Mediterranean diet, omega-3, or antioxidants) where participants had a reduction in pain outcomes [84,86]. Commonalities among all of these interventions include a focus on improving diet quality and nutrient density. This is supported by another systematic review of 71 studies (evidence level 1b) [85], which found that studies that used a dietary intervention to alter overall intake, particularly vegetarian or Mediterranean diets, or the quality of a specific nutrient such as fat or protein, achieved statistically significant reductions in pain intensity [85].

Three other reviews, collectively including 218 studies (evidence level 2b) have also explored the role of nutrition in CNCP. However, these studies include a large number of mechanism-based studies, and have summarised the literature, rather than provided a synthesis of results [35,87,88]. When comparing the summaries provided in these reviews to the results from the systematic reviews outlined above, it is still evident that the literature points towards optimising diet quality, increasing consumption of core foods such as fruit, vegetables, breads and cereals, meat, dairy, and their alternatives and reducing energy-dense nutrient-poor foods such as confectionary, sugar sweetened beverages, and processed meats.

Among the systematic reviews conducted in this area, many share limitations, with substantial heterogeneity among pain "conditions" and dietary interventions. Intervention studies that include participants with multiple types of CNCP are rare and it is more common to find studies which explore the impact of nutrition on sub-types such as arthritis, musculoskeletal pain, fibromyalgia, or gastrointestinal pain (e.g., inflammatory bowel disease (IBD) and irritable bowel syndrome (IBS)). There is a challenge in balancing nutritional recommendations relevant to the breadth of people with CNCP with a focus on more specific recommendations for particular diseases or individuals. The majority of the studies included in these systematic reviews were also of low methodological quality and used unidimensional tools to measure pain outcomes. This indicates the need for more and higher quality studies that use multidimensional tools to measure pain outcomes to ensure all aspects of pain are considered.

Given that this is an emerging field of research, there are also a number of expert consensus papers (evidence level 5b) on this topic that should be considered. A common aspect of all of these papers (n = 4) is the focus on systemic inflammation [19,22,79,89]. Consequently, these papers suggest, consistent with healthy eating principles for chronic disease reduction, that dietary intake should include fruits and vegetables, food rich in antioxidant nutrients (in particular polyphenols), olive oil, nuts, legumes, and adequate intake of micronutrients (omega-3, vitamin B12, vitamin D and magnesium) [19,22,79,89]. These papers also acknowledge the challenges people with CNCP face in achieving healthy dietary patterns and behaviours. There is a need to consider socioeconomic and cultural differences, food availability and psychological or physical difficulties.

Nutrition interventions are highly variable in clinical settings. The availability of dietitians is often a significant limiting factor. Other allied health professionals have variable nutrition training and consumers are often left to seek dietary advice on their own. The following section will provide appropriate evidence-based recommendations for a range of health professionals.

2.2. Recommendations for Clinicians

2.2.1. Dietary Assessment

Dietary assessment is extremely important, as acknowledged in Philpot et al. (evidence level 5b). Pain services would benefit from working with dietitians to access their skills in dietary assessment [79]. Dietary screeners which assess diet quality (e.g., The Healthy Eating Quiz) [78] along with an assessment of psychological, physical and medical issues allows clinicians to look at the relationship between diet and pain experiences and diet-related risk factors with other chronic diseases. This also allows clinicians to identify some of the socioeconomic, physical, and psychological barriers to healthy eating that are common in people experiencing CNCP [22,79].

A common theme arising in the evidence is the potential role of vitamin and mineral deficiencies, such as Vitamin D, Vitamin B12, and magnesium, in pain experiences [22,79,88]. The only non-invasive way to determine if a patient has a micronutrient deficiency is through systematic dietary assessment that reflects usual dietary intake conducted by a dietitian. Some practical tips on dietary assessment and identification of micronutrient deficiencies are available in Appendix A.

2.2.2. Optimise Diet Quality

All the systematic reviews exploring the role of nutrition in pain management (evidence level 1b) emphasised optimising diet quality [82–86]. Poor diet quality is associated with high consumptions of energy-dense nutrient foods that lack key nutrients found in core foods such as fruits, vegetables, breads and cereals, meat, dairy, and their alternatives. Globally, poor dietary intake is the one of the top modifiable risk factors for morbidity and mortality [90]. Specifically, high sodium intake and low intake of whole grains, fruit, nuts, and seeds are the top three leading risk factors [90]. In line with the evidence presented in this paper, these foods contain fibre, vitamins, and antioxidants that are associated with reducing pain experiences [89]. Given that over 90% of Australians and Americans do not follow their respective country's evidence-based dietary guidelines [91,92], the first step to improving diet quality is to increase adherence to national dietary guidelines. While national dietary guidelines are not specific to CNCP management, they promote healthy eating and lifestyle behaviours which may better translate for those experiencing CNCP.

2.2.3. Consume Fruit and Vegetables Rich in Phytonutrients to Reduce Oxidative Stress

All of the systematic reviews (level 1b) included a large number of studies that used plant-rich eating (e.g., vegetarian or vegan dietary patterns), anti-inflammatory, and Mediterranean diets [82–86]. A major component of all of these dietary patterns are fruits, vegetables, and whole grains, which contain phytonutrients with antioxidant properties. To maximise consumption of phytonutrients and polyphenols it is important to consume a wide range of different coloured fruits and vegetables [89]. However, as acknowledged in some of the expert review evidence (level 5b), there are additional considerations that may impact someone's ability to include a wide range of fresh and colourful fruit and vegetables in their diet [22,79,89]. This can include potential exacerbation of pain through preparation and cooking, and/or lack of motivation to shop and cook [89]. Practical tips to address this are found in Appendix A.

2.2.4. Consume Long Chain and Monounsaturated Fats (e.g., Omega-3 and Olive Oil)

A number of experimental studies included in the systematic reviews (level 1b) that have been synthesised for this paper have shown that long chain and monounsaturated fats, especially omega-3 fats and olive oil reduce pain [82–86]. Suggestions on how to increase omega-3 fats and olive oil can be found in Appendix A.

2.2.5. Increase Fibre and Water Intake

Fibre is essential for proper digestion and maintenance of a healthy microbiome. Fibre and fluid work together to promote bowel health. It is important that when your patient increases their fibre intake, they also increase their fluid intake. Fibre is found in fruits, vegetables, and whole grains, which are the main components of the plant rich dietary interventions included in the systematic reviews that make up the evidence for this paper.

2.2.6. Reduce and Limit Ultra-Processed Food and Added Sugar Intake

Ultra-processed and sugar-dense foods and drinks contain very high amounts of energy and negligible amounts of beneficial nutrients. These foods are often high in fat, salt, and sugar, and in the case of beverages, caffeine, which can impact sleep. Some examples include soft drinks, sweet or savoury packaged snacks, confectionary, and reconstituted meat products. These foods are often high in fat, salt, and sugar, and in the case of beverages, caffeine. These nutrients can have a number of effects including increasing circulating inflammatory markers and oxidation [11,93] and impacting sleep. In relation to sugar consumption, the World Health Organisation (WHO) recommends that adults limit intake of 'free sugar' including table sugar, honey, syrups, and sugar-sweetened beverages to less than 10% of total energy [94].

2.2.7. Other Nutritional Considerations

As shown in Figure 1, nutrition also encompasses other dietary factors such as caffeine and alcohol. Caffeine is commonly consumed in tea and coffee, and evidence shows that low to moderate consumption of coffee is associated with reduced mortality [95]. Tea and coffee contain other phytonutrients such as polyphenols, and it may be that these are responsible for their health benefits [95]. Coffee consumption later in the day or in high doses (>200 mg/serve or >400 mg/day) may increase anxiety and reduce quality of sleep, both of which can negatively influence pain experiences [95]. Decaffeinated options are a good alternative to avoid increased anxiety or sleep issues. Other sources of caffeine or guarana such as soft drinks and energy drinks should be avoided, as they contain large quantities of added sugars and lack nutrients [95]. Energy drinks are also associated with cardiac and psychological issues [95].

Evidence suggests that excessive alcohol intake can dysregulate descending inhibitory pathways and reward network circuitry, which can lead to hyperalgesia [96]. Alcohol also disrupts REM sleep, which can feed into the cyclic relationship between poor sleep and poor eating habits [74,97]. Resveratrol, an antioxidant with anti-inflammatory properties that can be found in red wine may play a role in reducing pain severity [98]. The best advice is to follow national alcohol guidelines such as the National Health and Medical Research Council guidelines in Australia to consume no more than 10 standard drinks per week [99].

2.3. Nutrition Considerations for Vulnerable Groups

2.3.1. Older People

Advancing age is major risk factor for developing CNCP. Approximately 20% of adults in the Western world experience CNCP; however, this almost doubles in those aged over 65 years [2,4]. It is also estimated that up to 93% of residents in aged care experience CNCP [100]. As the population ages, the prevalence is expected to increase over time, which will lead to increased healthcare burden and costs.

Malnutrition and dehydration are highly prevalent among older people, especially those in residential aged care facilities. See Table 2 for strategies on how prevent these issues. These nutrition-related issues are also associated with increased risk of experiencing pain [100]. Approximately 50% of older people in Australia are malnourished or at risk of malnutrition, and up to 68% are at risk of dehydration [100]. In addition to an increased risk of experiencing pain, these issues also result in decreased quality of life and increased risk of falls and fractures, sarcopenia, confusion, constipation, and fatigue, all of which further impact the morbidity and mortality of older people [100]. Older people experiencing pain who are malnourished or dehydrated should be referred to a dietitian for medical nutrition therapy [100]. Malnutrition is also associated with deconditioning. This leads to a loss of muscle mass and strength. Consumption of high quality protein combined with resistance and strengthening exercises assist in building muscle mass and strength [101]. In Australia, guidelines state that those aged 70 years and over should consume approximately 1 g protein per kilogram of body weight per day [102]. Consuming high quality protein sources (e.g., lean meat, eggs, nuts, and legumes) across 2–3 meals per day optimises muscle protein synthesis [103].

Table 2. Nutrition-related tips and strategies to assist older people in managing pain experiences [100].

Monitor Signs for Malnutrition and Risk of Malnutrition	Monitor Signs for Reduced Fluid Intake and Risk of Dehydration	Stimulate Appetite	Increase Fluid Intake	Improve Eating Experience	Reduce Constipation
- Assess and regularly screen older people to determine their nutrition status - Identify changes in weight, food and drink intake and appetite - Identify gastrointestinal symptoms - Monitor changes in mobility and function - Identify psychological disease and/or dementia	- Ongoing pain and dementia may reduce ability and memory - Not feeling thirsty - Inconvenience - Medication side effects - Unable to access drinks - Fluid restrictions	- Offer smaller portions more frequently throughout the day - Increase fat, protein and/or flavour content - Ensure meals are appealing	- Offer small frequent drinks between meals - Offer foods with higher water content (e.g., soup, fruit, and yoghurt) - Ensure drinks are clearly and easily accessible - Ensure adequate support for drinking and toileting is available if needed - Contraindications: heart failure and fluid restrictions	- Ensure older people have choices at meal times - Find out food preferences and incorporate into meals - Provide eating assistance, where needed - Ensure dining environment is appealing - Do not rush meals	- Encourage high fibre foods, e.g., keep the skin on fruit, high fibre breakfast cereals - Dietary supplements (e.g., psyllium husk) can be added to foods if needed - Laxative and/or stool softening agents may be needed. Increased fluid is also required for these to be effective - Beverages containing sorbitol (e.g., prune or pear juice)

2.3.2. Culturally and Linguistically Diverse Populations

CNCP disproportionally affects culturally and linguistically diverse populations (CALD), migrants, and refugees [3]. In a cross-sectional study conducted by Kurita 2012 et al., it was reported that the prevalence of CNCP in Danish-born participants was 26%, compared to non-Western born participants in whom the prevalence was 40% [3]. Several studies conducted in Sweden, Switzerland, and Denmark show that immigrants, especially from non-Western backgrounds, have more diagnosed musculoskeletal conditions, higher pain intensity, healthcare utilisation, and increased risk of poor mental health [104]. CALD populations are also less likely to engage in treatment options and have poorer outcomes [104] Systematic reviews frequently limit literature searches to studies published in English and observational and experimental studies often exclude non-English speaking people [104].

There are a variety of complex biopsychosocial and lifestyle factors that influence pain experiences and nutrition practices and beliefs for CALD populations. Some cultures may put different emphases on the relationship between nutrition and the biomedical contribution to pain experiences.

Different cultures have varying beliefs around different foods and their potential role in healing and pain. For example, arthritis may be considered a "hot" condition that needs to be treated with "cooling" foods. In some cultures, food preparation may be a major part of identity, and the loss of ability to express this identity may cause significant distress and worsen an individual's pain. The impact of language can also directly affect nutrition quality, making it more difficult to shop and read labels, while experiencing pain may also make it more difficult to be able to study and participate in a new culture and language. Culture also affects the types of food eaten, and the manner and volume of eating. In addition, food is frequently an important component of traditions and celebrations.

3. Future Directions for Clinical Practice

In order to optimise therapeutic outcomes, pain services should incorporate nutrition screening, assessment, and treatment alongside treatments from other allied health professionals. These should be developed and implemented in conjunction with dietitians and integrated into current pain management practice. Evidence shows that a clinically meaningful reduction in pain can be achieved with personalised dietary advice for patients experiencing CNCP [53]. The whole-person approach to pain management can be strengthened with the inclusion of a person-centred dietary assessment and intervention. Similarly, multidisciplinary teams can also be strengthened with the inclusion of a registered or accredited dietitian to provide this service. It should be acknowledged that while there is dietary advice that can be given to anyone experiencing pain, it is not always a one-size-fits-all approach and dietitians are best placed to provide individualised medical nutrition therapy where needed. In services where this may not be possible, another option is establishing a consultative relationship with a dietitian outside the service. The dietitian can provide their expertise by leading nutrition professional development for clinicians and nutrition programs for individuals and patient groups.

In contemporary practice, dietary assessment of patients attending pain services is uncommon and, therefore, there is very limited information about the dietary intakes and behaviours of patients outside of research studies. To effectively translate research findings from nutrition-based studies, it would be helpful to have a greater understanding of the nutritional status of patients. Collaborations and networks exist to collect data from pain services around the world to assist with benchmarking, but this data does not currently include dietary information.

Exploring the role of telehealth in providing treatments to patients, nutrition-related or otherwise, is also something that should be considered, given some of the barriers patients face in attending face to face appointments [105]. These may include travel time, cost, and accessibility to services. This would extend the reach of dietary treatment to patients who may not currently be able to access it. Contingent upon a viable funding model, nutrition education and behaviour change can easily be delivered via telehealth and there is evidence to support its use for many chronic health conditions [105].

Advocacy needs to continue for the role of nutrition in CNCP management. This can be done at a local, national, or international level through pain services, national pain societies, government prevention strategies and strategic plans, dietetic organisations, consumer groups, and the International Association for the Study of Pain.

4. Future Directions for Research

It is evident from the included studies that gaps exist in research that has been undertaken to explore the relationships between nutrition and pain management. The systematic reviews found that the heterogeneity among studies made it difficult to draw strong conclusions. Future intervention studies need to include larger, higher powered sample sizes and test both the efficacy and effectiveness of the intervention. It would also be valuable to include other outcomes such as physical function, psychological measures, biomarkers of inflammation, blood glucose, blood lipids, and blood pressure to determine the effect of interventions on comorbid mental and physical health conditions.

Another limitation of current evidence is the lack of information provided on the intervention components and methods of the included studies. It is therefore difficult to extract precise information on intervention content, mode and frequency of delivery, and the qualifications of the person who delivered the intervention. For example, interventions may be categorised as vegetarian or vegan without specifying critical components such as amounts of sugar and/or refined grains. All of this information is required in order to replicate interventions and translate findings into clinical practice. If future studies better report methodologies and results it would lead to more consistent analysis and synthesis of outcomes and more meaningful interpretation.

The implementation of routine dietary assessment is another important consideration for chronic pain trials. Use of consistent and comprehensive assessment tools is key. Participant burden can be reduced by utilising tools which incorporate technology such as image-based food records. Many of the studies included in the systematics reviews used a unidimensional measure of pain, such as a visual analogue scale. Multidimensional tools that incorporate pain interference and pain self-efficacy provide a more comprehensive measure of pain outcomes, especially in the context of the whole-person approach.

When translating the research into clinical settings, one should consider using co-production or co-design methods to engage and include stakeholders in the development and undertaking of research studies to ensure that the intervention is feasible and acceptable to the local context. Engaging stakeholders will also ensure that the intervention is appropriate and relevant for their needs and wants. With an increased focus on knowledge translation and implementation science, these types of studies are required to ensure that interventions work in the real world.

5. Conclusions

Diet should play a pivotal role in pain management. There is a strong link between diet and systemic inflammation and other chronic health conditions associated with CNCP. Best evidence pain management incorporates active strategies that target biopsychosocial and lifestyle factors such as biomedical, mind–body connection, physical activity, sleep, and nutrition. These factors are of variable importance in different individuals and complex inter-relationships exist between them. Nutrition is an area that traditionally has not received sufficient attention in CNCP management. This state-of-the-art paper summarises the relationships between diet, inflammation, comorbidities, and pain management, and uses the current literature to provide recommendations on improving the dietary habits and behaviours of those experiencing CNCP. The paper also proposes future directions for practice and clinical research in this space.

Author Contributions: All authors contributed to the conceptualization, writing—original draft preparation and writing—review and editing. All authors have read and agreed to the published version of the manuscript.

Funding: This research received no external funding.

Institutional Review Board Statement: Not applicable.

Informed Consent Statement: Not applicable.

Data Availability Statement: Not applicable.

Conflicts of Interest: The authors declare no conflict of interest.

Appendix A. Key Messages and Practical Nutrition Tips for Pain Management

(adapted from Brain et al., 2020 [89])

Key Messages:

1. People with chronic non-cancer pain (CNCP) should be encouraged to consume:
    a. A wide range of nutrient-dense foods (e.g., fruits, vegetables, whole grain breads and cereals, meat, dairy, and their alternatives) to ensure they are meeting their nutritional requirements.

- b. The recommended amount of fruit and vegetables should be based on your country's dietary guidelines and to focus on consuming a rainbow of colors every day.
- c. Long chain and monounsaturated fats (e.g., omega-3 and olive oil).
- d. More fibre and fluid. Adult females should consume 25 g/day of fibre and adult males 30 g/day. Adults should aim for 2–3 L of water per day.
- e. Less ultra-processed foods and foods containing added sugars.

2. Find resources and strategies through your country's dietetic organisation such as Dietitian Australia, the Academy of Nutrition and Dietetics, The European Federation of the Associations of Dietitians, or the British Dietetics Association that support this information and that you can provide to patients that will assist them.

Practical Tips for Conducting Dietary Assessments:

- Assist patients to screen their diet quality using tools such as the Healthy Eating Quiz
- If you are concerned about potential nutritional deficiencies consider referring patients to a dietitian for a comprehensive dietary assessment and personalised advice and support.

Practical Tips to Optimize Diet Quality

- Become familiar and learn about your country's dietary guidelines.
- Use an inclusive approach, emphasise important foods that should be added (e.g., vegetables), rather than focusing on foods that should be removed (e.g., energy-dense snack foods).
- Ensure that nutrition-based education is aimed at improving diet quality, as this will address systemic inflammation and enhance pain management.
- Be aware that this is a broad approach and there may be individualized variation. For personalized dietary advice patients should be referred to a dietitian.
- Educate patients on the role of vitamins and minerals in pain management and food sources of these nutrients. For example, good dietary-sources of Vitamin D include fish and eggs, good sources of Vitamin B12 are meat, fish, and dairy, and magnesium can be found in green leafy vegetables and whole grains.
- Encourage patients to spend some time outside to obtain Vitamin D from sun exposure. For most people, 10–15 min of sun on the arms and legs most days of the week will provide most of the Vitamin D required. However, this will vary based on location and the time of year.

Practical Tips for Fruit and Vegetable Consumption Which are Rich in Phytonutrients to Reduce Oxidative Stress

- Educate your patients on the important role of fruits and vegetables in pain management.
- Encourage your patients to buy in-season fruits and vegetables and to try a new fruit or vegetable each week where possible.
- If preparation and cooking is an issue for your patients, encourage them to include variety by using frozen mixed vegetables or reduced-salt canned vegetables (e.g., tomatoes and lentils), which can be easily incorporated into meals such as stir-frys, stews, or pasta dishes. Frozen fruits and vegetables are a great option as they maintain their nutritional quality.
- Work with your patient to come up with ways to incorporate fruit and vegetables into their daily routine, e.g., including vegetables as a snack throughout the day, ensuring half their plate is covered in vegetables at main meals, using frozen berries as a snack, or the addition of yoghurt or cereal.

Practical Tips for Consuming Long Chain and Monounsaturated Fats (e.g., Omega-3 and Olive Oil)

- Educate patients on the role of omega-3 and olive oil in pain management.
- Communicate, motivate and encourage patients to consume foods high in omega-3 and olive oil.

- ○ Consume oily fish (e.g., salmon and sardines), flax seed oil or canola oil, linseed, and walnuts to boost omega-3 intake. Aim for a minimum of 2–3 servings of oily fish per week.
- ○ Use extra virgin olive oil as the preferred oil in cooking and salad dressings.
- ○ Reduce saturated and trans fats (e.g., butter, processed foods, and hydrogenated vegetable oils).
- ○ Limit polyunsaturated fats high in omega-6 such as sunflower and safflower oils.
- Supplements: It is preferable to focus on diet quality through food intake rather than via supplements. Seek advice from a dietitian or medical professional if your patient is considering high doses of fish oil supplements. Evidence suggests that 3000 mg of omega-3, over a 3-month period reduces pain experiences, especially in rheumatoid arthritis [106]. There are two types of omega-3 fats in fish oil supplements, EPA and DHA. Supplements which have a ratio of EPA/DHA of ≥ 1.5 are most beneficial. Suggest good quality brands which contain high doses of omega-3.

Practical Tips to Increase Fibre and Water Consumption
- Encourage patients to consume the recommended serves of fruits and vegetables to increase fibre intake.
- Provide practical suggestions such as switching to whole meal or whole grain breads, pasta, and breakfast cereals. Keep the skin on fruits and incorporate a variety of mixed vegetables and lentils into meals. Add psyllium husk or bran to meals at breakfast time.
- Fill a large (1.5 L) drinking bottle with water every day and set a goal to consume it throughout the day.

Practical Tips to Reduce and Limit Ultra-Processed Food and Added Sugar Intake
- Work with patients to swap sugary and energy drinks for water or mineral water flavoured with fresh fruit.
- Encourage consumption of healthy convenient snacks such as fruit, vegetable sticks, or yoghurt.
- Incorporate strategies to help patients cook meals at home rather than relying on highly processed conveniently prepared or take away foods.
- Recommend cooking meals in bulk and freezing the leftovers so patients have a quick, easy, and healthy meal they can have when they have a flare up and do not feel like cooking.

Practical Nutrition Tips for Vulnerable Populations
Older People

Clinicians and aged care facilities should monitor for signs of malnutrition and dehydration. Assist older people and their families to optimise their food and fluid intake to reduce pain experiences in older people. Some practical tips and strategies can be found in Table 2.

People from CALD Backgrounds
- Be aware of eating patterns and beliefs of the cultural group you are working with (recognising individual variation).
- Adapt your practice accordingly and include family and community where possible.
- Culturally informed approaches enhance engagement [107].

References

1. Classification of Chronic Pain. Descriptions of chronic pain syndromes and definitions of pain terms. Prepared by the International Association for the Study of Pain, Subcommittee on Taxonomy. *Pain Suppl.* **1986**, *3*, S1–S226.
2. Croft, P.; Blyth, F.M.; van der Windt, D. The global occurrence of chronic pain: An introduction. In *Chronic Pain Epidemiology: From Aetiology to Public Health*; Academic Press: Cambridge, MA, USA, 2010; pp. 9–18.
3. Kurita, G.P.; Sjøgren, P.; Juel, K.; Højsted, J.; Ekholm, O. The burden of chronic pain: A cross-sectional survey focussing on diseases, immigration, and opioid use. *Pain* **2012**, *153*, 2332–2338. [CrossRef]
4. Deloitte Access Economics. *The Cost of Pain in Australia*; Deloitte Access Economics: Sydney, Australia, 2019.
5. Gaskin, D.J.; Richard, P. The Economic Costs of Pain in the United States. *J. Pain* **2012**, *13*, 715–724. [CrossRef]
6. Allingham, S.; Blanchard, M.; Tardif, H.; Quinsey, K.; Bryce, M.; Cameron, K.; White, J.; Damm, S.; Eagar, K. *Electronic Persistent Pain Outcomes Collaboration Annual Data Report 2019*; University of Woolongong: Wollongong, Australia, 2020.
7. Hayes, C.; Hodson, F.J. A Whole-Person Model of Care for Persistent Pain: From Conceptual Framework to Practical Application. *Pain Med.* **2011**, *12*, 1738–1749. [CrossRef]
8. Hayes, C.; Naylor, R.; Egger, G. Understanding Chronic Pain in a Lifestyle Context: The Emergence of a Whole-Person Ap-proach. *Am. J. Lifestyle Med.* **2012**, *6*, 421–428. [CrossRef]
9. Holliday, S.; Hayes, C.; Jones, L.; Gordon, J.; Harris, N.; Nicholas, M. Prescribing wellness: Comprehensive pain management outside specialist services. *Aust. Prescr.* **2018**, *41*, 86–91. [CrossRef] [PubMed]
10. Hansen, K.A.; McKernan, L.C.; Carter, S.D.; Allen, C.; Wolever, R.Q. A Replicable and Sustainable Whole Person Care Model for Chronic Pain. *J. Altern. Complement. Med.* **2019**, *25* (Suppl. 1), S86–S94. [CrossRef] [PubMed]
11. Blaak, E.E.; Antoine, J.; Benton, D.; Björck, I.; Bozzetto, L.; Brouns, F.; Diamant, M.; Dye, L.; Hulshof, T.; Holst, J.J.; et al. Impact of postprandial glycaemia on health and prevention of disease. *Obes. Rev.* **2012**, *13*, 923–984. [CrossRef] [PubMed]
12. Wiebe, N.; Ye, F.; Crumley, E.T.; Bello, A.; Stenvinkel, P.; Tonelli, M. Temporal Associations Among Body Mass Index, Fasting Insulin, and Systemic Inflammation: A Systematic Review and Meta-analysis. *JAMA Netw. Open* **2021**, *4*, e211263. [CrossRef]
13. Chambers, E.S.; Byrne, C.S.; Morrison, D.; Murphy, K.G.; Preston, T.; Tedford, C.; Garcia-Perez, I.; Fountana, S.; Serrano-Contreras, J.I.; Holmes, E.; et al. Dietary supplementation with inulin-propionate ester or inulin improves insulin sensitivity in adults with overweight and obesity with distinct effects on the gut microbiota, plasma metabolome and systemic inflammatory responses: A randomised cross-over trial. *Gut* **2019**, *68*, 1430–1438. [CrossRef] [PubMed]
14. Marion-Letellier, R.; Savoye, G.; Ghosh, S. Polyunsaturated fatty acids and inflammation. *IUBMB Life* **2015**, *67*, 659–667. [CrossRef]
15. Raphael, W.; Sordillo, L.M. Dietary Polyunsaturated Fatty Acids and Inflammation: The Role of Phospholipid Biosynthesis. *Int. J. Mol. Sci.* **2013**, *14*, 21167–21188. [CrossRef]
16. Simopoulos, A.P.; DiNicolantonio, J.J. The importance of a balanced ω-6 to ω-3 ratio in the prevention and management of obesity. *Open Hear.* **2016**, *3*, e000385. [CrossRef]
17. Bendsen, N.T.; Stender, S.; Szecsi, P.; Pedersen, S.B.; Basu, S.; Hellgren, L.; Newman, J.; Larsen, T.M.; Haugaard, S.B.; Astrup, A. Effect of industrially produced trans fat on markers of systemic inflammation: Evidence from a randomized trial in women. *J. Lipid Res.* **2011**, *52*, 1821–1828. [CrossRef] [PubMed]
18. Oteng, A.-B.; Kersten, S. Mechanisms of Action of trans Fatty Acids. *Adv. Nutr.* **2020**, *11*, 697–708. [CrossRef]
19. Nijs, J.; Yilmaz, S.T.; Elma, Ö.; Tatta, J.; Mullie, P.; Vanderweeën, L.; Clarys, P.; Deliens, T.; Coppieters, I.; Weltens, N.; et al. Nutritional intervention in chronic pain: An innovative way of targeting central nervous system sensitization? *Expert Opin. Ther. Targets* **2020**, *24*, 793–803. [CrossRef]
20. Ji, R.R.; Nackley, A.; Huh, Y.; Terrando, N.; Maixner, W. Neuroinflammation and Central Sensitization in Chronic and Widespread Pain. *Anesthesiology* **2018**, *129*, 343–366. [CrossRef]
21. Rizzetto, L.; Fava, F.; Tuohy, K.M.; Selmi, C. Connecting the immune system, systemic chronic inflammation and the gut microbiome: The role of sex. *J. Autoimmun.* **2018**, *92*, 12–34. [CrossRef] [PubMed]
22. Bjørklund, G.; Aaseth, J.; Doşa, M.D.; Pivina, L.; Dadar, M.; Pen, J.J.; Chirumbolo, S. Does diet play a role in reducing nociception related to inflammation and chronic pain? *Nutrition* **2019**, *66*, 153–165. [CrossRef] [PubMed]
23. Manach, C.; Scalbert, A.; Morand, C.; Rémésy, C.; Jiménez, L. Polyphenols: Food sources and bioavailability. *Am. J. Clin. Nutr.* **2004**, *79*, 727–747. [CrossRef] [PubMed]
24. Chai, S.C.; Davis, K.; Zhang, Z.; Zha, L.; Kirschner, K.F. Effects of Tart Cherry Juice on Biomarkers of Inflammation and Ox-idative Stress in Older Adults. *Nutrients* **2019**, *11*, 228. [CrossRef] [PubMed]
25. Kelley, D.S.; Adkins, Y.; Laugero, K.D. A Review of the Health Benefits of Cherries. *Nutrients* **2018**, *10*, 368. [CrossRef] [PubMed]
26. Kent, K.; Charlton, K.; Roodenrys, S.; Batterham, M.; Potter, J.; Traynor, V.; Gilbert, H.; Morgan, O.; Richards, R. Consumption of anthocyanin-rich cherry juice for 12 weeks improves memory and cognition in older adults with mild-to-moderate dementia. *Eur. J. Nutr.* **2017**, *56*, 333–341. [CrossRef]
27. Schell, J.; Scofield, R.H.; Barrett, J.R.; Kurien, B.T.; Betts, N.; Lyons, T.J.; Zhao, Y.D.; Basu, A. Strawberries Improve Pain and Inflammation in Obese Adults with Radiographic Evidence of Knee Osteoarthritis. *Nutrients* **2017**, *9*, 949. [CrossRef] [PubMed]
28. Guan, V.X.; Mobasheri, A.; Probst, Y.C. A systematic review of osteoarthritis prevention and management with dietary phytochemicals from foods. *Maturitas* **2019**, *122*, 35–43. [CrossRef] [PubMed]

29. Brain, K.; Burrows, T.; Rollo, M.E.; Hayes, C.; Hodson, F.J.; Collins, C.E. Population Characteristics in a Tertiary Pain Service Cohort Experiencing Chronic Non-Cancer Pain: Weight Status, Comorbidities, and Patient Goals. *Healthcare* **2017**, *5*, 28. [CrossRef] [PubMed]
30. Bruggink, L.; Hayes, C.; Lawrence, G.; Brain, K.; Holliday, S. Chronic pain: Overlap and specificity in multimorbidity management. *Aust. J. Gen. Pract.* **2019**, *48*, 689–692. [CrossRef]
31. Minihane, A.M.; Vinoy, S.; Russell, W.R.; Baka, A.; Roche, H.M.; Tuohy, K.M.; Teeling, J.L.; Blaak, E.E.; Fenech, M.; Vauzour, D.; et al. Low-grade inflammation, diet composition and health: Current research evidence and its translation. *Br. J. Nutr.* **2015**, *114*, 999–1012. [CrossRef]
32. Furman, D.; Campisi, J.; Verdin, E.; Carrera-Bastos, P.; Targ, S.; Franceschi, C.; Ferrucci, L.; Gilroy, D.W.; Fasano, A.; Miller, G.W.; et al. Chronic inflammation in the etiology of disease across the life span. *Nat. Med.* **2019**, *25*, 1822–1832. [CrossRef]
33. Naylor, R.; Hayes, C.; Egger, G. The Relationship Between Lifestyle, Metaflammation, and Chronic Pain: A Systematic Review. *Am. J. Lifestyle Med.* **2012**, *7*, 130–137. [CrossRef]
34. Aghasafari, P.; George, U.; Pidaparti, R. A review of inflammatory mechanism in airway diseases. *Inflamm. Res.* **2019**, *68*, 59–74. [CrossRef] [PubMed]
35. Kaushik, A.S.; Strath, L.J.; Sorge, R.E. Dietary Interventions for Treatment of Chronic Pain: Oxidative Stress and Inflammation. *Pain Ther.* **2020**, *9*, 487–498. [CrossRef]
36. Charles-Messance, H.; Mitchelson, K.A.; Castro, E.D.M.; Sheedy, F.J.; Roche, H.M. Regulating metabolic inflammation by nutritional modulation. *J. Allergy Clin. Immunol.* **2020**, *146*, 706–720. [CrossRef] [PubMed]
37. Potenza, M.A.; Nacci, C.; De Salvia, M.A.; Sgarra, L.; Collino, M.; Montagnani, M. Targeting endothelial metaflammation to counteract diabesity cardiovascular risk: Current and perspective therapeutic options. *Pharmacol. Res.* **2017**, *120*, 226–241. [CrossRef]
38. Donnelly, C.R.; Andriessen, A.S.; Chen, G.; Wang, K.; Jiang, C.; Maixner, W.; Ji, R.-R. Central Nervous System Targets: Glial Cell Mechanisms in Chronic Pain. *Neurotherapeutics* **2020**, *17*, 846–860. [CrossRef] [PubMed]
39. Kaur, N.; Chugh, H.; Sakharkar, M.K.; Dhawan, U.; Chidambaram, S.B.; Chandra, R. Neuroinflammation Mechanisms and Phytotherapeutic Intervention: A Systematic Review. *ACS Chem. Neurosci.* **2020**, *11*, 3707–3731. [CrossRef]
40. Malta, I.; Moraes, T.; Rodrigues, G.; Franco, P.; Galdino, G. The role of oligodendrocytes in chronic pain: Cellular and molecular mechanisms. *J. Physiol. Pharmacol.* **2019**, *70*, 70.
41. Robinson, W.H.; Lepus, C.M.; Wang, Q.; Raghu, H.; Mao, R.; Lindstrom, T.M.; Sokolove, J. Low-grade inflammation as a key mediator of the pathogenesis of osteoarthritis. *Nat. Rev. Rheumatol.* **2016**, *12*, 580–592. [CrossRef] [PubMed]
42. Bjurström, M.F.; Bodelsson, M.; Montgomery, A.; Harsten, A.; Waldén, M.; Janelidze, S.; Hall, S.; Hansson, O.; Irwin, M.R.; Mattsson-Carlgren, N. Differential expression of cerebrospinal fluid neuroinflammatory mediators depending on osteoarthritis pain phenotype. *Pain* **2020**, *161*, 2142–2154. [CrossRef]
43. Barnett, K.; Mercer, S.; Norbury, M.; Watt, G.; Wyke, S.; Guthrie, B. Epidemiology of multimorbidity and implications for health care, research, and medical education: A cross-sectional study. *Lancet* **2012**, *380*, 37–43. [CrossRef]
44. Ohayon, M.M.; Stingl, J. Prevalence and comorbidity of chronic pain in the German general population. *J. Psychiatr. Res.* **2012**, *46*, 444–450. [CrossRef]
45. Oliveira, C.B.; Maher, C.G.; Franco, M.R.; Kamper, S.J.; Williams, C.; Silva, F.G.; Pinto, R.Z. Co-occurrence of Chronic Musculoskeletal Pain and Cardiovascular Diseases: A Systematic Review with Meta-analysis. *Pain Med.* **2019**, *21*, 1106–1121. [CrossRef] [PubMed]
46. Pozzobon, D.; Ferreira, P.H.; Dario, A.B.; Almeida, L.; Vesentini, G.; Harmer, A.R.; Ferreira, M.L. Is there an association be-tween diabetes and back pain? A systematic review with meta-analyses. *PLoS ONE* **2019**, *14*, e0212030. [CrossRef] [PubMed]
47. Hitt, H.C.; McMillen, R.C.; Thornton-Neaves, T.; Koch, K.; Cosby, A.G. Comorbidity of obesity and pain in a general popu-lation: Results from the Southern Pain Prevalence Study. *J. Pain* **2007**, *8*, 430–436. [CrossRef]
48. Stone, A.A.; Broderick, J. Obesity and Pain Are Associated in the United States. *Obesity* **2012**, *20*, 1491–1495. [CrossRef]
49. Dean, E.; Hansen, R.G. Prescribing Optimal Nutrition and Physical Activity as "First-Line" Interventions for Best Practice Management of Chronic Low-Grade Inflammation Associated with Osteoarthritis: Evidence Synthesis. *Arthritis* **2012**, *2012*, 1–28. [CrossRef] [PubMed]
50. VanDenKerkhof, E.G.; Macdonald, H.M.; Jones, G.T.; Power, C.; Macfarlane, G. Diet, Lifestyle and Chronic Widespread Pain: Results from the 1958 British Birth Cohort Study. *Pain Res. Manag.* **2011**, *16*, 87–92. [CrossRef]
51. Collins, C.E.; Young, A.F.; Hodge, A. Diet quality is associated with higher nutrient intake and self-rated health in mid-aged women. *J. Am. Coll. Nutr.* **2008**, *27*, 146–157. [CrossRef]
52. Meleger, A.L.; Froude, C.K.; Walker, J., 3rd. Nutrition and eating behavior in patients with chronic pain receiving long-term opioid therapy. *PM&R* **2014**, *6*, 7–12.e1.
53. Brain, K.; Burrows, T.L.; Rollo, M.E.; Hayes, C.; Hodson, F.J.; Collins, C.E. The Effect of a Pilot Dietary Intervention on Pain Outcomes in Patients Attending a Tertiary Pain Service. *Nutrients* **2019**, *11*, 181. [CrossRef]
54. National Health and Medical Research Council. *Australian Dietary Guidelines*; National Health and Medical Research Council: Canberra, Australia, 2013.
55. National Health and Medical Research Council. *Eat for Health*; National Health and Medical Research Council: Canberra, Australia, 2013.

56. Wiss, D. A Biopsychosocial Overview of the Opioid Crisis: Considering Nutrition and Gastrointestinal Health. *Front. Public Health* **2019**, *7*, 193. [CrossRef] [PubMed]
57. Bjarnason, I.; Scarpignato, C.; Holmgren, E.; Olszewski, M.; Rainsford, K.D.; Lanas, A. Mechanisms of Damage to the Gastrointestinal Tract from Nonsteroidal Anti-Inflammatory Drugs. *Gastroenterology* **2018**, *154*, 500–514. [CrossRef]
58. Wang, X.; Tang, Q.; Hou, H.; Zhang, W.; Li, M.; Chen, D.; Gu, Y.; Wang, B.; Hou, J.; Liu, Y.; et al. Gut Microbiota in NSAID Enteropathy: New Insights from Inside. *Front. Cell. Infect. Microbiol.* **2021**, *11*, 572. [CrossRef] [PubMed]
59. Jahromi, S.R.; Togha, M.; Fesharaki, S.H.; Najafi, M.; Moghadam, N.B.; Kheradmand, J.A.; Kazemi, H.; Gorji, A. Gastrointestinal adverse effects of antiepileptic drugs in intractable epileptic patients. *Seizure* **2011**, *20*, 343–346. [CrossRef] [PubMed]
60. Oliva, V.; Lippi, M.; Paci, R.; Del Fabro, L.; Delvecchio, G.; Brambilla, P.; De Ronchi, D.; Fanelli, G.; Serretti, A. Gastrointestinal side effects associated with antidepressant treatments in patients with major depressive disorder: A systematic review and meta-analysis. *Prog. Neuro-Psychopharmacol. Biol. Psychiatry* **2021**, *109*, 110266. [CrossRef]
61. Camilleri, M.; Drossman, D.A.; Becker, G.; Webster, L.R.; Davies, A.N.; Mawe, G.M. Emerging treatments in neurogastroenterology: A multidisciplinary working group consensus statement on opioid-induced constipation. *Neurogastroenterol. Motil.* **2014**, *26*, 1386–1395. [CrossRef]
62. Kumar, L.; Barker, C.; Emmanuel, A. Opioid-Induced Constipation: Pathophysiology, Clinical Consequences, and Management. *Gastroenterol. Res. Pract.* **2014**, *2014*, 1–6. [CrossRef]
63. Bannon, S.; Greenberg, J.; Mace, R.A.; Locascio, J.J.; Vranceanu, A.-M. The role of social isolation in physical and emotional outcomes among patients with chronic pain. *Gen. Hosp. Psychiatry* **2021**, *69*, 50–54. [CrossRef]
64. Karayannis, N.V.; Baumann, I.; Sturgeon, J.; Melloh, M.; Mackey, S. The Impact of Social Isolation on Pain Interference: A Longitudinal Study. *Ann. Behav. Med.* **2019**, *53*, 65–74. [CrossRef]
65. Menec, V.H.; Newall, N.E.; Mackenzie, C.S.; Shooshtari, S.; Nowicki, S. Examining social isolation and loneliness in combi-nation in relation to social support and psychological distress using Canadian Longitudinal Study of Aging (CLSA) data. *PLoS ONE* **2020**, *15*, e0230673. [CrossRef]
66. Amy Janke, E.; Kozak, A.T. "The more pain I have, the more I want to eat": Obesity in the context of chronic pain. *Obesity* **2012**, *20*, 2027–2034. [CrossRef]
67. Gibson-Smith, D.; Bot, M.; Brouwer, I.A.; Visser, M.; Penninx, B.W. Diet quality in persons with and without depressive and anxiety disorders. *J. Psychiatr. Res.* **2018**, *106*, 1–7. [CrossRef]
68. Teasdale, S.B.; Ward, P.; Samaras, K.; Firth, J.; Stubbs, B.; Tripodi, E.; Burrows, T.L. Dietary intake of people with severe mental illness: Systematic review and meta-analysis. *Br. J. Psychiatry* **2019**, *214*, 251–259. [CrossRef]
69. Wirt, A.; Collins, C.E. Diet quality—What is it and does it matter? *Public Health Nutr.* **2009**, *12*, 2473–2492. [CrossRef]
70. Bigand, T.; Wilson, M. Overeating during painful episodes among adults with chronic pain: A preliminary study. *Appetite* **2019**, *137*, 99–103. [CrossRef] [PubMed]
71. Masheb, R.M.; Douglas, M.; Kutz, A.M.; Marsh, A.G.; Driscoll, M. Pain and emotional eating: Further investigation of the Yale Emotional Overeating Questionnaire in weight loss seeking patients. *J. Behav. Med.* **2020**, *43*, 479–486. [CrossRef]
72. Emami, A.S.; Woodcock, A.; Swanson, H.E.; Kapphahn, T.; Pulvers, K. Distress tolerance is linked to unhealthy eating through pain catastrophizing. *Appetite* **2016**, *107*, 454–459. [CrossRef] [PubMed]
73. Agency for Clinical Innovation Pain: Lifestyle and Nutrition. Available online: https://www.aci.health.nsw.gov.au/chronic-pain/for-everyone/pain-lifestyle-and-nutrition (accessed on 19 September 2021).
74. Fenton, S.; Burrows, T.L.; Skinner, J.A.; Duncan, M.J. The influence of sleep health on dietary intake: A systematic review and meta-analysis of intervention studies. *J. Hum. Nutr. Diet.* **2020**, *34*, 273–285. [CrossRef] [PubMed]
75. Haack, M.; Simpson, N.; Sethna, N.; Kaur, S.; Mullington, J. Sleep deficiency and chronic pain: Potential underlying mecha-nisms and clinical implications. *Neuropsychopharmacology* **2020**, *45*, 205–216. [CrossRef]
76. Depner, C.M.; Stothard, E.R.; Wright, K.P. Metabolic Consequences of Sleep and Circadian Disorders. *Curr. Diabetes Rep.* **2014**, *14*, 1–9. [CrossRef] [PubMed]
77. Michie, S.; Van Stralen, M.M.; West, R. The behaviour change wheel: A new method for characterising and designing behaviour change interventions. *Implement. Sci.* **2011**, *6*, 42. [CrossRef] [PubMed]
78. Williams, R.L.; Rollo, M.E.; Schumacher, T.; Collins, C.E. Diet Quality Scores of Australian Adults Who Have Completed the Healthy Eating Quiz. *Nutrients* **2017**, *9*, 880. [CrossRef] [PubMed]
79. Philpot, U.; Johnson, M. Diet therapy in the management of chronic pain: Better diet less pain? *Pain Manag.* **2019**, *9*, 335–338. [CrossRef]
80. Towery, P.; Guffey, J.S.; Doerflein, C.; Stroup, K.; Saucedo, J.; Taylor, J. Chronic musculoskeletal pain and function improve with a plant-based diet. *Complement. Ther. Med.* **2018**, *40*, 64–69. [CrossRef] [PubMed]
81. The Joanna Briggs Institute Levels of Evidence and Grades of Recommendation Working Party Joanna Briggs Institute Levels of Evidence and Grades of Recommendation. Available online: https://jbi.global/sites/default/files/2019--05/JBI-Levels-of-evidence_2014_0.pdf (accessed on 19 September 2021).
82. Field, R.; Pourkazemi, F.; Turton, J.; Rooney, K. Dietary Interventions Are Beneficial for Patients with Chronic Pain: A Sys-tematic Review with Meta-Analysis. *Pain Med.* **2021**, *22*, 694–714. [CrossRef]
83. Elma, Ö.; Yilmaz, S.T.; Deliens, T.; Coppieters, I.; Clarys, P.; Nijs, J.; Malfliet, A. Do Nutritional Factors Interact with Chronic Musculoskeletal Pain? A Systematic Review. *J. Clin. Med.* **2020**, *9*, 702. [CrossRef]

84. Genel, F.; Kale, M.; Pavlovic, N.; Flood, V.M.; Naylor, J.M.; Adie, S. Health effects of a low-inflammatory diet in adults with arthritis: A systematic review and meta-analysis. *J. Nutr. Sci.* **2020**, *9*, 37. [CrossRef]
85. Brain, K.; Burrows, T.L.; Rollo, M.E.; Chai, L.K.; Clarke, E.D.; Hayes, C.; Hodson, F.J.; Collins, C.E. A systematic review and meta-analysis of nutrition interventions for chronic noncancer pain. *J. Hum. Nutr. Diet.* **2018**, *32*, 198–225. [CrossRef]
86. Silva, A.R.; Bernardo, A.; Costa, J.; Cardoso, A.; Santos, P.; De Mesquita, M.F.; Patto, J.V.; Moreira, P.; Silva, M.L.; Padrão, P. Dietary interventions in fibromyalgia: A systematic review. *Ann. Med.* **2019**, *51* (Suppl. 1), 2–14. [CrossRef] [PubMed]
87. Dragan, S.; Șerban, M.C.; Damian, G.; Buleu, F.; Valcovici, M.; Christodorescu, R. Dietary Patterns and Interventions to Al-leviate Chronic Pain. *Nutrients* **2020**, *12*, 2510. [CrossRef]
88. Rondanelli, M.; Faliva, M.A.; Miccono, A.; Naso, M.; Nichetti, M.; Riva, A.; Guerriero, F.; De Gregori, M.; Peroni, G.; Perna, S. Food pyramid for subjects with chronic pain: Foods and dietary constituents as anti-inflammatory and antioxidant agents. *Nutr. Res. Rev.* **2018**, *31*, 131–151. [CrossRef]
89. Brain, K.; Burrows, T.L.; Rollo, M.; Collins, C. Nutrition and Chronic Pain. Available online: https://www.iasp-pain.org/resources/fact-sheets/nutrition-and-chronic-pain/ (accessed on 19 September 2021).
90. Health effects of dietary risks in 195 countries, 1990–2017: A systematic analysis for the Global Burden of Disease Study 2017. *Lancet* **2019**, *393*, 1958–1972. [CrossRef]
91. Krebs-Smith, S.M.; Guenther, P.M.; Subar, A.F.; Kirkpatrick, S.I.; Dodd, K.W. Americans do not meet federal dietary recommendations. *J. Nutr.* **2010**, *140*, 1832–1838. [CrossRef]
92. Australian Institute of Health and Welfare (AIHW). *Diet*; AIHW: Canberra, Australia, 2020.
93. Elizabeth, L.; Machado, P.; Zinöcker, M.; Baker, P.; Lawrence, M. Ultra-Processed Foods and Health Outcomes: A Narrative Review. *Nutrients* **2020**, *12*, 1955. [CrossRef]
94. *World Health Organisation Guideline: Sugar Intake for Adults and Children*; World Health Organisation: Geneva, Switzerland, 2015.
95. Van Dam, R.M.; Hu, F.B.; Willett, W.C. Coffee, Caffeine, and Health. *N. Engl. J. Med.* **2020**, *383*, 369–378. [CrossRef]
96. Witkiewitz, K.; Vowles, K.E. Alcohol and Opioid Use, Co-Use, and Chronic Pain in the Context of the Opioid Epidemic: A Critical Review. *Alcohol. Clin. Exp. Res.* **2018**, *42*, 478–488. [CrossRef] [PubMed]
97. Roehrs, T.; Roth, T. Sleep, Sleepiness, and Alcohol Use. *Alcohol Res. Health* **2001**, *25*, 101–109. [PubMed]
98. Marouf, B.H.; Hussain, S.A.; Ali, Z.S.; Ahmmad, R.S. Resveratrol Supplementation Reduces Pain and Inflammation in Knee Osteoarthritis Patients Treated with Meloxicam: A Randomized Placebo-Controlled Study. *J Med Food* **2018**, *21*, 1253–1259. [CrossRef]
99. Commonwealth of Australia. *Australian Guidelines to Reduce Health Risks from Drinking Alcohol*; National Health and Medical Research Council: Canberra, Australia, 2020.
100. Schumacher, T.; Burrows, T.L.; Rollo, M.; Collins, C. Pain and nutrition. In *Pain in Residential Aged Care Guidelines*, 2nd ed.; Gouke, R., Ed.; Australian Pain Society: Sydney, Australia, 2018; pp. 125–134.
101. Carbone, J.W.; Pasiakos, S.M. Dietary Protein and Muscle Mass: Translating Science to Application and Health Benefit. *Nutrients* **2019**, *11*, 1136. [CrossRef]
102. National Health and Medical Research Council; New Zealand Ministry of Health. *Nutrient Reference Values for Australia and New Zealand*; National Health and Medical Research Council: Canberra, Australia, 2006.
103. Loenneke, J.P.; Loprinzi, P.D.; Murphy, C.H.; Phillips, S.M. Per meal dose and frequency of protein consumption is associated with lean mass and muscle performance. *Clin Nutr* **2016**, *35*, 1506–1511. [CrossRef] [PubMed]
104. Brady, B.; Veljanova, I.; Chipchase, L. Are multidisciplinary interventions multicultural? A topical review of the pain literature as it relates to culturally diverse patient groups. *Pain* **2016**, *157*, 321–328. [CrossRef] [PubMed]
105. Kelly, J.T.; Allman-Farinelli, M.; Chen, J.; Partridge, S.R.; Collins, C.; Rollo, M.; Haslam, R.; Diversi, T.; Campbell, K.L. Dietitians Australia position statement on telehealth. *Nutr. Diet* **2020**, *77*, 406–415. [CrossRef] [PubMed]
106. Senftleber, N.K.; Nielsen, S.M.; Andersen, J.R.; Bliddal, H.; Tarp, S.; Lauritzen, L.; Furst, D.E.; Suarez-Almazor, M.E.; Lyddiatt, A.; Christensen, R. Marine Oil Supplements for Arthritis Pain: A Systematic Review and Meta-Analysis of Randomized Trials. *Nutrients* **2017**, *9*, 42. [CrossRef] [PubMed]
107. Brady, B.; Veljanova, I.; Schabrun, S.; Chipchase, L. Integrating culturally informed approaches into physiotherapy assessment and treatment of chronic pain: A pilot randomised controlled trial. *BMJ Open* **2018**, *8*, 021999. [CrossRef] [PubMed]

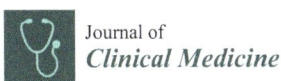

Journal of
Clinical Medicine

Review

Associates of Insomnia in People with Chronic Spinal Pain: A Systematic Review and Meta-Analysis

Thomas Bilterys [1,2,3], Carolie Siffain [1], Ina De Maeyer [1], Eveline Van Looveren [1,2,3], Olivier Mairesse [4,5], Jo Nijs [1,3,6], Mira Meeus [2,3,7], Kelly Ickmans [1,3,6,8], Barbara Cagnie [2], Dorien Goubert [2], Lieven Danneels [2], Maarten Moens [9,10] and Anneleen Malfliet [1,3,6,8,*]

[1] Pain in Motion Research Group (PAIN), Department of Physiotherapy, Human Physiology and Anatomy, Faculty of Physical Education and Physiotherapy, Vrije Universiteit Brussel, 1090 Brussels, Belgium; thomas.bilterys@vub.be (T.B.); carolie18@hotmail.com (C.S.); Ina_dm@hotmail.com (I.D.M.); Eveline.VanLooveren@UGent.be (E.V.L.); jo.nijs@vub.be (J.N.); kelly.ickmans@vub.be (K.I.)
[2] Department of Rehabilitation Sciences and Physiotherapy, Faculty of Medicine & Health Sciences, Ghent University, 9000 Ghent, Belgium; Mira.Meeus@UGent.be (M.M.); barbara.cagnie@ugent.be (B.C.); goubertdorien@gmail.com (D.G.); lieven.danneels@ugent.be (L.D.)
[3] Pain in Motion International Research Group, 1090 Brussels, Belgium
[4] Experimental and Applied Psychology, Faculty of Psychology and Educational Sciences, Vrije Universiteit Brussel, 1050 Brussels, Belgium; olivier.mairesse@vub.be
[5] Sleep Laboratory and Unit for Chronobiology, Brugmann University Hospital, 1020 Brussels, Belgium
[6] Department of Physical Medicine and Physiotherapy, University Hospital Brussels, 1090 Brussels, Belgium
[7] Department of Rehabilitation Sciences and Physiotherapy (MOVANT), Faculty of Medicine and Health Sciences, University of Antwerp, 2610 Antwerpen, Belgium
[8] Research Foundation Flanders (FWO), 1000 Brussels, Belgium
[9] Department of Neurosurgery and Radiology, University Hospital Brussels, 1090 Brussels, Belgium; maarten.TA.moens@vub.be
[10] Center for Neuroscience, Vrije Universiteit Brussel, 1090 Brussels, Belgium
* Correspondence: anneleen.malfliet@vub.be

Citation: Bilterys, T.; Siffain, C.; De Maeyer, I.; Van Looveren, E.; Mairesse, O.; Nijs, J.; Meeus, M.; Ickmans, K.; Cagnie, B.; Goubert, D.; et al. Associates of Insomnia in People with Chronic Spinal Pain: A Systematic Review and Meta-Analysis. *J. Clin. Med.* **2021**, *10*, 3175. https://doi.org/10.3390/jcm10143175

Academic Editor: Markus W. Hollmann

Received: 18 June 2021
Accepted: 14 July 2021
Published: 19 July 2021

Publisher's Note: MDPI stays neutral with regard to jurisdictional claims in published maps and institutional affiliations.

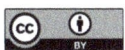

Copyright: © 2021 by the authors. Licensee MDPI, Basel, Switzerland. This article is an open access article distributed under the terms and conditions of the Creative Commons Attribution (CC BY) license (https://creativecommons.org/licenses/by/4.0/).

Abstract: Insomnia is a major problem in the chronic spinal pain (CSP) population and has a negative impact on health and well-being. While insomnia is commonly reported, underlying mechanisms explaining the relation between sleep and pain are still not fully understood. Additionally, no reviews regarding the prevention of insomnia and/or associated factors in people with CSP are currently available. To gain a better understanding of the occurrence of insomnia and associated factors in this population, we conducted a systematic review of the literature exploring associates for insomnia in people with CSP in PubMed, Web of Science and Embase. Three independent reviewers extracted the data and performed the quality assessment. A meta-analysis was conducted for every potential associate presented in at least two studies. A total of 13 studies were found eligible, which together identified 25 different potential associates of insomnia in 24,817 people with CSP. Twelve studies had a cross-sectional design. Moderate-quality evidence showed a significantly higher rate for insomnia when one of the following factors was present: high pain intensity, anxiety and depression. Low-quality evidence showed increased odds for insomnia when one of the following factors was present: female sex, performing no professional activities and physical/musculoskeletal comorbidities. Higher healthcare use was also significantly related to the presence of insomnia. One study showed a strong association between high levels of pain catastrophizing and insomnia in people with chronic neck pain. Last, reduced odds for insomnia were found in physically active people with chronic low back pain compared to inactive people with chronic low back pain. This review provides an overview of the available literature regarding potential associates of insomnia in people with CSP. Several significant associates of insomnia were identified. These findings can be helpful to gain a better understanding of the characteristics and potential origin of insomnia in people witch CSP, to identify people with CSP who are (less) likely to have insomnia and to determine directions of future research in this area.

Keywords: back pain; neck pain; associates; socio-demographic factors; psychosocial factors; lifestyle factors; sleep–wake disorders; systematic review

1. Introduction

Chronic spinal pain (CSP) is a highly prevalent and debilitating condition associated with poor quality of life and high socioeconomic impact [1–5]. Furthermore, CSP can coexist with many comorbidities (like other chronic diseases), which generally leads to larger negative effects on physical and mental functioning, a reduced treatment response, higher levels of disability and higher costs compared to CSP alone [6–8].

Insomnia, defined as the presence of a long sleep latency, frequent nocturnal awakenings, prolonged periods of wakefulness during the sleep period or early awakenings, is common in people with CSP [9–12]. Up to 59% report insomnia, making it one of the most reported comorbidities in CSP [9–12]. Moreover, people with chronic low back pain are 18 times more likely to experience insomnia compared to people without chronic low back pain [11]. If left untreated, insomnia negatively impacts mood, physical symptoms, pain sensitivity, fatigue and health-related quality of life [13,14]. Additionally, insomnia is related to less productivity and increased work absenteeism [15]. Considering all of the above, co-occurring CSP and insomnia present a serious public health challenge which is currently rarely addressed in treatment [11].

Currently, underlying mechanisms explaining the relation between sleep and pain are still not fully understood [16]. A recent review provided an overview of the available evidence regarding investigated putative mediating variables on the pathway between sleep variables and pain intensity [17]. Based on the available body of research, they speculated that psychological and physiological components of emotional experience and attentional processes are likely mediators. However, this review focusses on the factors influencing the link between sleep and pain (i.e., mediators) in the general pain population. None of the included studies investigated mediators or associated factors specifically in people with CSP. Additionally, the review did not include studies which investigated potential associated factors if no formal test of mediation or a test of the significance of mediated effects was conducted.

A clear overview of factors (including socio-demographic, psycho-social and lifestyle factors) associated with insomnia in people with CSP could lead to a better understanding, a change in decision making and further improvement of preventive and treatment strategies (i.e., targeting possible identified factors). Yet, since such an overview is currently unavailable, the purpose of this systematic review and meta-analysis is to provide an overview of associates of insomnia in people with CSP. The primary aim of this review is to determine which factors are associated with insomnia in people with CSP. The secondary aim is to determine the strength of association for these factors.

2. Methods

This systematic review was conducted in accordance with the PRISMA guidelines and initially registered in the PROSPERO database (registry number CRD42018116710) [18]. A search for eligible studies was performed in three electronic databases, i.e., PubMed, Web of Science and Embase. The last search was conducted on 12 September 2019.

2.1. Identification and Selection of Studies
2.1.1. Eligibility Criteria

Studies were eligible when meeting the following criteria: (1) including adults (>18 years) suffering from non-specific CSP (i.e., low back pain or neck pain not attributable to a specific pathology) for at least 3 months, (2) reporting insomnia-related outcomes [19,20], such as variables described in terms of sleep disturbances, sleep difficulties, sleep problems, restless sleep, disturbed sleep and sleep continuity;,(3) presenting data to identify associated factors with insomnia (i.e., odds ratios (ORs) or sufficient data to calculate the ORs) and (4) being written in English, French or Dutch.

The next criteria were applied for exclusion of studies: (1) abstracts, case reports, reviews, meta-analysis, letters and editorials, and (2) studies including participants diagnosed with specific medical conditions that can explain CSP (e.g., neck or back surgery in the past three years, osteoporotic vertebral fractures or rheumatologic diseases), diagnosed with chronic widespread pain (fibromyalgia or chronic fatigue syndrome), being shift workers, suffering from severe underlying sleep-related comorbidities or being pregnant or were pregnant in the preceding year.

2.1.2. Information Sources

A systematic search was conducted in PubMed, Web of Science and Embase. The search in PubMed was performed using MeSH terms and free keywords based on the PECO-acronym, in which the "population" (P) was represented as people with CSP, the "exposure" (E) as potential associates and the "outcome" (O) as insomnia. Since studies without comparison groups were eligible, no search terms for "comparison group" (C) were used in the final search. Using free keywords, a comparable search was performed in Web of Science and Embase. No search filters were used. An overview of the applied search terms can be found in Table S1. Full search strategies of all databases are presented in Supplementary file S1. Additionally, reference lists of the relevant articles were hand-searched for additional eligible papers.

2.1.3. Study Selection

After removing duplicates, three reviewers (C.S., I.D. and T.B.) independently screened all retrieved records to determine the eligibility. First, all records were screened by title and abstract in a blinded standardized manner using Rayyan software [21]. Studies that presented relevant data in accordance with the review question were included, even if the main research question was not relevant for this review. All discrepancies were resolved by consensus among the three researchers. When no agreement could be reached through discussion, a fourth author (A.M.) made the final decision. Reasons for exclusion were registered in all phases.

2.2. Data Collection Process

Three authors (C.S., I.D. and T.B) extracted the relevant data independently using a self-created data extraction form containing the following items: (1) author, (2) year of publication, (3) study design, (4) sample size, (5) nature of the sample, (6) age (years ± standard deviation), (7) assessment methods of insomnia, (8) prevalence rate of insomnia and (9) investigated or determinable potential associates. Data of factors/variables investigated in each study were extracted and presented in the tables, figures and meta-analyses of this review if ORs could be determined. Variables presented in the included studies without sufficient data to determine ORs were not included. One reviewer (T.B.) checked the extracted data and resolved any disagreement.

2.3. Risk of Bias Assessment of Individual Studies

Three reviewers (C.S., I.D. and T.B.) evaluated the methodological quality and risk of bias by using an adapted form of the Newcastle-Ottawa Scale (NOS), independently [22,23]. The NOS assesses the quality of studies in three main areas, i.e., selection, comparability and outcome or exposure, and leads to a maximum total score of 10. The quality of individual studies was rated as high, moderate and low based on designated thresholds [24]. Studies with a score of ≥ 7 out of 10 were considered high quality, studies with at least a score of 5 were rated as moderate quality and a score lower than 5 was considered low quality. Strict scoring criteria were determined a priori based on findings in the literature [25–29]. The response-rate was considered "satisfactory" when it reached $\geq 80\%$ [25]. The sample size was considered "justified and satisfactory" if the number of needed participants was reached based on a sample size calculation, or when the study is a national or epidemiological study. For the section "comparability", two points were possibly awarded: one for controlling for age or sex, and one for controlling for any other factor. Since age and sex differences in sleep are common [26–29], both factors were considered to be the most important factors to be controlled for. When an item was not described, a score of zero was given for that particular item. Overall risk of bias was considered "high" if the total score was 4 or lower. A score of at least 7 was considered as a "low" risk of bias. Uncertainties were solved by consensus among the three reviewers. The used NOS-version with details about the scoring criteria is provided in Supplementary file S2.

2.4. Summary Measures

The primary outcome measures were ORs with 95% confidence intervals (CIs). For every meta-analysis, a pooled OR (OR_p) with 95% CI and *p*-value is presented. The statistical significance level (alpha) was set at 0.05.

2.5. Methods of Analysis

The number of subjects within the investigated subgroups (exposed subgroup and unexposed subgroup to the potential associated factor) with and without insomnia were collected to calculate ORs for each factor using Revman software (Review manager 5.3). Subsequently, random effects meta-analyses were performed for all the factors which were presented in at least two of the included studies [30]. The heterogeneity (I^2) was assessed by the method proposed by Higgins et al. [30]. To determine the significance of the heterogeneity amongst studies, a Chi-squared (X^2) test was conducted with an alpha set at 0.05 [31,32]. When a high heterogeneity ($I^2 > 50\%$) between studies was present [33], subgroup analyses (based on NOS-score, study design, pain location and used measurement tools) were performed to possibly clarify the underlying systematic differences and reduce the substantial heterogeneity.

2.6. Quality of Evidence

A modified version of the Grading of Recommendations Assessment, Development and Evaluation (GRADE) criteria was used to assess the quality of evidence for all analyses [34]. The criteria were modified to make them more suitable and relevant. The quality of evidence was downgraded from high by one level based on: phase of investigation (cross-sectional), study limitations (>25% of participants from studies with high risk of bias), inconsistency of results ($I^2 > 50\%$), imprecision (sample size < 400 participants), indirectness (e.g., inclusion of different populations and interventions) and publication bias (funnel plot and the Egger test if ≥ 10 studies [35]). Evidence was upgraded when there was at least a moderate effect size (OR > 2.5), or evidence of an exposure-response gradient.

3. Results

3.1. Study Selection

The systematic search resulted in a total of 953 articles on PubMed, 1790 articles on Web of Science and 1647 articles on Embase. A total of 13 articles were included after the removal of duplicates, title and abstract screening and full-text eligibility assessment. No additional records were identified through hand-searching. The selection process is illustrated in Figure 1. An overview of the excluded articles assessed at full text and the reason for exclusion is presented in Table S2.

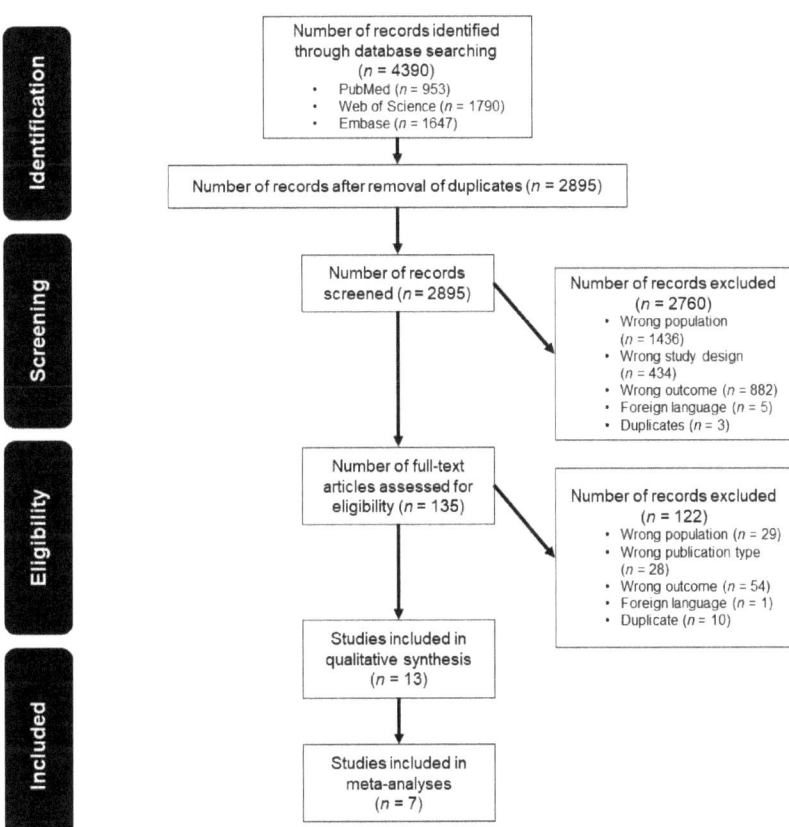

Figure 1. Flow diagram illustrating the study selection process.

3.2. Study Characteristics

Twelve out of thirteen included studies were cross-sectional studies [11,12,36–45]. One included study was a cohort study [46]. A total of 24,817 participants were included across all studies, with sample sizes ranging from 70 to 10,849 participants [11,41]. The prevalence rate of insomnia across the studies ranged from 11% to 92% [12,38]. Nine studies used a validated questionnaire to retrieve information regarding the presence of insomnia [11,12,36,39,40,42,44–46]. Three other studies used a self-designed questionnaire [38,41,43] and one study made use of a health database [37]. A detailed overview of the characteristics of the included studies can be found in Table 1.

Table 1. Characteristics of the included studies.

Author	Design	Sample Size (N)	Nature of the Sample	Age (Range and/or Years ± SD)	Pain Duration	Sleep Outcome	Prevalence Rates of Insomnia	Investigated Factors
Aili et al. 2015	C	1408	Care seeking CLBP and CNP, community sample	Range: 20–59 y	≥6 mo	Karolinska Sleep Questionnaire	NM	Sex, age, other physical illness, professional activity
Blay et al. 2007	CS	2997	CLBP, population-based sample	Range: 60–81 y	≥6 mo	Short Psychiatric Evaluation Schedule	42.5% sleep disturbance	Professional activity, income, medical consultation, hospitalizations, self-rated health, physical activity
Dimarco et al. 2018	CS	709	CLBP, sample in clinical setting	34.9 ± 11.9 y	Opioid naïve: 26.04 ± 50.21 mo Prior opioid users: 22.64 ± 46.26 mo	Data extracted from Military Health System Data Repository	19% insomnia	Prior opioid use
Ho et al. 2019	CS	6559	CLBP, community sample	52.2 ± 15.2 y Range: 19.1–95.9 y	≥3 mo	Modified insomnia criteria from DSM-5	10.9% insomnia	High CRP level
Kim et al. 2015	CS	218	CNP, sample in clinical setting	52.8 ± 14.3 y Range: 20–83 y	≥3 mo	Insomnia Severity Index	53.7% mild to severe insomnia	Sex, age, BMI, pain duration, pain score, spine surgery history, shoulder or arm pain, neck mobility problems, myofascial pain components, anxiety, depression, headache, comorbid musculoskeletal conditions
Majid et al. 2017	CS	358	CLBP, sample in clinical setting	NM	≥3 mo	Insomnia Severity Index	58.7% sleep disturbance	Sex
Marin et al. 2006	CS	268	CLBP, sample in clinical setting	47 y ± NM Range: 18–89 y	≥6 mo	Pittsburgh Sleep Quality Index	92% sleep disturbances	Sleep medication intake after pain
Mork et al. 2013	CS	10,849	CLBP and CNP, community sample	43.0 ± 13.9 y	≥3 mo	Self-Reported Questionnaire	NM	Sex, physical activity, BMI
Park et al. 2016	CS	256	CNP, sample in clinical setting	52.8 ± 14.7 y Range: 20–84 y	≥3 mo	Insomnia Severity Index	24.22% clinical insomnia	Pain catastrophizing
Ris et al. 2017	CS	200	CNP, sample in clinical setting	Traumatic: 43.5 ± 11.4 y Non-traumatic: 47.5 ± 11.3 y	≥6 mo	Self-reported Disturbed nights/week	19.5% sleep disturbances	Traumatic Onset
Shmagel et al. 2016	CS	700	CLBP, community sample	Range: 20–69 y	≥3 mo	NAHANS Questionnaires	52.7% sleep disturbances	Healthcare Use
Tang et al. 2007	CS	70	CLBP, sample in clinical setting	46 ± 10.9 y Range: 18–65 y	≥6 mo	Insomnia Severity Index	53% with moderate or severe insomnia	Sex, race
Wang et al. 2016	CS	225	CLBP	40.7 ± 11.4 y	≥3 mo	Insomnia Severity Index	25.8% clinical insomnia	Depression, anxiety, severity of CLBP

Abbreviations: BMI, body mass index; C, cohort; CLBP, chronic low back pain; CNP, chronic neck pain; CRP, C-reactive protein; CS, cross-sectional; DSM-5, the Diagnostic and Statistical Manual of Mental Disorders 5th Edition; mo, month; NHANES, National Health and Nutrition Examination Survey; NM, not mentioned; y, year.

3.3. Risk of Bias within Studies

The overall methodological quality of the included studies is moderate to high, with scores ranging from 5 to 8 out of 10. Five out of thirteen studies were rated high quality, implying a "low" risk of bias. The other seven studies were rated as moderate quality, implying a "moderate" risk of bias. The main weakness was the relatively low response rate and the lack of comparison between the non-respondents and respondents (11 studies). The second most common source of bias was the lack of control for confounders (6 studies). The results of the quality assessment are presented in Table 2.

Table 2. Quality assessment by the Adapted Newcastle–Ottawa scale.

Studies	Selection				Comparability	Outcome			Total
	Representativeness of the Sample (Maximum 1 star)	Sample Size (Maximum 1 Star)	Non-Respondents (Maximum 1 Star)	Ascertainment of the Exposure (Factor) (Maximum 2 Stars)	Confounding Factors (Maximum 2 Stars)	Assessment of the Outcome (Maximum 2 Stars)	Statistical Test (Maximum 1 Star)		Mean = 6.23 Median = 6
Aili et al. 2015	☆	☆		☆☆	☆☆	☆	☆		8
Blay et al. 2007	☆	☆	☆	☆		☆	☆		6
Dimarco et al. 2019	☆			☆	☆☆	☆☆	☆		7
Ho et al. 2019	☆	☆		☆☆	☆☆	☆	☆		8
Kim et al. 2015	☆			☆☆		☆	☆		5
Majid et al. 2017	☆	☆		☆☆		☆			5
Marin et al. 2006	☆	☆		☆		☆	☆		5
Mork et al. 2014	☆	☆		☆	☆	☆	☆		6
Park et al. 2016	☆	☆		☆☆		☆	☆		6
Ris et al. 2017	☆	☆		☆		☆	☆		5
Shmagel et al. 2016	☆	☆		☆	☆☆	☆	☆		7
Tang et al. 2007	☆			☆☆	☆	☆	☆		6
Wang et al. 2016	☆			☆☆	☆☆	☆	☆		7

The quality of the included studies is scored in three main areas, i.e., selection, comparability and outcome or exposure. Every star represents one point, which leads to a maximum total score of 10. The quality of individual studies were rated as high, moderate and low based on designated thresholds [24]. Studies with a score of ≥7 out of 10 were considered high quality. Studies with at least a score of 5 were rated as moderate quality studies. A score lower than 5 was considered low quality. Overall risk of bias was considered "high" if the total score was 4 or lower. A score of at least 7 was consider as "low" risk of bias.

3.4. Synthesis of Results

In total, 25 different potential associates across 13 studies were identified. An overview of all included studies, including the identified factors and related ORs, is presented in Table 3. A meta-analysis was conducted for all the following factors which were presented in at least two of the included studies: sex (being female) [11,39–41,46], age (older age) [39,46], body mass index (BMI) [39,41], physical activity [36,41], professional activity [36,46], comorbidities [39,46], high pain intensity [39,45], depression [39,45] and anxiety [39,45]. No significant heterogeneity was found between studies analyzed for sex ($I^2 = 17\%$, $p = 0.30$), age ($I^2 = 0\%$, $p = 0.99$), BMI ($I^2 = 0\%$, $p = 0.43$), professional activity ($I^2 = 0\%$, $p = 0.78$), pain intensity ($I^2 = 0\%$, $p = 0.92$), depression ($I^2 = 0\%$, $p = 0.98$) and anxiety ($I^2 = 0\%$, $p = 0.59$). The assessment of the overall quality of the evidence for each analysis can be found in Table S3. Moderate-quality evidence was found for the factors pain intensity, anxiety and depression. Low- or very-low-quality evidence was found for the other examined factors.

3.5. Sex

Five studies reported on biological sex as a potential associated factor with insomnia ($n = 12,722$) [11,39–41,46]. The combined data indicates that female patients are more likely to have insomnia compared to male patients (OR_p 1.45, 95% CI = (1.22–1.71), $p < 0.0001$, low-quality evidence) (Figure 2A).

3.6. Age

Age was studied in 2 articles ($n = 1626$) [39,46]. No significant intergroup difference in insomnia prevalence was observed between older and younger people with CSP (OR_p 1.08, 95% CI = (0.87–1.33), $p = 0.49$, low-quality evidence) (Figure 2B).

3.7. Body Mass Index

Two studies reported on BMI ($n = 10,886$) [39,41]. No significant association was found between the presence of insomnia and a higher BMI (OR_p 1.12, 95% CI = (0.94–1.35), $p = 0.21$, low-quality evidence) (Figure 2C).

Table 3. Overview of included studies with the potential associates and related odds ratios.

Author	Factor	Number of Participants with Insomnia (n)	Number of Participants without Insomnia (n)	Number of Participants in Reference and Investigated Subgroup (n)	(Adjusted) Odds Ratio [95% CI]
Aili et al. 2015	Sex	529	879		
	- Women	380	515	895	1.80 [1.43–2.27]
	- Men	149	364	513	1.0
	Age	529	879		
	- ≥45 years	234	373	607	1.08 [0.87–1.34]
	- <45 years	295	506	801	1.0
	Other physical illness	529	879		
	- Yes	120	133	253	1.65 [1.25–2.17]
	- No	409	746	1155	1.0
	Professional activity	529	879		
	- Not working	76	81	157	1.65 [1.18–2.31]
	- Working	453	798	1251	1.0
Blay et al. 2007	Professional activity	1274	1723		
	- Yes	115	231	346	1.0
	- No	1159	1492	2651	1.56 [1.23–1.98]
	Income	1274	1723		
	- High	312	631	943	0.56 [0.48–0.66]
	- Low	962	1092	2054	1.0
	Medical Consultation	1274	1723		
	- Yes	1041	1299	2340	1.46 [1.22–1.74]
	- No	233	424	657	1.0
	Hospitalizations	1274	1723		
	- >1	359	323	682	1.70 [1.43–2.02]
	- ≤1	915	1400	2315	1.0
	Self-rated health	1274	1723		
	- Impaired	1117	1170	2287	3.36 [2.77–4.09]
	- Not impaired	157	553	710	1.0
	Physical activity	1274	1723		
	- Yes	410	665	1075	0.75 [0.65–0.88]
	- No	864	1058	1922	1.0
Dimarco et al. 2018	Opioid user	112	592		
	- Yes	93	391	484	2.52 [1.49–4.24]
	- No	19	201	220	1.0
Ho et al. 2019	CRP Level	719	5840		
	- Elevated or very high	205	1390	1595	1.27 [1.07–1.52]
	- Very high	37	256	296	1.25 [0.88–1.79]
	- Elevated	168	1134	1302	1.28 [1.06–1.54]
	- Normal	514	4450	4964	1.0

Table 3. Cont.

Author	Factor	Number of Participants with Insomnia (n)	Number of Participants without Insomnia (n)	Number of Participants in Reference and Investigated Subgroup (n)	(Adjusted) Odds Ratio [95% CI]
Kim et al. 2015	Sex	50	168		
	- Women	30	94	124	1.18 [0.62–2.25]
	- Men	20	74	94	1.0
	Age	50	168		
	- ≥65 years	12	38	50	1.08 [0.51–2.27]
	- <65 years	38	130	168	1.0
	BMI	50	168		
	- ≥25 kg/m^2	17	44	61	1.45 [0.74–2.86]
	- <25 kg/m^2	33	124	157	1.0
	Pain duration	50	168		
	- ≥1 year	28	78	106	1.47 [0.78–2.77]
	- <1 year	22	90	112	1.0
	Pain score	50	168		
	- ≥7 NRS	31	60	91	2.94 [1.53–5.64]; Adj. 2.46 [1.12–5.40]
	- <7 NRS	19	108	127	1.0
	History of spine surgery	50	168		
	- Yes	7	15	22	1.74 [0.50–6.04]
	- No	43	153	196	1.0
	Shoulder or arm pain	50	168		
	- Yes	31	99	130	1.14 [0.60–2.18]
	- No	19	69	88	1.0
	Neck mobility problems	50	168		
	- Yes	13	43	56	1.02 [0.50–2.10]
	- No	37	125	162	1.0
	Comorbid musculoskeletal pain conditions	50	168		
	- Yes	24	35	59	3.51 [1.80–6.84]; Adj. 2.82 [1.22–6.54]
	- No	26	133	159	1.0
	Comorbid neuropathic pain component	50	168		
	- Yes	16	24	40	2.824 [1.354–5.887]
	- No	34	144	178	1.0
	Myofascial pain components	50	168		
	- Yes	20	50	70	1.57 [0.82–3.03]
	- No	30	118	148	1.0

Table 3. Cont.

Author	Factor	Number of Participants with Insomnia (n)	Number of Participants without Insomnia (n)	Number of Participants in Reference and Investigated Subgroup (n)	(Adjusted) Odds Ratio [95% CI]
	Anxiety	50	168		
	- HADS-A $\geq$ 8	23	32	55	3.62 [1.84–7.12]; Adj. 1.42 [0.58–3.48]
	- HADS-A < 8	27	136	163	1.0
	Depression	50	168		
	- HADS-D $\geq$ 8	29	33	62	5.65 [2.87–11.13]; Adj. 3.69 [1.57–8.67]
	- HADS-D < 8	21	135	156	1.0
	Headache	50	168		
	- Yes	13	35	48	1.34 [0.64–2.78]
	- No	37	133	170	1.0
Majid et al. 2017	Sex	210	148		
	- Women	131	82	213	1.33 [0.87–2.05]
	- Men	79	66	145	1.0
Marin et al. 2006	Sleep medication intake after pain	230	18		
	- Yes	130	4	134	4.55 [1.45–14.25]
	- No	100	14	114	1.0
Mork et al. 2013	Sex				
	Low back pain	181	4203		
	- Women	119	2260	2379	1.50 [1.09–2.05]
	- Men	62	1762	1824	1.0
	Neck pain	265	6200		
	- Women	161	3412	3573	1.26 [0.98–1.63]
	- Men	104	2788	2892	1.0
	Activity Level: leisure time physical exercise				
	Low back pain	135	2955		
	- Inactive	80	1717	1797	1.0
	- Active	55	1238	1293	0.95 [0.67–1.35]
	Neck pain	195	4514		
	- Inactive	110	2659	2769	1.0
	- Active	85	1855	1940	1.11 [0.83–1.48]
	BMI				
	Low back pain	181	4022		
	- $\geq$25 kg/cm^3	86	1693	1779	1.25 [0.92–1.68]
	- <25 kg/cm^3	95	2329	2424	1.0
	Neck pain	265	6200		
	- $\geq$25 kg/cm^3	113	2627	2740	1.01 [0.79–1.30]
	- <25 kg/cm^3	152	3573	3725	1.0

Table 3. Cont.

Author	Factor	Number of Participants with Insomnia (n)	Number of Participants without Insomnia (n)	Number of Participants in Reference and Investigated Subgroup (n)	(Adjusted) Odds Ratio [95% CI]
Park et al. 2016	Pain catastrophizing	62	194		
	- High	42	44	86	7.16 [3.81–13.43]
	- Low	20	150	170	1.0
Ris et al. 2017	Traumatic onset	39	161		
	- Yes	19	101	120	0.56 [0.28–1.14]
	- No	20	60	80	1.0
Shmagel et al. 2016	Healthcare use	172	528		
	- ≥10 healthcare visits/year	124	246	370	2.96 [2.03–4.31]
	- <10 visits/year	48	282	330	1.0
Tang et al. 2007	Sex	37	33		
	- Women	25	24	49	0.78 [0.28–2.19]
	- Men	12	9	21	1.0
	Race	37	33		
	- Caucasian	26	20	46	1.54 [0.57–4.14]
	- Non-Caucasian	11	13	24	1.0
Wang et al. 2016	Depression (Diagnosis of major depressive episode)	58	167		
	- Yes	13	8	21	5.74 [2.24–14.71]
	- No	45	159	204	1.0
	Anxiety (Diagnosis of an anxiety disorder)	58	167		
	- Yes	22	30	52	2.79 [1.44–5.41]
	- No	36	137	173	1.0
	Pain score	58	167		
	- VAS ≥ 7	32	51	83	2.80 [1.52–5.17]
	- VAS < 7	26	116	142	1.0

Abbreviations: Adj., adjusted; BMI, body mass index; CI, confidence interval; HADS, Health Anxiety and Depression Scale; LBP, low back pain; PE, patients exposed; VAS, Visual Analogue Scale.

3.8. Physical Activity

Physical activity was studied in two studies (n = 10,796) [36,41]. No significant association was found between physical activity and the presence of insomnia in people with CSP (OR$_p$ 0.90, 95% CI = (0.70–1.17), p = 0.43, very-low-quality evidence). A significant heterogeneity was observed (I^2 = 66%, p = 0.43). Since Mork et al. examined chronic neck and back pain patients and reported both separately, a subgroup analysis including only the data regarding people with low back pain was performed [41]. This subgroup analysis resulted in an improvement of the heterogeneity (I^2 = 30%, p = 0.23). Consequently, OR$_p$ decreased to 0.80 (95% CI = (0.66–0.98), p = 0.03, low-quality evidence), indicating that insomnia is less common in physically active, chronic low back pain patients (Figure 2D).

3.9. Professional Activity

Two studies reported on professional activity (n = 4405) [36,46]. The pooled data showed that people with CSP without any professional activity are more likely to have insomnia compared to people with CSP who perform a job (OR$_p$ 1.59, 95% CI = (1.31–1.93), p < 0.001, low-quality evidence) (Figure 2E).

3.10. Comorbidities

Physical or musculoskeletal comorbidities were studied in two studies (n = 1626) [39,46]. A significant intergroup difference (OR$_p$ 2.25, 95% CI = (1.09–4.68), p = 0.03, very-low-quality evidence) with a significant heterogeneity (I^2 = 76%, p = 0.04) was observed. Despite high heterogeneity, no subgroup analyses could be performed as comorbidities were only discussed in two articles. Furthermore, a subgroup analysis seems unnecessary due to the results of both studies being in the same direction (Figure 2F).

3.11. Pain Intensity

Pain intensity was considered as a putatively associated factor with insomnia in two studies (n = 443) [39,45]. The meta-analysis revealed that people with CSP with high pain intensity levels (VAS/NRS $\geq$ 7) are more likely to have insomnia compared to those with lower pain intensity levels (OR$_p$ 2.86, 95% CI = (1.83–4.48), p < 0.001, moderate-quality evidence) (Figure 2G).

3.12. Depression

Two studies reported on depression as a factor (n = 443) [39,45]. The odds for insomnia were 5.68 times higher in people with CSP with depression compared to those without depression (OR$_p$ 5.68, 95% CI = (3.28–9.85), p < 0.001, moderate-quality evidence) (Figure 2H).

3.13. Anxiety

Two studies discussed anxiety as a factor (n = 443) [39,45]. The pooled data demonstrated that people with CSP with anxiety are more likely to have insomnia compared to people with CSP without anxiety (OR$_p$ 3.17, 95% CI = (1.98–5.09), p < 0.001, moderate-quality evidence) (Figure 2I).

3.14. Other

Each of the following factors were only discussed in one included article: income [36], medical consultation [36], hospitalization [36], self-rated health [36], prior opioid use [37], high C-reactive protein blood levels [38], pain duration [39], spine surgery history [39], shoulder/arm pain [39], neck mobility problems [39], myofascial pain [39], headache [39], use of sleep medication [14], pain catastrophizing [42], traumatic onset [43], healthcare use [44] and race [13]. A detailed overview of all included studies with the identified factors and their related ORs is presented in Table 3.

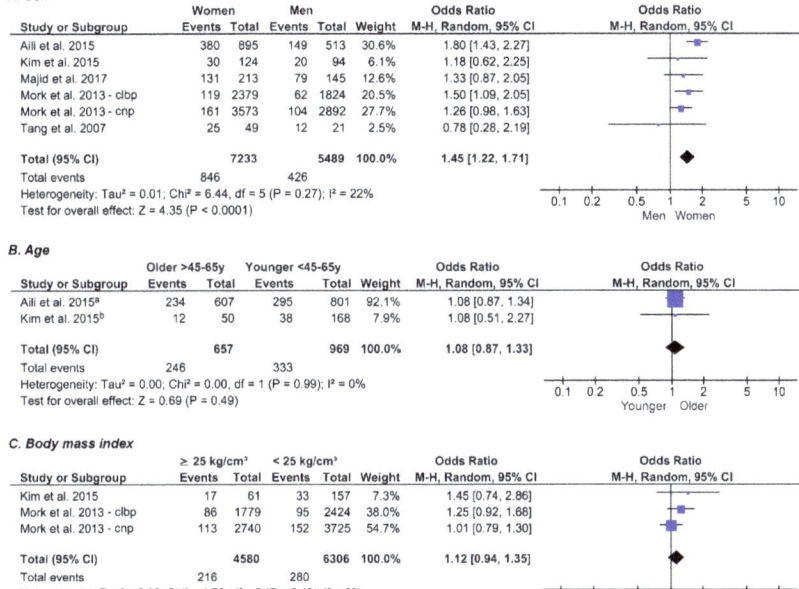

Figure 2. Cont.

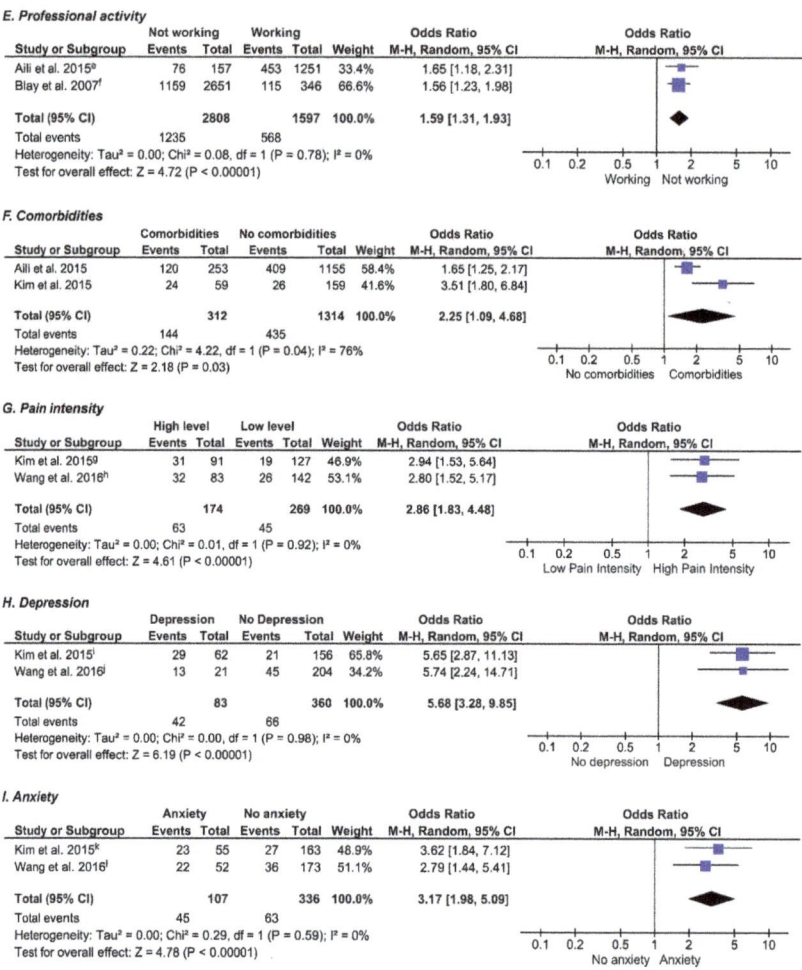

Figure 2. Forest plots showing odds ratios of several potential associated factors with insomnia in people with chronic spinal pain. A meta-analysis is conducted for the factors sex (n = 12,722), age (n = 1626), body mass index (n = 10,886), physical activity (n = 10,796), professional activity (n = 4405), comorbidities (n = 1626), pain intensity (n = 443), depression (n = 443) and anxiety (n = 443). Every blue box represents the observed odds ratio of the corresponding study. The size of every blue box is proportional to the weight of the study in the meta-analysis. The confidence intervals are represented by the horizontal lines through the blue boxes. The pooled odds ratio is represented by a black diamond, with the lateral tips of the diamond representing the associated confidence interval. Abbreviations: CNP, chronic neck pain; CLBP, chronic low back pain. [a] Aili et al. defined younger participants as people < 45 years [46]. [b] Kim et al. defined younger participants as people < 65 years [39]. [c] Blay et al. dichotomized physical activity in Yes/No but did not provide any detail about the level of physical activity used as a cut-off [36]. [d] Mork et al. defined physically active people as people performing more than one (accumulated) hour of exercise per week [41]. [e] Aili et al. defined performing no professional activity as "Unemployed for the last year/not working" [46]. [f] Blay at al. dichotomized professional activity as active/non-active but did not provide any further details [36]. [g] Kim et al. defined a high pain score as NRS ≥ 7 [39]. [h] Wang et al. defined a high pain score as VAS ≥ 7 [45]. [i] Kim et al. defined depression as a score of at least 8 on the HADS-D [39]. [j] Participants in the study of Wang et al. were screened by a board-certified psychiatrist for the presence of a current major depressive episode [45]. [k] Kim et al. defined depression as a score of at least 8 on the HADS-A [39]. [l] Participants in the study of Wang et al. were screened by a board-certified psychiatrist for the presence of any anxiety disorders [45].

4. Discussion

The purpose of this systematic review and meta-analysis was to identify factors associated with the presence and development of insomnia in people with nonspecific CSP. A total of 13 studies were included, which together described 25 different potential associates of insomnia [11,12,36–46]. It was possible to carry out a meta-analysis for nine factors. Sex (being female), professional activity (not performing any professional activities), the presence of comorbidities, depression, anxiety and high pain intensity were significantly associated with elevated odds for insomnia. A significant heterogeneity was found for the factors of physical activity and comorbidities. A subgroup analysis was only possible for the factor physical activity, which became significant for people with chronic low back pain. Age and BMI could not be identified as associates.

Included studies looked into the possibility of the factors sex and age as associates of insomnia in people with CSP. The pooled data regarding sex as an associate showed that the odds for insomnia were 1.45 times higher for females compared to males (low-quality evidence). Similar results are found in the general population, with woman being almost 1.5 times more likely to develop insomnia compared to men [28]. It is suggested that this higher rate of insomnia in females might be explained by a higher prevalence of anxiety and depression, potentially indirectly induced by genetic factors [28]. However, underlying reasons for these sex differences still remain unclear since insomnia could not be solely explained by the higher prevalence of anxiety and depression alone. Different to the CSP population, age does appear to be associated with insomnia in the general population, with older adults showing a higher prevalence of insomnia [28,47]. As people get older, normal changes occur in our sleep architecture (e.g., more light sleep and fragmentation) [48]. However, these changes can contribute to the development of insomnia. Besides these natural changes of sleep, other comorbidities and specific sleep pathologies which can negatively influence sleep are also more common as people get older [49,50]. Furthermore, sleep difficulties in older adults seem to be more related to age-related conditions rather than to age itself [51,52]. Not finding this relation with age in people with CSP can be explained by the possible dominating influence of the characteristics of the pain condition. It is likely that pain is the predominant reason for insomnia in people with CSP, which could potentially overshadow or negate the effect of age on sleep. Another explanation might be the low number of included studies. Additional studies might increase the precision of the OR_p. However, it is likely that age has a negligible influence on the presence of insomnia in CSP since the 95% CI is relatively small and the OR_p is very close to one. Yet, as age and sex are fixed factors, that cannot be targeted in therapy, focusing on other modifiable factors (such as comorbidities, pain intensity, depression and anxiety) seems more clinically relevant.

This systematic review with meta-analysis demonstrates that people with CSP with high pain severity (NRS/VAS $\geq$ 7) are almost 3 times more likely to have insomnia (moderate-quality evidence). However, since only 2 studies were included in the meta-analysis, some caution is warranted regarding the strength of the results. Nevertheless, the results are in accordance with the findings of a recent review investigating relationships, comorbidities and treatments in chronic pain and sleep disturbances, which indicated that sleep problems in people with chronic pain are associated with greater pain severity [53]. Evidence strongly suggests a bidirectional relationship, with pain and sleep co-existing and impacting each other [54,55]. Insomnia and pain seem to share similar pathways, such as mesolimbic dopaminergic pathways and serotoninergic pathways [16,56]. Generally, pain is associated with an increased stress-response and elevated levels of arousal [57], which can negatively affect sleep [58]. Furthermore, people with chronic pain are prone to start worrying about their health, which can further aggravate poor sleep [11,59–61]. Additionally, even a limited amount of sleep loss appears to have a de-activating effect on several analgesic systems, while activating hyperalgesic systems [16]. Furthermore, impaired sleep can result in low-grade inflammatory responses [62,63], which is found to potentially affect brain function [64] and increase pain sensitivity [63,65,66]. This bidirectional relationship creates a vicious cycle which can perpetuate and amplify sleep problems and pain (i.e., increasing pain disrupting the sleep and sleep disturbances exacerbating the pain). Taking all findings into account, the results of our analysis regarding pain intensity seems to be in line with the current research findings of the general chronic pain population, indicating that pain intensity has a clear impact on sleep. However, underlying mechanisms explaining the relation between sleep and pain are still not fully understood [16]. Addressing the vicious pain–sleep cycle in the evaluation and treatment of CSP seems to be essential to deliver the best possible care.

Similar to the link with pain intensity, the presence of depression and/or anxiety in CSP is linked to the prevalence of insomnia according to our results (moderate-quality evidence). However, since only two studies were included in the meta-analysis of both anxiety and depression, some caution is warranted regarding the strength of the results. Nevertheless, the strong associations of both factors do not come as a surprise since depression and anxiety are considered as the most prevalent comorbidities of both pain [67,68] and insomnia [69]. Furthermore, people with co-occurring pain and sleep problems appear to be more likely to present comorbid depression, catastrophizing, anxiety and suicidal ideation [53]. Moreover, previous research has demonstrated complex interactions between pain, sleep and depression, without a clear causal ordering [53,54]. Similarly, anxiety is found to be closely related with pain and insomnia, but the direction and underlying mechanisms of these relations are still unclear [68,70]. Given their relationship with pain and insomnia, addressing both depression and anxiety symptoms as an integral part of the evaluation and treatment of people with CSP and comorbid insomnia seems warranted.

Two studies looked at physical activity, which was found to be a non-significant associate after pooling (very-low-quality evidence). However, one could expect that inactivity would be an associate since there is sufficient evidence that physical activity has small but still positive effects on sleep in the general population [71]. Furthermore, physical activity has been identified as a strong "Zeitgeber" (i.e., a cue that helps to synchronize our biological rhythm to a 24 h cycle) [72]. Moreover, evidence shows that physical activity is beneficial, and therefore recommended, in people with CSP [73–76]. Importantly, our analysis showed that statistical heterogeneity was present, indicating a discrepancy between the data of both studies. After applying a subgroup analysis based on pain location, the heterogeneity improved, and physical activity became a small but significant protective factor for insomnia in people with chronic low back pain (low-quality evidence). This implies that physically active back pain patients are less likely to have insomnia.

A notable significant OR of 7.16 was found for pain catastrophizing, indicating that people with CSP with high levels of catastrophizing are much more likely to have insomnia [42]. However, pain catastrophizing was only investigated by one study, which only included people with chronic neck pain [42]. Therefore, the strength of the relation between insomnia and pain catastrophizing is rather indicative. It might be that studies that investigated anxiety and depression as factors considered catastrophizing as a part of the anxiety/depression complex since they share common elements and are closely related [77]. While there is some overlap with other cognitive and emotional processes, it is clear that catastrophizing is a unique construct [77]. Nevertheless, pain catastrophizing can be considered a clinically important psychological factor on its own given the high OR and its central role in the development of chronic disabling pain [42,78,79]. Therefore, targeting and reducing pain catastrophizing should be considered in CSP management.

Lastly, several studies investigating different aspects of healthcare use (i.e., medical consultations, number of hospitalizations, number of healthcare visits/year and opioid use) were included in this review [36,37,44]. Since each reported healthcare-related factor embodied a specific element of healthcare use and different thresholds for dichotomizations were used, the decision was made to not pool the data. However, all factors related to healthcare use show significantly higher odds (ranging from 1.45 to 2.96), indicating that people with CSP and comorbid insomnia are making significantly more use of the healthcare system compared to the average person with CSP.

Since the majority of chronic neck pain and chronic back pain (about 90%) can be considered non-specific/idiopathic [80,81], the investigated target population of this review were people with non-specific CSP. This implies that the presented results regarding several factors and their association with insomnia may vary in people with a specific diagnosis. However, a study by Kim et al. investigating risk factors for insomnia in a mixed sample of people with chronic low back pain with varying diagnoses (including lumbar disc herniation, spinal stenosis, spondylolisthesis, musculoskeletal back pain and mixed cases) showed similar results [82]. The study indicated that people with chronic low back pain with high pain intensity levels (VAS $\geq$ 7), comorbid musculoskeletal pain conditions and neuropathic pain components anxiety (HADS-A $\geq$ 8) and/or depression (HADS-D $\geq$ 8) were more likely to have insomnia (respectively 2.57, 14.71, 3.42, 3.14 and 5.58 times more likely), which is in accordance with the results of our review. In this study, sex, age and BMI were not identified as associates. However, a similar OR was found for sex (OR 1.40, 95% CI = (0.88–2.23)). A study of Yun et al. investigated associated factors with insomnia in a sample of 194 people diagnosed with failed back surgery syndrome [83]. Pain intensity (VAS $\geq$ 7), catastrophizing ($\geq$30 PCS), anxiety (HADS-A $\geq$ 8) and depression (HADS-D $\geq$ 8) were found to be significantly related to insomnia. Compared to our results in people with non-specific CSP, higher ORs were found for all these factors in this sample of people with failed back surgery (respectively 5.01, 11.70, 8.09 and 9.53), suggesting an even stronger relation between these factors and insomnia in people diagnosed with failed back surgery syndrome. In contrast with our results, sex and comorbid musculoskeletal pain were not identified as risk factors. This suggests, despite some similarities, that associates and their strength of association with insomnia probably vary between non-specific CSP and CSP with a specific origin. Furthermore, associates might also vary between people with different CSP diagnoses. Nevertheless, the results of this review can serve as a basis since the majority of chronic low back and chronic neck pain is non-specific.

4.1. Strengths and Limitations

To our knowledge, this is the first systematic review with meta-analysis which provides a clear overview of associates of insomnia in people with CSP. This review has several strengths, including a rigorous methodology. First, this review was conducted in accordance with the PRISMA guidelines, which ensures a transparent, stepwise and complete approach. Second, we were able to perform several meta-analyses and one subgroup analysis which overcomes the issue of small sample sizes and makes it possible to draw more reliable and valid conclusions. Third, several comprehensive search strategies were used, including the screening of three different databases and additional hand-searching. Fourth, the screening and quality assessment has been conducted individually by three independent researchers. This improves the overall strength of the review by reducing the chance of making errors and missing an eligible study. Lastly, this review was a priori registered in the PROSPERO database, which avoids unplanned duplication, promotes transparency and reduces potential bias.

Despite the methodology used in this review and meta-analysis, a few limitations should be acknowledged. First, most included studies were cross-sectional in nature, implying that the results cannot provide information on causality, but rather provide an indication of association between the factors and insomnia. However, these ORs do indicate that insomnia is more prevalent in the presence of specific characteristics and can help to construct causal hypotheses. When translated to clinical practice, this means that the identified factors cannot predict whether a person with CSP will develop insomnia, yet they can help to identify those people with CSP that are very likely to suffer from insomnia. Second, most factors were only reported by less than four studies (except for sex). If more studies for each factor were available, the power and the generalizability of the meta-analyses would increase. According to recent research, five or more studies would be required to sufficiently power random-effects meta-analyses [84]. Despite the low number of studies for each factor, clear significant results were found for several factors. However, obtained results (i.e., ORs) would be a more precise representation if more studies were available. Additionally, more factors might become significant if more studies were available. However, most non-significant factors that potentially can become significant with increased number (and quality) of studies will be less relevant compared to the factors (with high ORs) that are clearly related to insomnia. Third, an adapted NOS for cross-sectional studies was used to assess the methodological quality, which was also applied for the included longitudinal cohort study [46], since no other valid alternative was available with the same point spread. However, the cohort study only measured sleep disturbances at baseline. Therefore, the extracted data to determine OR from this study could be considered as cross-sectional data. Last, the heterogeneity for the factors of "comorbidities" and "physical activity" was rather high. A possible explanation for this might be a different definition for physical activity and comorbidities, the use of different assessment methods and/or the use of different cut-off values. Regarding physical activity, for example, Blay et al. included people suffering from back pain who were aged 60 years or more, and used physical activity in a dichotomized manner (yes/no) [36]. On the other hand, Mork et al. focused on adults suffering from neck/shoulder and back pain, and classified participants as physically active when they performed more than one (accumulated) hour of exercise per week [41]. Furthermore, insomnia was also measured in different ways across all studies, which could have led to an increase in heterogeneity. Nevertheless, no significant heterogeneity was found in seven out of nine factors.

Taking these limitations into consideration, future studies should aim for large sample sizes and a rigorous methodology to ensure high-quality studies with strong and exact results. Furthermore, more factors that are targetable by different therapies (such as social-, psychological-, environmental-, contextual- and behavioral-related factors) should be investigated to make it possible to well-anticipate these associated factors and deliver the best possible care. Researchers should also implement a longitudinal design which makes it possible to draw conclusions regarding factors related to the development of insomnia in people with CSP. This would enable clinicians to make better predictions as to whether a patient with CSP is at risk of developing insomnia or not. Consequently, this will also help to develop preventive strategies or at least lead to early identification. Besides, future research should also focus on investigating and unravelling the underlying mechanisms explaining the relation between sleep and pain. This will help to gain a better understanding of the bidirectional relation and the underlying mechanisms. Complementary findings of future research regarding associated factors and underlying mechanisms can lead to an improvement of pharmacological and non-pharmacological approaches for the management of CSP comorbid with sleep disturbances and preventive strategies for insomnia.

4.2. Clinical Implications

While insomnia is a common and important issue in people with CSP, it is rarely addressed in the treatments for CSP. The results of this study can be helpful for clinicians to identify people with CSP early, who are very or less likely to have or develop insomnia based on the presence of several identified associated factors and the strength of the association. Based on the results, people with high pain intensity scores, who report depressive symptoms, who have anxiety and who catastrophize pain, have the highest chance of displaying insomnia. Furthermore, the identified associated factors might be a starting point to improve future treatment approaches. Nevertheless, more longitudinal research is needed to make firm conclusions regarding causality, the predictive value of the associated factors and the effectiveness of new treatment approaches, specifically targeting these associated factors.

This systematic review with meta-analysis shows that insomnia is relatively common in people with CSP. Several significant factors associated with insomnia in CSP were identified: moderate-quality evidence was found for the factors high pain intensity scores (NRS/VAS $\geq$ 7), depressive symptoms (HADS-D $\geq$ 8) and anxiety (HADS-A $\geq$ 8), and low-quality evidence was found for the factors female sex, the presence of comorbidities, performing no professional activities, pain catastrophizing and higher healthcare use. Low-quality evidence suggested that physically active low back pain patients are also less likely to suffer from insomnia. Having knowledge of these factors can help clinicians to identify patients who are (less) likely to have insomnia.

Supplementary Materials: The following are available online at https://www.mdpi.com/article/10.3390/jcm10143175/s1, Supplementary file S1, Supplementary file S2, Table S1: Search Terms, Table S2: Overview excluded articles screened on full text, Table S3: Quality of Evidence - Modified version of the Grading of Recommendations Assessment, Development, and Evaluation criteria.

Author Contributions: T.B.: conceptualization, methodology, formal analysis, investigation, writing—original draft, writing—review and editing, visualization, project administration; C.S.: investigation, writing—review and editing; I.D.M.: investigation, writing—review and editing; E.V.L.: writing—review and editing; O.M.: writing—review and editing; J.N.: writing—review and editing; M.M. (Mira Meeus): writing—review and editing; K.I.: writing—review and editing; B.C.: writing—review and editing; D.G.: writing—review and editing, funding acquisition; L.D.: writing—review and editing; M.M. (Maarten Moens): writing—review and editing; A.M.: investigation, writing—review and editing, supervision, project administration. All authors have read and agreed to the published version of the manuscript.

Funding: Anneleen Malfliet is funded by the Research Foundation Flanders (FWO), Belgium. Eveline Van Looveren and Thomas Bilterys are both funded by the Applied Biomedical Research Program (TBM) of the Agency for Innovation by Science and Technology (IWT) and the Research Foundation Flanders (FWO), Belgium. The funding agencies had no influence in the design of the study, the data collection, the analysis or the interpretation of the data and decisions regarding publication.

Institutional Review Board Statement: Not applicable.

Informed Consent Statement: Not applicable.

Data Availability Statement: Not applicable.

Acknowledgments: The authors give their sincere thanks to Laurence Leysen of the Pain in Motion Research Group (PAIN), Department of Physiotherapy, Human Physiology and Anatomy at the Vrije Universiteit Brussel for her assistance in teaching how to perform meta-analyses.

Conflicts of Interest: The authors declare no conflict of interest.

References

1. Murray, C.J.; Vos, T.; Lozano, R.; Naghavi, M.; Flaxman, A.D.; Michaud, C.; Ezzati, M.; Shibuya, K.; Salomon, J.A.; Abdalla, S.; et al. Disability-adjusted life years (DALYs) for 291 diseases and injuries in 21 regions, 1990-2010: A systematic analysis for the Global Burden of Disease Study 2010. *Lancet* **2012**, *380*, 2197–2223. [CrossRef]
2. Balague, F.; Mannion, A.F.; Pellise, F.; Cedraschi, C. Non-specific low back pain. *Lancet* **2012**, *379*, 482–491. [CrossRef]
3. Gore, M.; Tai, K.S.; Sadosky, A.; Leslie, D.; Stacey, B.R. Use and costs of prescription medications and alternative treatments in patients with osteoarthritis and chronic low back pain in community-based settings. *Pain Pract. Off. J. World Inst. Pain* **2012**, *12*, 550–560. [CrossRef]
4. Hoy, D.; Bain, C.; Williams, G.; March, L.; Brooks, P.; Blyth, F.; Woolf, A.; Vos, T.; Buchbinder, R. A systematic review of the global prevalence of low back pain. *Arthritis Rheum.* **2012**, *64*, 2028–2037. [CrossRef]
5. Fejer, R.; Kyvik, K.O.; Hartvigsen, J. The prevalence of neck pain in the world population: A systematic critical review of the literature. *Eur. Spine J.* **2006**, *15*, 834–848. [CrossRef]
6. Von Korff, M.; Crane, P.; Lane, M.; Miglioretti, D.L.; Simon, G.; Saunders, K.; Stang, P.; Brandenburg, N.; Kessler, R. Chronic spinal pain and physical-mental comorbidity in the United States: Results from the national comorbidity survey replication. *Pain* **2005**, *113*, 331–339. [CrossRef] [PubMed]
7. Hartvigsen, J.; Natvig, B.; Ferreira, M. Is it all about a pain in the back? *Best Pract. Res. Clin. Rheumatol.* **2013**, *27*, 613–623. [CrossRef]
8. Hartvigsen, J.; Hancock, M.J.; Kongsted, A.; Louw, Q.; Ferreira, M.L.; Genevay, S.; Hoy, D.; Karppinen, J.; Pransky, G.; Sieper, J.; et al. What low back pain is and why we need to pay attention. *Lancet* **2018**, *391*, 2356–2367. [CrossRef]

9. Alsaadi, S.M.; McAuley, J.H.; Hush, J.M.; Maher, C.G. Prevalence of sleep disturbance in patients with low back pain. *Eur. Spine J.* **2011**, *20*, 737–743. [CrossRef] [PubMed]
10. Bahouq, H.; Allali, F.; Rkain, H.; Hmamouchi, I.; Hajjaj-Hassouni, N. Prevalence and severity of insomnia in chronic low back pain patients. *Rheumatol. Int.* **2013**, *33*, 1277–1281. [CrossRef]
11. Tang, N.K.; Wright, K.J.; Salkovskis, P.M. Prevalence and correlates of clinical insomnia co-occurring with chronic back pain. *J. Sleep Res.* **2007**, *16*, 85–95. [CrossRef]
12. Marin, R.; Cyhan, T.; Miklos, W. Sleep disturbance in patients with chronic low back pain. *Am. J. Phys. Med. Rehabil.* **2006**, *85*, 430–435. [CrossRef]
13. Institute of Medicine Committee on Sleep Medicine and Research. The National Academies Collection: Reports funded by National Institutes of Health. In *Sleep Disorders and Sleep Deprivation: An Unmet Public Health Problem*; Colten, H.R., Altevogt, B.M., Eds.; National Academies Press (US), National Academy of Sciences: Washington, DC, USA, 2006.
14. Sayar, K.; Arikan, M.; Yontem, T. Sleep quality in chronic pain patients. *Can. J. Psychiatry* **2002**, *47*, 844–848. [CrossRef]
15. Daley, M.; Morin, C.M.; LeBlanc, M.; Gregoire, J.P.; Savard, J. The economic burden of insomnia: Direct and indirect costs for individuals with insomnia syndrome, insomnia symptoms, and good sleepers. *Sleep* **2009**, *32*, 55–64.
16. Haack, M.; Simpson, N.; Sethna, N.; Kaur, S.; Mullington, J. Sleep deficiency and chronic pain: Potential underlying mechanisms and clinical implications. *Neuropsychopharmacology* **2020**, *45*, 205–216. [CrossRef]
17. Whibley, D.; AlKandari, N.; Kristensen, K.; Barnish, M.; Rzewuska, M.; Druce, K.L.; Tang, N.K.Y. Sleep and Pain: A Systematic Review of Studies of Mediation. *Clin. J. Pain* **2019**, *35*, 544–558. [CrossRef]
18. Liberati, A.; Altman, D.G.; Tetzlaff, J.; Mulrow, C.; Gotzsche, P.C.; Ioannidis, J.P.; Clarke, M.; Devereaux, P.J.; Kleijnen, J.; Moher, D. The PRISMA statement for reporting systematic reviews and meta-analyses of studies that evaluate health care interventions: Explanation and elaboration. *J. Clin. Epidemiol.* **2009**, *62*, e1–e34. [CrossRef]
19. Schutte-Rodin, S.; Broch, L.; Buysse, D.; Dorsey, C.; Sateia, M. Clinical guideline for the evaluation and management of chronic insomnia in adults. *J. Clin. Sleep Med.* **2008**, *4*, 487–504.
20. American Psychiatric Association. *Diagnostic and Statistical Manual of Mental Disorders*, 5th ed.; American Psychiatric Association: Washington, DC, USA, 2013.
21. Elmagarmid, A.; Fedorowicz, Z.; Hammady, H.; Ilyas, I.; Khabsa, M.; Ouzzani, M. Rayyan: A systematic reviews web app for exploring and filtering searches for eligible studies for Cochrane Reviews. In Proceedings of the 22nd Cochrane Colloquium, Evidence-informed public health: Opportunities and challenges, Hyderabad, India, 21–25 September 2014; pp. 21–26.
22. Stang, A. Critical evaluation of the Newcastle-Ottawa scale for the assessment of the quality of nonrandomized studies in meta-analyses. *Eur. J. Epidemiol.* **2010**, *25*, 603–605. [CrossRef]
23. Modesti, P.A.; Reboldi, G.; Cappuccio, F.P.; Agyemang, C.; Remuzzi, G.; Rapi, S.; Perruolo, E.; Parati, G. Panethnic Differences in Blood Pressure in Europe: A Systematic Review and Meta-Analysis. *PLoS ONE* **2016**, *11*, e0147601. [CrossRef]
24. McPheeters, M.L.; Kripalani, S.; Peterson, N.B.; Idowu, R.T.; Jerome, R.N.; Potter, S.A.; Andrews, J.C. Closing the quality gap: Revisiting the state of the science (vol. 3: Quality improvement interventions to address health disparities). *Evid. Rep. Technol. Assess. (Full Rep.)* **2012**, *3*, 1–475.
25. Fincham, J.E. Response rates and responsiveness for surveys, standards, and the Journal. *Am. J. Pharm. Educ.* **2008**, *72*, 43. [CrossRef]
26. Reyner, L.A.; Horne, J.A.; Reyner, A. Gender- and age-related differences in sleep determined by home-recorded sleep logs and actimetry from 400 adults. *Sleep* **1995**, *18*, 127–134.
27. Suh, S.; Cho, N.; Zhang, J. Sex Differences in Insomnia: From Epidemiology and Etiology to Intervention. *Curr. Psychiatry Rep.* **2018**, *20*, 69. [CrossRef]
28. Zhang, B.; Wing, Y.K. Sex differences in insomnia: A meta-analysis. *Sleep* **2006**, *29*, 85–93. [CrossRef]
29. Van Eycken, S.; Neu, D.; Newell, J.; Kornreich, C.; Mairesse, O. Sex-Related Differences in Sleep-Related PSG Parameters and Daytime Complaints in a Clinical Population. *Nat. Sci. Sleep* **2020**, *12*, 161–171. [CrossRef]
30. Higgins, J.P.; Thompson, S.G.; Deeks, J.J.; Altman, D.G. Measuring inconsistency in meta-analyses. *BMJ* **2003**, *327*, 557–560. [CrossRef]
31. Deeks, J.J.; Higgins, J.P.; Altman, D.G.; Group, C.S.M. Analysing data and undertaking meta-analyses. *Cochrane Handb. Syst. Rev. Interv.* **2019**, 241–284. [CrossRef]
32. Higgins, J.P.; Green, S. *Cochrane Handbook for Systematic Reviews of Interventions*; John Wiley & Sons: Hoboken, NJ, USA, 2011; Volume 4.
33. Higgins, J.P.; Thompson, S.G. Quantifying heterogeneity in a meta-analysis. *Stat. Med.* **2002**, *21*, 1539–1558. [CrossRef]
34. Huguet, A.; Hayden, J.A.; Stinson, J.; McGrath, P.J.; Chambers, C.T.; Tougas, M.E.; Wozney, L. Judging the quality of evidence in reviews of prognostic factor research: Adapting the GRADE framework. *Syst. Rev.* **2013**, *2*, 71. [CrossRef]
35. Sterne, J.A.; Gavaghan, D.; Egger, M. Publication and related bias in meta-analysis: Power of statistical tests and prevalence in the literature. *J. Clin. Epidemiol.* **2000**, *53*, 1119–1129. [CrossRef]
36. Blay, S.L.; Andreoli, S.B.; Gastal, F.L. Chronic painful physical conditions, disturbed sleep and psychiatric morbidity: Results from an elderly survey. *Ann. Clin. Psychiatry* **2007**, *19*, 169–174. [CrossRef]

37. DiMarco, L.A.; Ramger, B.C.; Howell, G.P.; Serrani, A.M.; Givens, D.L.; Rhon, D.I.; Cook, C.E. Differences in Characteristics and Downstream Drug Use Among Opioid-Naive and Prior Opioid Users with Low Back Pain. *Pain Pract. Off. J. World Inst. Pain* **2019**, *19*, 149–157. [CrossRef]
38. Ho, K.K.N.; Simic, M.; Cvancarova Smastuen, M.; de Barros Pinheiro, M.; Ferreira, P.H.; Bakke Johnsen, M.; Heuch, I.; Grotle, M.; Zwart, J.A.; Nilsen, K.B. The association between insomnia, c-reactive protein, and chronic low back pain: Cross-sectional analysis of the HUNT study, Norway. *Scand. J. Pain* **2019**. [CrossRef]
39. Kim, S.H.; Lee, D.H.; Yoon, K.B.; An, J.R.; Yoon, D.M. Factors Associated with Increased Risk for Clinical Insomnia in Patients with Chronic Neck Pain. *Pain Physician* **2015**, *18*, 593–598. [PubMed]
40. Majid, B.; Arif, M.A.; Saeed, R.; Ahmad, A.; Fatima, M. Frequency and severity of insomnia in chronic low back pain. *Rawal Med. J.* **2017**, *42*, 528–530.
41. Mork, P.J.; Vik, K.L.; Moe, B.; Lier, R.; Bardal, E.M.; Nilsen, T.I. Sleep problems, exercise and obesity and risk of chronic musculoskeletal pain: The Norwegian HUNT study. *Eur. J. Public Health* **2014**, *24*, 924–929. [CrossRef]
42. Park, S.J.; Lee, R.; Yoon, D.M.; Yoon, K.B.; Kim, K.; Kim, S.H. Factors associated with increased risk for pain catastrophizing in patients with chronic neck pain: A retrospective cross-sectional study. *Med. (Baltim.)* **2016**, *95*, e4698. [CrossRef]
43. Ris, I.; Juul-Kristensen, B.; Boyle, E.; Kongsted, A.; Manniche, C.; Sogaard, K. Chronic neck pain patients with traumatic or non-traumatic onset: Differences in characteristics. A cross-sectional study. *Scand. J. Pain* **2017**, *14*, 1–8. [CrossRef] [PubMed]
44. Shmagel, A.; Foley, R.; Ibrahim, H. Epidemiology of Chronic Low Back Pain in US Adults: Data From the 2009-2010 National Health and Nutrition Examination Survey. *Arthritis Care Res. (Hoboken)* **2016**, *68*, 1688–1694. [CrossRef]
45. Wang, H.Y.; Fu, T.S.; Hsu, S.C.; Hung, C.I. Association of depression with sleep quality might be greater than that of pain intensity among outpatients with chronic low back pain. *Neuropsychiatr. Dis. Treat.* **2016**, *12*, 1993–1998. [CrossRef]
46. Aili, K.; Nyman, T.; Hillert, L.; Svartengren, M. Sleep disturbances predict future sickness absence among individuals with lower back or neck-shoulder pain: A 5-year prospective study. *Scand. J. Public Health* **2015**, *43*, 315–323. [CrossRef] [PubMed]
47. Roth, T. Insomnia: Definition, prevalence, etiology, and consequences. *J. Clin. Sleep Med.* **2007**, *3*, S7–S10. [CrossRef]
48. Scullin, M.K.; Bliwise, D.L. Sleep, cognition, and normal aging: Integrating a half century of multidisciplinary research. *Perspect. Psychol. Sci.* **2015**, *10*, 97–137. [CrossRef]
49. Senaratna, C.V.; Perret, J.L.; Lodge, C.J.; Lowe, A.J.; Campbell, B.E.; Matheson, M.C.; Hamilton, G.S.; Dharmage, S.C. Prevalence of obstructive sleep apnea in the general population: A systematic review. *Sleep Med. Rev.* **2017**, *34*, 70–81. [CrossRef]
50. Patel, D.; Steinberg, J.; Patel, P. Insomnia in the Elderly: A Review. *J. Clin. Sleep Med.* **2018**, *14*, 1017–1024. [CrossRef]
51. Ancoli-Israel, S. Sleep and its disorders in aging populations. *Sleep Med.* **2009**, *10* (Suppl. 1), S7–S11. [CrossRef]
52. Smagula, S.F.; Stone, K.L.; Fabio, A.; Cauley, J.A. Risk factors for sleep disturbances in older adults: Evidence from prospective studies. *Sleep Med. Rev.* **2016**, *25*, 21–30. [CrossRef]
53. Husak, A.J.; Bair, M.J. Chronic Pain and Sleep Disturbances: A Pragmatic Review of Their Relationships, Comorbidities, and Treatments. *Pain Med.* **2020**. [CrossRef]
54. Finan, P.H.; Goodin, B.R.; Smith, M.T. The association of sleep and pain: An update and a path forward. *J. Pain* **2013**, *14*, 1539–1552. [CrossRef]
55. Cheatle, M.D.; Foster, S.; Pinkett, A.; Lesneski, M.; Qu, D.; Dhingra, L. Assessing and Managing Sleep Disturbance in Patients with Chronic Pain. *Anesthesiol. Clin.* **2016**, *34*, 379–393. [CrossRef]
56. Nijs, J.; Mairesse, O.; Neu, D.; Leysen, L.; Danneels, L.; Cagnie, B.; Meeus, M.; Moens, M.; Ickmans, K.; Goubert, D. Sleep Disturbances in Chronic Pain: Neurobiology, Assessment, and Treatment in Physical Therapist Practice. *Phys. Ther.* **2018**, *98*, 325–335. [CrossRef]
57. Wall, P.D.; Melzack, R.; Bonica, J.J. *Textbook of Pain*; Churchill Livingstone: Edinburgh, Scotland, UK, 1999; Volume 994.
58. Kim, E.J.; Dimsdale, J.E. The effect of psychosocial stress on sleep: A review of polysomnographic evidence. *Behav. Sleep Med.* **2007**, *5*, 256–278. [CrossRef] [PubMed]
59. Crombez, G.; Vlaeyen, J.W.; Heuts, P.H.; Lysens, R. Pain-related fear is more disabling than pain itself: Evidence on the role of pain-related fear in chronic back pain disability. *Pain* **1999**, *80*, 329–339. [CrossRef]
60. Gatchel, R.J.; Neblett, R.; Kishino, N.; Ray, C.T. Fear-Avoidance Beliefs and Chronic Pain. *J. Orthop. Sports Phys. Ther.* **2016**, *46*, 38–43. [CrossRef] [PubMed]
61. Kroenke, K.; Outcalt, S.; Krebs, E.; Bair, M.J.; Wu, J.; Chumbler, N.; Yu, Z. Association between anxiety, health-related quality of life and functional impairment in primary care patients with chronic pain. *Gen. Hosp. Psychiatry* **2013**, *35*, 359–365. [CrossRef]
62. Mullington, J.M.; Simpson, N.S.; Meier-Ewert, H.K.; Haack, M. Sleep loss and inflammation. *Best Pract. Res. Clin. Endocrinol. Metab.* **2010**, *24*, 775–784. [CrossRef]
63. Haack, M.; Lee, E.; Cohen, D.A.; Mullington, J.M. Activation of the prostaglandin system in response to sleep loss in healthy humans: Potential mediator of increased spontaneous pain. *Pain* **2009**, *145*, 136–141. [CrossRef]
64. Pollmacher, T.; Haack, M.; Schuld, A.; Reichenberg, A.; Yirmiya, R. Low levels of circulating inflammatory cytokines–do they affect human brain functions? *Brain Behav. Immun.* **2002**, *16*, 525–532. [CrossRef]
65. Wodarski, R.; Schuh-Hofer, S.; Yurek, D.A.; Wafford, K.A.; Gilmour, G.; Treede, R.D.; Kennedy, J.D. Development and pharmacological characterization of a model of sleep disruption-induced hypersensitivity in the rat. *Eur. J. Pain* **2015**, *19*, 554–566. [CrossRef]

66. Schuh-Hofer, S.; Wodarski, R.; Pfau, D.B.; Caspani, O.; Magerl, W.; Kennedy, J.D.; Treede, R.D. One night of total sleep deprivation promotes a state of generalized hyperalgesia: A surrogate pain model to study the relationship of insomnia and pain. *Pain* **2013**, *154*, 1613–1621. [CrossRef]
67. Staner, L. Comorbidity of insomnia and depression. *Sleep Med. Rev.* **2010**, *14*, 35–46. [CrossRef] [PubMed]
68. Pereira, F.G.; Franca, M.H.; Paiva, M.C.A.; Andrade, L.H.; Viana, M.C. Prevalence and clinical profile of chronic pain and its association with mental disorders. *Rev. Saude Publica* **2017**, *51*, 96. [CrossRef]
69. Bair, M.J.; Robinson, R.L.; Katon, W.; Kroenke, K. Depression and pain comorbidity: A literature review. *Arch. Intern. Med.* **2003**, *163*, 2433–2445. [CrossRef]
70. Dunietz, G.L.; Swanson, L.M.; Jansen, E.C.; Chervin, R.D.; O'Brien, L.M.; Lisabeth, L.D.; Braley, T.J. Key insomnia symptoms and incident pain in older adults: Direct and mediated pathways through depression and anxiety. *Sleep* **2018**, *41*. [CrossRef]
71. Kredlow, M.A.; Capozzoli, M.C.; Hearon, B.A.; Calkins, A.W.; Otto, M.W. The effects of physical activity on sleep: A meta-analytic review. *J. Behav. Med.* **2015**, *38*, 427–449. [CrossRef]
72. Quante, M.; Mariani, S.; Weng, J.; Marinac, C.R.; Kaplan, E.R.; Rueschman, M.; Mitchell, J.A.; James, P.; Hipp, J.A.; Cespedes Feliciano, E.M.; et al. Zeitgebers and their association with rest-activity patterns. *Chronobiol. Int.* **2019**, *36*, 203–213. [CrossRef]
73. Gordon, R.; Bloxham, S. A Systematic Review of the Effects of Exercise and Physical Activity on Non-Specific Chronic Low Back Pain. *Healthcare* **2016**, *4*, 22. [CrossRef]
74. Malfliet, A.; Ickmans, K.; Huysmans, E.; Coppieters, I.; Willaert, W.; Bogaert, W.V.; Rheel, E.; Bilterys, T.; Wilgen, P.V.; Nijs, J. Best Evidence Rehabilitation for Chronic Pain Part 3: Low Back Pain. *J. Clin. Med.* **2019**, *8*, 1063. [CrossRef]
75. Palmlof, L.; Holm, L.W.; Alfredsson, L.; Magnusson, C.; Vingard, E.; Skillgate, E. The impact of work related physical activity and leisure physical activity on the risk and prognosis of neck pain—A population based cohort study on workers. *BMC Musculoskelet. Disord.* **2016**, *17*, 219. [CrossRef]
76. Geneen, L.J.; Moore, R.A.; Clarke, C.; Martin, D.; Colvin, L.A.; Smith, B.H. Physical activity and exercise for chronic pain in adults: An overview of Cochrane Reviews. *Cochrane Database Syst. Rev.* **2017**, *4*, Cd011279. [CrossRef] [PubMed]
77. Quartana, P.J.; Campbell, C.M.; Edwards, R.R. Pain catastrophizing: A critical review. *Expert Rev. Neurother.* **2009**, *9*, 745–758. [CrossRef]
78. Boersma, K.; Linton, S.J. Psychological processes underlying the development of a chronic pain problem: A prospective study of the relationship between profiles of psychological variables in the fear-avoidance model and disability. *Clin. J. Pain* **2006**, *22*, 160–166. [CrossRef] [PubMed]
79. Walton, D.M.; Macdermid, J.C.; Giorgianni, A.A.; Mascarenhas, J.C.; West, S.C.; Zammit, C.A. Risk factors for persistent problems following acute whiplash injury: Update of a systematic review and meta-analysis. *J. Orthop. Sports Phys. Ther.* **2013**, *43*, 31–43. [CrossRef] [PubMed]
80. Koes, B.W.; van Tulder, M.W.; Thomas, S. Diagnosis and treatment of low back pain. *BMJ* **2006**, *332*, 1430–1434. [CrossRef] [PubMed]
81. Stanton, T.R.; Leake, H.B.; Chalmers, K.J.; Moseley, G.L. Evidence of Impaired Proprioception in Chronic, Idiopathic Neck Pain: Systematic Review and Meta-Analysis. *Phys. Ther.* **2016**, *96*, 876–887. [CrossRef] [PubMed]
82. Kim, S.H.; Sun, J.M.; Yoon, K.B.; Moon, J.H.; An, J.R.; Yoon, D.M. Risk factors associated with clinical insomnia in chronic low back pain: A retrospective analysis in a university hospital in Korea. *Korean J. Pain* **2015**, *28*, 137–143. [CrossRef]
83. Yun, S.Y.; Kim, D.H.; Do, H.Y.; Kim, S.H. Clinical insomnia and associated factors in failed back surgery syndrome: A retrospective cross-sectional study. *Int. J. Med. Sci.* **2017**, *14*, 536–542. [CrossRef]
84. Jackson, D.; Turner, R. Power analysis for random-effects meta-analysis. *Res. Synth. Methods* **2017**, *8*, 290–302. [CrossRef]

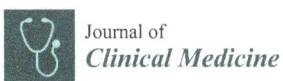

Review

Specific versus Non-Specific Exercises for Chronic Neck or Shoulder Pain: A Systematic Review

Lirios Dueñas [1,2,†], Marta Aguilar-Rodríguez [1,*,†], Lennard Voogt [3,4], Enrique Lluch [1,2,4], Filip Struyf [5], Michel G. C. A. M. Mertens [4,5], Kayleigh De Meulemeester [4,6] and Mira Meeus [4,5,6]

1. Department of Physiotherapy, Faculty of Physiotherapy, University of Valencia, 46010 Valencia, Spain; lirios.duenas@uv.es (L.D.); enrique.lluch@uv.es (E.L.)
2. Physiotherapy in Motion, Multi-Specialty Research Group (PTinMOTION), Department of Physiotherapy, University of Valencia, 46010 Valencia, Spain
3. Research Centre for Health Care Innovations, Rotterdam University of Applied Sciences, 3015 GG Rotterdam, The Netherlands; l.p.voogt@hr.nl
4. Pain in Motion Research Group (PAIN), Department of Physiotherapy, Human Physiology and Anatomy, Faculty of Physical Education & Physiotherapy, Vrije Universiteit Brussel, 1050 Brussels, Belgium; michel.mertens@uantwerpen.be (M.G.C.A.M.M.); Kayleigh.DeMeulemeester@UGent.be (K.D.M.); mira.meeus@uantwerpen.be (M.M.)
5. MOVANT Research Group, Department of Rehabilitation Sciences and Physiotherapy, Faculty of Medicine and Health Sciences, University of Antwerp, 2000 Antwerp, Belgium; filip.struyf@uantwerpen.be
6. Department of Rehabilitation Sciences and Physiotherapy, Faculty of Medicine and Health Sciences, Ghent University, 9000 Ghent, Belgium
* Correspondence: marta.aguilar@uv.es; Tel.: +34-963851308
† These two authors contributed equally to this work.

Abstract: The current systematic review aimed to compare the effect of injury-focused (specific) exercises versus more general (non-specific) exercises on pain in patients with chronic neck or shoulder pain. We searched PubMed, EMBASE, and Web of Science. Two reviewers screened and selected studies, extracted outcomes, assessed risk of bias, and rated the quality of evidence. A total of nine eligible studies, represented in 13 articles, were identified, with a considerable risk of bias. One article investigated the acute effect of single bouts of exercise on pain and reported an immediate pain reduction after non-specific exercise. Regarding short-term effects, seven out of the nine studies found no differences in pain between interventions, with inconsistent results among two other studies. Concerning the long-term effects, while pain reduction seems to be favored by specific exercises (two out of four articles), the best format is still unclear. Based on the acute effects, a single bout of non-specific exercise seems to be a better option for pain-relief for patients with chronic neck or shoulder pain. For short-term effects, there are no differences in pain between specific and non-specific exercises. Regarding long-term effects, specific exercises seem to be the best option. Nevertheless, more studies are warranted.

Keywords: chronic pain; musculoskeletal pain; exercise therapy; neck pain; shoulder pain; systematic review

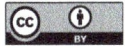

1. Introduction

The prevalence of neck pain has steadily increased during the past two decades [1] and is now, second to back pain, the most common musculoskeletal disorder [2,3]. Additionally, shoulder pain is responsible for approximately 16% of all musculoskeletal complaints [4], with a yearly incidence of 15 new episodes per 1.000 patients seen in primary care settings [5]. Neck and shoulder symptoms are often persistent and recurrent, with from 40% to 50% of patients reporting persistent symptoms after 6 to 12 months [6] and 14% of patients continuing care after 2 years [7].

Successfully treating patients with chronic neck or shoulder pain (CNSP) is a challenging issue for clinicians. Exercise therapy is found to be an effective treatment strategy to relieve pain and improve patient's level of functioning in daily activities in various chronic musculoskeletal pain disorders, including chronic neck pain [8–11] and chronic shoulder pain [12,13]. However, although the evidence for exercise therapy is strong, it is still difficult to demonstrate the superiority of one exercise approach over another in chronic pain populations [14].

Exercise interventions aim to correct biomechanical disturbances, but can also be directed to specific psychological and behavioural characteristics of chronic pain problems [14]. Naugle et al. [15] summarized the neurophysiological and hypoalgesic, effects of acute bouts of exercise in healthy and chronic pain populations in a meta-analytic review. In healthy populations, the evidence suggests that different types of acute bouts of exercise decrease the perception of experimentally induced pain. However, in patients with local muscular pain (e.g., shoulder myalgia), exercising non-painful muscles (non-specific exercises (NSE)) seems to activate generalized endogenous hypoalgesia, but exercising painful muscles (specific exercises (SE)) increases pain sensitivity in both the exercising muscle and distant locations [15,16]. While healthy people present exercise-induced hypoalgesia, regardless of the type of exercise, this mechanism seems to fail in subgroups of chronic pain patients. Among these patients, a bout of exercise can even result in a hyperalgesic response, indicating that exercise therapy should be tailored to prevent symptom flares. Nevertheless, the long-term responses to exercise therapy seem to be effective for a wide variety of chronic pain diagnoses (for a review, see Kroll, 2015 [14]).

Considering this, designing an optimal, tailor-made, exercise program for a person with CNSP requires an understanding of the underlying working mechanisms of different exercise interventions [14,17]. Additionally, the differences between the acute effects of one bout of exercise and training effects (acute, short-term, and long-term effects) should be taken into account when addressing exercise for chronic pain patients. Based on the state-of-the-art, as summarized above, the question remains as to which type of exercise, specific or non-specific, is more convenient for pain relief in people with CNSP. The aim of this systematic review was to provide a constructive overview of the existing literature reporting pain experience, following specific versus non-specific exercise therapy in CNSP patients.

2. Materials and Methods

2.1. Data Sources and Searches

This systematic review is registered in the PROSPERO register of systematic reviews (registration number: CRD42020145234) and is in accordance with the PRISMA guidelines [18]. An extensive search was conducted of the online databases PubMed, Web of Science, and Embase. Databases were searched within a 2-day period, retrospective of inception, to May 2020, with a subsequent update to January 2021. The search strategy was based on the Population, Intervention, Comparison, Outcome, Study Design (PICOS) framework and was conducted to find controlled studies (S) evaluating the effect of specific exercise programs, including neck or shoulder exercises (I), on pain (O) in CNSP patients (P), compared to non-specific exercise programs (i.e., exercises that do not specifically involve the affected region) (C). Key words from these groups were combined. The construct of the search strategy is presented in Table 1.

Table 1. Search strategy.

	Keywords
Group 1 (Population)	"Arthralgia"(MeSH) OR "Bursitis"(MeSH) OR "Cervical vertebrae"(MeSH) OR "Chronic pain"(MeSH) OR "Hernia"(MeSH) OR "Intervertebral Disc Displacement"(MeSH) OR "Musculoskeletal System"(MeSH) OR "Myalgia"(MeSH) OR "Myofascial Pain Syndromes"(MeSH) OR "Neck"(MeSH) OR "Neck Pain"(MeSH) OR "Osteoarthritis"(MeSH) OR "Pain, intractable"(MeSH) OR "Rotator cuff"(MeSH) OR "Shoulder Impingement Syndrome"(MeSH) OR "Shoulder Pain"(MeSH) OR "Shoulder"(MeSH) OR "Tendinopathy"(MeSH) OR "Whiplash Injuries"(MeSH) OR (Chronic pain OR Intractable pain OR Joint Pain OR Muscle Pain OR Musculoskeletal pain OR Myalgia OR Myofascial pain OR Osteoarthritis OR Persistent pain OR Severe pain OR Tendinopathy) AND (Neck OR Shoulder OR Cervical OR Adhesive capsulitis OR Frozen shoulder OR Impingement OR Rotator cuff OR Spinal disc herniation OR Spinal pain OR Whiplash)
Group 2 (Intervention)	"Exercise"(MeSH) OR "Exercise Therapy"(MeSH) OR "Cervical Vertebrae"(MeSH) OR "Functional Laterality"(MeSH) OR "Isometric Contraction"(MeSH) OR "Isotonic Contraction"(MeSH) OR "Muscle Strength"(MeSH) OR "Muscle Stretching Exercises"(MeSH) OR "Neck"(MeSH) OR "Plyometric Exercise"(MeSH) OR "Proprioception"(MeSH) OR "Resistance Training"(MeSH) OR "Shoulder"(MeSH) OR "Visual Motor Coordination"(MeSH) OR "Weight Lifting"(MeSH) OR "Weight-Bearing Exercise Program"(MeSH) OR Exercise AND (Shoulder OR Cervical OR Neck OR Abduction OR Adduction OR Balls OR Bands OR Concentric OR Coordination OR Dynamic OR Eccentric OR Extension OR External Rotation OR Flexibility OR Flexion OR Free weights OR Internal rotation OR Isometric OR Isotonic OR Kettlebell OR Motor control OR Plyometric OR Proprioception OR Red cord OR Resistance training OR Resisted OR Static OR Strength OR Strength training equipment OR Stretching OR Thera-band OR Weight-bearing exercise program OR Weights)
Group 3 (Comparison)	"Exercise"(MeSH) OR "Exercise Movement Techniques"(MeSH) OR "Exercise Therapy"(MeSH) OR "Bicycling"(MeSH) OR "Dancing"(MeSH) OR "Hydrotherapy"(MeSH) OR "Jogging"(MeSH) OR "Muscle Stretching Exercises"(MeSH) OR "Physical Fitness"(MeSH) OR "Physical Endurance"(MeSH) OR "Resistance Training"(MeSH) OR "Running"(MeSH) OR "Swimming"(MeSH) OR "Walking"(MeSH) OR "Yoga"(MeSH) OR Exercise AND (Non-specific exercise OR Non-specific training OR Aspecific OR Activity program OR Aerobic OR Alexander technique OR Aquatic exercise OR Bicycling OR Cycling OR Dancing OR Endurance OR Fitness OR General exercise OR Generic exercise OR Hydrotherapy OR Jogging OR Physical activity OR Resistance training OR Rowing OR Running OR Stretching OR Swimming OR Tai chi OR Training OR Walking OR Yoga)
Group 4 (Outcome)	"Pain"(MeSH) OR "Pain Measurement"(MeSH) OR "Analgesia"(MeSH) OR "Central Nervous System Sensitization"(MeSH) OR "Hyperalgesia"(MeSH) OR "Hypersensitivity"(MeSH) OR "Nociceptors"(MeSH) OR "Pain Management"(MeSH) OR "Pain Threshold"(MeSH) OR "Pain Perception"(MeSH) OR "Pain, Intractable"(MeSH) OR "Pain, Referred"(MeSH) OR "Somatosensory Disorders"(MeSH) OR "Visual Analogue Scale"(MeSH) OR Pain OR Pain measurement OR Algometry OR Analgesia OR Central nervous system sensitization OR Centrally mediated pain modulation OR Conditioned pain modulation OR Endogenous pain inhibition OR Endogenous pain-inhibitory mechanisms OR Exercise-induced hgperalgesia OR Hyperalgesia OR Hypersensitivity OR Hypoalgesia OR McGill OR Nociceptors OR Pain control OR Pain threshold OR Pain-relief OR Persistent pain OR Pressure pain thresholds OR Quantitative sensory testing OR Referred pain OR Sensitivity OR Somatosensory disorders OR Temporal summation OR Visual analogue scale OR Wind-up effect
Group 5 (Study design)	"Controlled Clinical Trials"(MeSH) OR Controlled clinical trials

Abbreviations: MeSH, Medical Subject Headings.

2.2. Study Selection

To be included in this review, studies had to meet the following inclusion criteria: (1) the study sample consisted of human adults (>18 years) with chronic (>3 months) neck and/or shoulder pain; (2) both treatments, SE (those focused on the neck or shoulder region) and NSE (including more generic training such as aerobic exercise, general fitness training, chain-stretching, body–mind, or other generic movement-related approaches), had to be compared in the study; (3) pain was measured as an outcome (both subjectively and objectively); (4) articles had to be written in English, Spanish, French, Dutch, or German; (5) full-text articles of original research had to be available; (6) only controlled clinical trials were allowed. Exclusion criteria determined that: (1) secondary research (reviews and meta-analysis) was not allowed; and (2) widespread pathologies and other co-morbidities could not be present.

The literature search was independently conducted, and the obtained articles were screened by two of the researchers (L.D. and M.A., both PhDs and experienced in chronic populations in a clinical setting), based on title and abstract. The full-text article was retrieved if the citation was considered potentially eligible and relevant. In the second phase, each full-text article was independently evaluated by the two researchers to see whether it fulfilled the inclusion criteria. If any of the eligibility criteria were not fulfilled, then the article was excluded. In case of disagreement, a third researcher was consulted (M.M., PhD, experienced in chronic pain research).

2.3. Data Extraction and Analysis

Important information from each study was selected and reported in an evidence table. The evidence table was composed of the following items: (1) reference; (2) participants' characteristics; (3) specific intervention(s); (4) non-specific intervention(s) and reference intervention if any; (5) outcome measures and timing; (6) main results. The results regarding training effects were clustered into acute, short-term, and long-term effects; for the first days of intervention, post-intervention, and after follow-up, respectively.

2.4. Quality Assessment and Data Synthesis

The Cochrane Collaboration's tool for assessing risk of bias was used (http://handbook.cochrane.org/, accessed on 24 May 2020) to assess the following domains: (1) the randomization process; (2) treatment allocation; (3) blinding of participants and personnel; (4) blinding of outcome assessors; (5) completeness of the outcome data; (6) reporting of results; (7) accounting for co-interventions; (8) other sources of bias. Item 8 was specifically focused on sample size calculation. With reference to a Cochrane review, sample size was considered inadequate if there were fewer than 50 participants per group and if power analysis was not applied and reported for relevant outcome measures [19].

After clustering the results based on exercise modes and timing of assessments, the overall quality of evidence per cluster was determined by applying the Grades of Recommendation, Assessment, Development, and Evaluation (GRADE) approach [20]. For every cluster, a GRADE summary statement is provided under the respective paragraph in italics.

Risk of bias assessment and grading of evidence was performed by two authors (L.D. and M.A.) independently, who were blinded from each other's assessment. After rating the selected articles/clusters, the results of both researchers were compared, and differences were analyzed. In case of disagreement, the reviewers assessed the article/cluster a second time to obtain a consensus. When consensus could not be reached, a third opinion was provided by the last author (M.M.).

3. Results

3.1. Search Results

The initial search of all databases resulted in 852 hits. Following two consecutive screening phases on title/abstract and full text, 10 eligible records remained. After manual searching of the reference lists, two more eligible articles were identified for inclusion. A recent update identified 57 new articles, leaving one of them for inclusion in the review, after the screening phases. Thus, a total of 13 articles, reporting the results of nine different randomized controlled trials, met the inclusion criteria. The corresponding flowchart is shown in Figure 1.

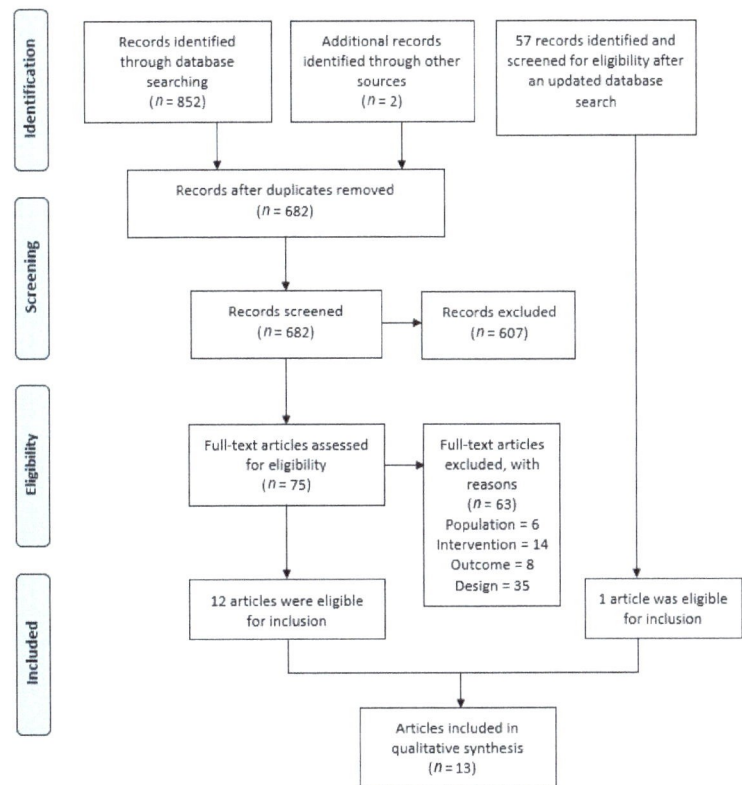

Figure 1. PRISMA flowchart of articles selection (adapted from Moher et al. [18]).

3.2. Risk of Bias and Quality of Evidence

Detailed information on the individual risk of bias can be found in Figure 2. In most cases (85.6% or 89 of 104 items), the two researchers agreed. After a comparison of the 15 differences, the reviewers reached a consensus for six items. The remaining nine points of discussion were solved after a third opinion. Nine of the 13 articles provided insufficient information about the allocation concealment [21–29]. None of the studies reported that the therapist was blinded. Additionally, blinding of the patients was impossible, given the nature of the therapy. In one study, the patients were kept naïve for the different interventions (specific or global stretching). This study was considered as having an unclear risk of bias, because the assumptions of patients were unclear [27]. Attrition and reporting bias were mainly low. Two of the 13 articles accounted for co-interventions by recording medications and other treatments received in a diary [30] and by registering medication type and frequency [27]; the other articles did not account for co-interventions. Five articles conducted a sample size calculation [23,26,27,30,31]. Two of the 13 articles [32,33] included more than 50 subjects per group.

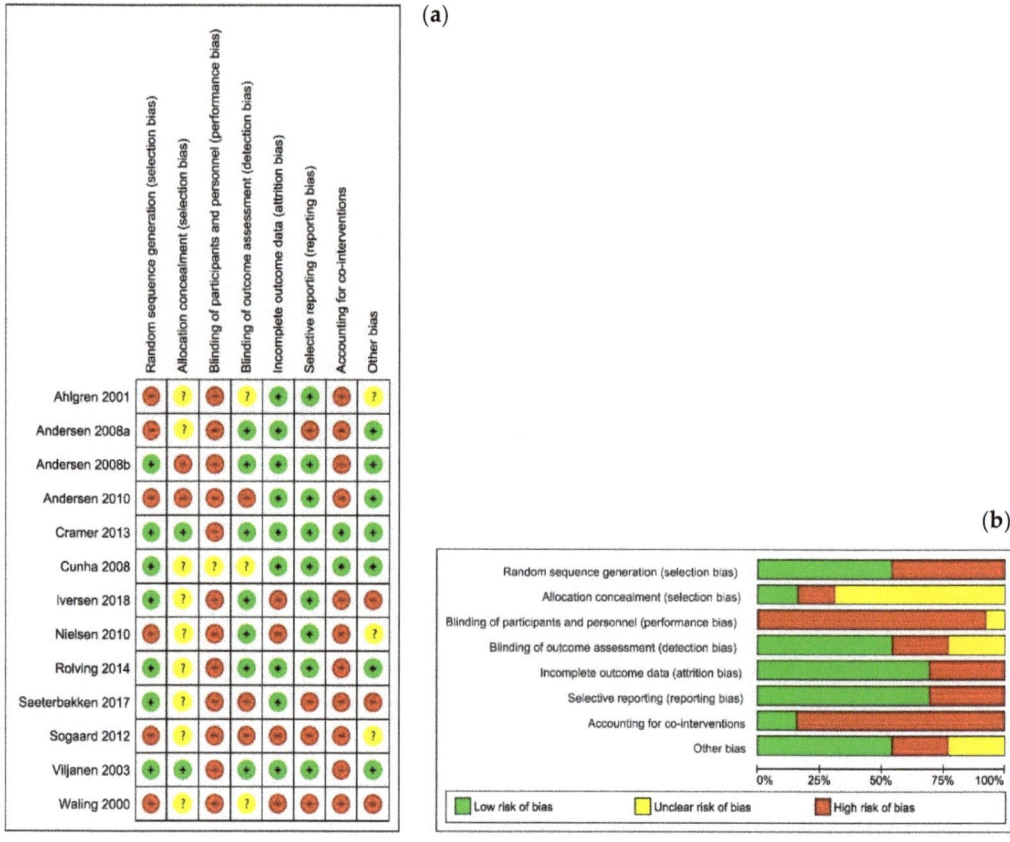

Figure 2. Risk of bias summary. These graphs illustrate the review authors' judgements about each risk of bias item for each included study (**a**) and presented as percentages across all included studies (**b**). Review Manager (RevMan) 5.3. [34]. Legend: (+) indicates "low risk of bias"; (?) indicates "unclear risk of bias"; (−) indicates "high risk of bias".

Information on risk of bias and the level of evidence, following the GRADE system, is presented per cluster in Table 2. Since none of the studies was double-blinded, all clusters started from a GRADE level of moderate.

Table 2. Risk of bias and grading the evidence per clusters based on exercise type and exercise effects over time OR follow-up (acute, short- and long-term effects).

1. SPECIFIC STRENGTH VS. NON-SPECIFIC AEROBIC

1.1. ACUTE EFFECTS

Study	VAS/NRS SI	VAS/NRS NSI	VAS/NRS REF	Risk of bias	GRADE
Andersen et al. [26]	↑ VAS in untrained patients; = VAS in trained patients	↓ VAS	ø		⊕⊕⊕⊖

1.2. SHORT-TERM EFFECTS

Study	SI	NSI	REF	Risk of bias	GRADE
Andersen et al. [32]	= pain (0–9 scale) in neck and shoulder pain patients		= pain (0–9 scale) in neck and shoulder pain patients		⊕⊕⊕⊖
Andersen et al. [26]	VAS in general ↓; VAS at worst ↓	VAS in general =; VAS at worst =			
Andersen et al. [33]	↓ pain (0–9 scale) > than REF		↓ pain (0–9 scale)		
Iversen et al. [21]	NRS =		ø		
Rolving et al. [23]	↓ NRS		ø		
Saeterbakken et al. [22]	VAS intensity ↓	VAS intensity ↓	VAS intensity =		
Søgaard et al. [24]	VAS at rest ↓ > than NSI and REF; VAS during repetitive and stress tasks =	VAS at rest =; VAS during repetitive tasks ↓ > than SI and REF	VAS at rest and during repetitive and stress tasks =		

1.3. LONG-TERM EFFECTS

Study	SI	NSI	REF	Risk of bias	GRADE
Andersen et al. [26]	VAS in general ↓; VAS at worst ↓ and keeps on, from short-term effects, stable and < than NSI and REF (therapy effects remained)	VAS in general =; VAS at worst = ø			⊕⊕⊕⊖
Saeterbakken et al. [22]	VAS intensity ↓		VAS intensity =		

2. SPECIFIC STRENGTH VS. BODY-MIND

2.1. ACUTE EFFECTS: no study

Table 2. *Cont.*

2.2.SHORT-TERM EFFECTS				
Ahlgren et al. [28]	Overall VAS ↓ ↓ VAS at worst > than REF	Overall VAS ↓	Overall VAS =	⊕⊕⊕
Cramer et al. [30]	VAS at motion ↓ VAS intensity =	VAS at motion ↓ VAS intensity ↓ > than SI	ø	⊕⊕⊕
Viljanen et al. [31]		= VAS		⊕⊕⊕
Waling et al. [29]	Pain at present = Pain in general = VAS at worst ↓ > than REF VAS at present and VAS at worst "exercisers" ↓ > than REF	Overall pain =	Overall pain =	⊕⊕⊕
2.3.LONG -TERM EFFECTS				
Viljanen et al. [31]		= VAS		⊕⊕⊕
3 -. SPECIFIC STRETCH VS. GENERAL STRETCH				
3.1.ACUTE EFFECTS: no study				
3.2.SHORT-TERM EFFECTS				
Cunha et al. [27]	↓ VAS		ø	⊕⊕⊕
3.3. LONG -TERM EFFECTS				
Cunha et al. [27]	↓ VAS (from baseline to 6 w follow-up post-intervention)		ø	⊕⊕⊕

Abbreviations: NRS, numerical rating scale; NSL non-specific intervention; REF, reference group; SI, specific intervention; VAS, visual analogical scale; W, week/s. Legend: ↑ indicates "increased/higher"; ↓ indicates "decreased/lower"; = indicates "no change"; (+) indicates "low risk of bias"; (−) indicates "high risk of bias". ø: not evaluated.

3.3. Study Characteristics

A total of 13 articles were reviewed, originating from nine data files (from now on referred to as studies). Although one study generally generated a single article, the results of three studies generated seven articles, whose differentiating aspects can be broadly disaggregated and conveyed as follows: (a) Andersen et al. [32,33], 2008 [32] referred to the short-term effects post-intervention with pain intensity as an outcome, while 2010 [33] referred to a higher sample size and pain regions as an additional outcome. (b) Andersen et al. [26], Nielsen et al. [25] and Søgaard et al. [24] varied their timeframes and outcomes. Andersen et al. [26] assessed the short-term effects post-intervention, similar to their counterparts, but included assessments halfway through the training period and after 10-week follow-up. An analysis was completed, looking at the acute effects after one session. Pain intensity was the outcome. Nielsen et al. [25] analyzed pressure-pain thresholds (PPTs), and Søgaard et al. [24] included repetitive and stressful work tasks as a test to evaluate the training effects on pain intensity. (c) Both Ahlgren et al. [28] and Waling et al. [29] evaluated the short-term effects post-intervention, varying in their assessed pain-related outcomes (pain intensity and PPTs and pain distribution, respectively).

The number of patients in each study varied from 33 to 616. Eight out of 13 articles only included women [22,24–29,31], whereas the other articles included both men and women. A total of 1229 women and 271 men were evaluated, with a mean age varying between 37.6 ± 6.1 years [28,29] and 50.3 ± 14.8 years [22] for the women and between 39.6 ± 9.2 years [23] and 49.0 ± 1.4 years for the men [32]. Most of the patients were office workers [22,24–26,31–33] and assembly line workers [24,26]. Six out of the 13 articles did not specify the patients jobs [21,23,27–30].

Out of 1500 patients, the vast majority (a total of 1269 patients) were diagnosed with non-specific chronic neck-shoulder pain [21–23,27,30–33]. The remaining 231 patients were diagnosed with trapezius myalgia [24–26,28,29]. No study analyzed patients with shoulder pain as a standalone disorder, and all were part of a sample of neck-shoulder pain patients.

Concerning the SE, strengthening exercises using dumbbells were used in six of the articles [24–26,31–33], followed by air machines [28,29], and elastic band [21–23] or isometric exercises using a towel [30]. One study included conventional auto-passive stretching as specific exercise [27].

The NSEs included in the studies were bicycle ergometer training [24–26], nordic walking [22], advice about staying physically active [21,23,32,33], global stretching [27], and body-mind therapies such as yoga [30], relaxation [21,31] or body awareness [21,28,29].

Most outcome measures concerned self-report pain measures. Visual analogue scales [22,24,26–31], 0–9 scales [32,33], and numeric rating scales [21,23] were used to evaluate pain. PPTs were measured in four of the included articles [21,25,29,30]. The other outcomes registered in the different articles were the body pain scale of the 36-item Short Form Health Survey (SF-36) [27,30], neck pain regions (n) [21,33], and pain drawings [21,29].

Frequency of therapies varied from 1 [33] to 5 times/week [30], with 3 times/week the most frequently used [21,23–26,28,29,31–33].

The total duration of the exercise program lasted from 6 weeks [27] to one year [32,33], with a modus of 9 to 10 weeks [22,24–26,28–30]. Follow-up varied between 6 weeks [27] and 9 months [31] after treatment ending.

All studies analyzed the short-term effects of exercise on pain. Four studies analyzed the long-term effects [22,26,27,31], and one study considered the acute effects after one exercise session [26].

Individual study results were clustered based on treatment types and follow-up effects: acute effects after one exercise session and training effects (acute, short-term, and long-term effects), as presented in Tables 3–5.

Table 3. Study characteristics. Specific strength vs. non-specific aerobic exercises.

Reference	Characteristics of Participants	Specific Intervention (SI)	Non-Specific Intervention (NSI) + Reference Intervention (REF)	Outcome Measures / Follow-Up Period	Main Results
Andersen et al. [32]	Office workers with neck or shoulder pain > 3/9 and ≥ 3 m Neck: n = 182, ♀(44 ± 0.9 y); ♂(49 ± 1.4 y) Shoulder: n = 94, ♀(44 ± 1.1 y); ♂(48 ± 1.4 y) SI group Neck: n = 61 Shoulder: n = 41 NSI group Neck: n = 59 Shoulder: n = 46 REF group Neck: n = 62 Shoulder: n = 37 ITT analysis	Specific neck-shoulder dynamic and static strengthening ex with dumbbells and inelastic strap - 20′ × 3/w for 1 y - 2/3 supervised - during working hours - Load ↑ when they performed > 15 reps/ex - Last 15″: high-speed dynamic power ex (kayaking or ergometer rowing)	**General fitness training** - 1 h/w during working hours for 1 y - Filled in a "contract", writing the ways to include + physical act in their lives - Swimming, fitness clubs, all-round strength and aerobic fitness lessons (1–4 visits/m), walking group sessions (step counters), group sessions of Nordic walking, aerobic fitness, etc. **REF group** - No physical act - Workplace ergonomics, stress management, etc. =supervision as SI and NSI	**Pain:** - Pain intensity during last 3 m (0–9 scale) ~baseline ~post-intervention (1 y)	**Short-term effects (post-intervention):** PAIN INTENSITY: - = SI, NSI and REF
Andersen et al. [33]	Same characteristics as Andersen et al. [32] n (at baseline) = 616 397 ♀(44.6 y); 219 ♂(45.7 y) (67 excluded/withdrew = 549) SI group n = 180 NSI group n = 187 REF group n = 182 ITT analysis			**Pain:** - Pain intensity during last 3 m (0–9 scale) - Pain regions (n = 0–11), with a VAS ≥ 3/9 ~baseline ~post-intervention (1 y)	**Short-term effects (post-intervention):** PAIN INTENSITY: - ↓ SI, NSI and REF - ΔSI and ΔNSI > ΔREF Pain regions (n): - ↓ SI and NSI; =REF

Table 3. *Cont.*

Reference	Characteristics of Participants	Specific Intervention (SI)	Non-Specific Intervention (NSI) + Reference Intervention (REF)	Outcome Measures / Follow-Up Period	Main Results
Andersen et al. [26]	♀office workers (30–60 y), assembly line or office workers, with CNSP (≥30 d in the last y), reporting pain ≥ 1 episode/w + pain intensities at T0 ≥ 3 (0–9 scale) + diagnosed as trapezius myalgia. $n = 48$ ♀ (end 43 ♀) 44 ± 8 y **SI group** $n = 18$ ♀, 44 ± 8 y **NSI group** $n = 16$ ♀, 49 ± 7 y **REF group** $n = 14$ ♀ (end 9 ♀) 48 ± 11 y	5 neck-shoulder specific strengthening ex with dumbbells - 20′ × 3/w supervised for 10 w - 3 sets (25–35″)/ex - High intensity (consecutive concentric and eccentric muscle contractions without pause or breaks) - Load progressively ↑ 12 → 8 RM; (~70 → 80% max intensity)	Bicycle ergometer training - 20′ × 3/w supervised for 10 w - High intensity - Intensity progressively ↑ 50 → 70% (Vo_{2max}) **REF group** - 1 h/w for 10 w - No physical act - Health counseling on group + on individual level (workplace ergonomics, diet, relaxation,...) - = supervision as SI and NSI	Pain (diary report): - General pain (VAS1) - Pain at worst (VAS2) - Pain immediately before the session (VAS3) - Pain immediately after the session (VAS4) ~baseline ~half of training period ~post-intervention (10 w) ~10 w follow-up	Acute effects after 1 ex session • 1st half of training period: - VAS4-VAS3: ↑ SI; ↓ NSI. Effects lasted for 2 h - ΔNSI > ΔSI and REF • 2nd half of training period: VAS4-VAS3: - ↓ NSI; = SI. Effects lasted for 2 h - ΔNSI > ΔSI and REF Short-term effects (post-intervention): VAS1,2: - ↓ SI; = NSI and REF - ΔSI > ΔNSI and REF Long-term effects (follow-up): VAS1,2: - ↓ SI; = NSI and REF - ΔSI > ΔNSI and REF
Nielsen et al. [25]				PPTs: - Painful trapezius (PPT1) - Non-painful tibialis anterior (PPT2) ~baseline ~post-intervention (10 w)	Short-term effects (post-intervention): PPT1: - ↑ SI; = NSI and REF - Δmyalgia < Δcontrols PPT2: - ↑ SI and NSI; = REF - Δmyalgia < Δcontrols
Søgaard et al. [24]	♀performing monotonous & repetitive work tasks + trapezius myalgia (30–60 y) $n = 47$ ♀ (end 39 ♀) **SI group** $n = 16$ ♀ 44.6 ± 8.5 y **NSI group** $n = 15$ ♀ 45.5 ± 8.0 y **REF group** $n = 16$ ♀ (end 8 ♀) 42.5 ± 11.1 y			Pain: - At rest (VAS1): measured prior to the repetitive task - During repetitive task (VAS2): pegboard work (40′), VAS every 5′. Changes in VAS slope (time curve) (mm/min)- VAS after 120′ rest immediately before a stressful Stroop task (VAS3). - VAS immediately after the stressful Stroop task (VAS4) ~baseline (2 d before the intervention) ~post-intervention (10 w)	Short-term effects (post-intervention): VAS1: - ↓ SI; = NSI and REF - ΔSI > ΔNSI and ΔREF VAS2: - ↓ NSI; = SI & REF - ΔNSI > ΔSI and ΔREF VAS3, 4: - ΔSI = ΔNSI = ΔREF

117

Table 3. Cont.

Reference	Characteristics of Participants	Specific Intervention (SI)	Non-Specific Intervention (NSI) + Reference Intervention (REF)	Outcome Measures / Follow-Up Period	Main Results
Iversen et al. [21]	Patients (16–70 y) + non-specific neck pain ≥ 3 m or ≥ 2 times ≥ 4 w in the past y and worst neck pain in last 2 w NRS ≥ 4 n = 59 (39 ♀ & 20 ♂) (end 31) **SI group** n = 29 (end 15) 20 ♀ & 9 ♂ 44.6 ± 8.1 y **NSI group** n = 30 (end 16) 19 ♀ & 11 ♂ 48.2 ± 10.6 y	MDR + 8 neck-shoulder specific strengthening ex. with elastic bands - 3 w MDR: patient education, stress management, group discussions - 9 w SI program: 3 times/w. Supervised at 1st and 3rd w - +1 session NSI - +3 group booster sessions - Yellow–gold Theraband® - Reps/ex until muscular failure - Load progressively ↑: sets/reps/band color - Diary for daily registration	MDR + General fitness training - 3 w MDR: patient education, stress management, group discussions - 9 w NSI program: 1st and 3rd w, 4 and 3 supervised sessions - Introduction to group-based and individual act (circle-training, endurance, low-intensity resistance, stretching) - +3 group booster sessions - Diary for daily registration	**Pain:** - Current neck pain (NRS1) - Pain at worst last 2 w (NRS2) - Pain at worst in last 4 w (NRS3) **PD:** Additional pain sites (n) **PPTs:** tibialis anterior muscle ~baseline ~post-intervention (12 w)	**Short-term effects (post-intervention):** NRS, pain sites and PPTs: - = SI and NSI - ΔSI = ΔNSI
Rolving et al. [23]	Patients on sick leave from work (4–16 w prior to study) due to non-specific neck pain (18–60 y) n = 83 (60 ♀ & 23 ♂) (end 71) **SI group** n = 43 (end 34) 27 ♀ & 16 ♂ 39.6 ± 9.2 y **NSI group** n = 40 (end 37) 33 ♀ & 7 ♂ 39.0 ± 11.0 y ITT analysis	General fitness training and 4 specific neck-shoulder-strengthening ex. With elastic band - 15–20′ supervised training ≥ 3 times/w for 12 w - Participants instructed to be physically active ≥ 30′/d, 3–4 h/w - 3 × 5 reps/ex - Load progressively ↑/2 w - Diary for daily registration	General fitness training - Participants instructed to be physically active ≥ 30′/d, 3–4 h/w for 12 w - Minimal supervision - Diary for daily registration	**Pain:** - Pain intensity during last w (0–10 scale) (NRS) ~baseline ~post-intervention (12 w)	**Short-term effects (post-intervention):** NRS: - ↓ SI and NSI - ΔSI = ΔNSI

Table 3. Cont.

Reference	Characteristics of Participants	Specific Intervention (SI)	Non-Specific Intervention (NSI) + Reference Intervention (REF)	Outcome Measures / Follow-Up Period	Main Results
Saeterbakken et al. [22]	♀ office workers with neck or shoulder pain ≥ 2 and ≥ 3 m, n = 34 ♀ (end 31 ♀) **SI group** n = 13 (end 12) 47.6 ± 11.9 y **NSI group** n = 10 (end 9) 41.0 ± 15.3 y **REF group** n = 11 (end 10) 50.3 ± 14.8 y	**5 neck-shoulder specific strengthening ex with elastic bands** - 30′ supervised training 2 times/w for 10 w - ≥ 2 d between sessions - 3 × 12 reps (3″/rep) - 1′ pause between ex. - Loads that allowed 12 reps, ending at or near to fatigue. When 17 reps, load progressively ↑	**Nordic walking** - 30′ supervised training 2 times/w for 10 w - ≥ 2 d between sessions - Moderate intensity. Progressively ↑ (Borg 6–20 scale) - Nordic walking poles: individually adjusted **REF group** - No physical act	**Pain:** - Pain intensity (last 5 days' mean) (VAS1) ~ baseline ~ post-intervention (10 w) ~ 10 w follow-up	**Short-term effects (post-intervention):** VAS 1: - ↓ SI and NSI; = REF - ΔSI = ΔNSI = ΔREF **Long-term effects (follow-up):** VAS1: - ↓ SI? (p = 0.058) and NSI; = REF - ΔSI = ΔNSI = ΔREF

Abbreviations: ′, minute/s; ″, second/s; ↑, increased/higher; ↓, decreased/lower; =, no change; ♂, male subjects; ♀, female subjects; ACT, activity/ies; D, day/s; EX, exercise/s; ITT, intention to treat analysis; M, month/s; n, number of subjects; NRS, numerical rating scale; NSI, non-specific intervention; PD, pain drawings; REF, reference group; REP/S, repetition/s; RM, repetition maximum; SI, specific intervention; VAS, visual analogical scale; W, week/s; Y, years.

Table 4. Study characteristics. Specific strength vs. body-mind exercises.

Reference	Characteristics of Participants	Specific Intervention (SI)	Non-Specific Intervention (NSI) + Reference Intervention (REF)	Outcome Measures / Follow-Up Period	Main Results
Ahlgren et al. [28]	♀ < 45 y with trapezius myalgia for ≥1 y + sick leave ≤ 1 m last y $n = 136$ ♀ (−34 excluded/withdrew = 102 ♀) 38.2 y **SI1 group** $n = 29$ ♀ 38.0 ± 6.0 y **SI2 group** $n = 28$ ♀ 38.5 ± 5.6 y **NSI group** $n = 25$ ♀ 37.6 ± 6.1 y **REF group** $n = 20$ ♀ 38.9 ± 5.4 y	- 3 × 1 h/w supervised for 10 w - 15′ general warm-up - Last 10′: stretching **SI1 group**: 4 neck-shoulder specific strengthening concentric ex with air machines - Load individualized to 2 × 12 RM - Load ↑ when 3 sets = comfortable **SI2 group**: endurance training with arm ergometer alternated with specific arm ex. with rubber expanders - 4 × 3′ arm ergometer (110–120 bpm) - Specific arm ex: 3′ - Expanders individually loaded to allow 30–35 RM/ex/set (3 sets)	**Body awareness** - 3 × 1 h/w supervised for 10 w - 15′ general warm-up - Muscular tension awareness and relaxation - Attention focused on balance, posture and breathing **REF group** - 1 × 2 h/w supervised for 10 w - No physical act. Learn and discuss stress management	**Pain:** - Pain at present (VAS1) - Pain in general (VAS2) - Pain at worst (VAS3) ~baseline ~post-intervention (10 w)	**Short-term effects (post-intervention):** VAS1: - ↓ SI1, SI2 and NSI; = REFVAS2: - ↓ SI1, SI2 and NSI; = REFVAS3: - ↓ SI1, SI2 and NSI; = REF- ΔSI1 & ΔSI2 > ΔREF
Waling et al. [29]				**PPTs**: 6 trigger points in the 3 portions of the trapezius (TP) muscle (TP2, TP4, TP5), 2 sides (R, L) **PD**: Pain distribution and pain character (% total body area)	**Short-term effects (post-intervention):** VAS 1: - ↓ SI1, SI2, NSI; = REF - ΔSI1 = ΔSI2 = ΔNSI = ΔREF - Δ "exercisers" (SI1 + SI2 + NSI) > ΔREF VAS 2: - ↓ SI1, SI2, NSI; = REF - ΔSI1 = Δ SI2 = ΔNSI = ΔREF VAS3: - ↓ SI1, SI2, NSI; = REF - ΔSI1 and ΔSI2 > ΔREF - Δ "exercisers" (SI1 + SI2 + NSI) > ΔREF PPTs: - ↑SI2 (in 2 trigger points); = SI1, NSI and REF - TP2L: ΔSI1 < ΔSI2 ΔSI2 > ΔREF - TP5L: ΔSI2 > ΔREF ΔNSI > ΔREF - TP2R, TP5R and TP5L: Δ "exercisers" (SI1 + SI2 + NSI) > ΔREF PD: - ΔSI1 = ΔSI2 = ΔNSI = ΔREF

Table 4. Cont.

Reference	Characteristics of Participants	Specific Intervention (SI)	Non-Specific Intervention (NSI) + Reference Intervention (REF)	Outcome Measures / Follow-Up Period	Main Results
Cramer et al. [30]	Patients (18–60 y) + non-specific neck pain VAS ≥ 4 and ≥ 3 m $n = 51$ 42 ♀ and 9 ♂ 47.8 ± 10.4 y VAS 4.5 ± 1.9 **SI group** $n = 26$ 21 ♀ and 5 ♂ 49.5 ± 9.5 y **NSI group** $n = 25$ 21 ♀ and 4 ♂ 46.2 ± 11.2 y	**Specific neck-shoulder posture awareness, stretching and strengthening ex** - 10′/d (home ex) for 9 w - Self-care manual - Sitting position - Use of a towel as an aid - Diary	**Yoga** - 90′ yoga session/w for 9 w: - 10–15 patients - 8–10 yoga postures/session - Last 15′ relaxation - Iyengar yoga type - 3 sitting + 3 standing postures - No previous experience in yoga + 10′/d (home ex) - Diary	**Pain:** - Pain at rest (VAS1) - Pain at motion (VAS2) (after 6 reps of head flex, ext, lateral flex R/L, rotation R/L) (mean pain intensity of the 6 movements) **SF36-BP** (bodily pain items) **PPTs:** - Maximal pain site (PPT) ~baseline ~post-intervention (9 w)	**Short-term effects (post-intervention):** VAS1: - ↓NSI; = SI - ΔNSI > ΔSI VAS2: - ↓ SI & NSI - ΔSI = ΔNSI SF36-BP: - ↑ NSI; = SI - ΔNSI > ΔSI PPTs: - ↑ NSI; = SI - ΔNSI > ΔSI
Viljanen et al. [31]	♀ office workers (30–60 y) with chronic non-specific neck pain ≥ 3 m $n = 393$ ♀ (end 340 ♀) **SI group** $n = 135$ ♀ (end 111 ♀) 45 ± 6.6 y **NSI group** $n = 128$ ♀ (end 110 ♀) 43 ± 7.3 y **REF group** $n = 130$ ♀ (end 119 ♀) 44 ± 7.4 y ITT analysis	**Specific neck-shoulder dynamic strengthening ex with dumbbells** - 3 times/w for 12 w + reinforcement training for 1 w: - Supervised groups ≤ 10 people - 1–3 kg according to RM test with 7.5 kg - Intensity progressively ↑ - Stretching after each ex	**Relaxation** - 3 times/w for 12 w + reinforcement training for 1 w: - Supervised groups ≤ 10 people - Progressive relaxation method, autogenic training, functional relaxation and systematic desensitisation - ≠ Techniques being incorporated through the 12 w **REF group** - Ordinary act - No supervision	**Pain:** - Pain intensity (VAS) ~Baseline ~post-intervention (13 w) ~3 m follow-up ~9 m follow-up	**Short-term effects (post-intervention):** VAS: - =SI, NSI and REF - ΔSI = ΔNSI = ΔREF **Long-term effects (both follow-up moments):** VAS: - =SI, NSI and REF - ΔSI = ΔNSI = ΔREF

Abbreviations: ′, minute/s; ↑, increased/higher; ↓, decreased/lower; =, no change; ≠, different; ♂, male subjects; ♀, female subjects; CI, confidence interval; D, day/s; EX, exercise/s; EXT, extension; FLEX, flexion; ITT, intention to treat analysis; KG, kilogram/s; L, left; M, month/s; n, number of subjects; NSI, Non-specific intervention; PD, pain drawings; R, right; REF, reference group; REPS, repetitions; RM, repetition maximum; SI, specific intervention; VAS, visual analogical scale; W, week/s; Y, years.

Table 5. Study characteristics. Specific stretch vs. general stretch.

Reference	Characteristics of Participants	Specific Intervention (SI)	Non-Specific Intervention (NSI) + Reference Intervention (REF)	Outcome Measures / Follow-Up Period	Main Results
Cunha et al. [27]	♀(35–60 y) with chronic neck pain lasting ≥ 3 m $n = 33$ ♀(end 31 ♀) **SI group** $n = 17$ (end 16) 48.7 ± 7.3 y **NSI group** $n = 16$ (end 15) 44.4 ± 7.8 y	**Static neck-shoulder stretching ex** - 60′ × 2/w for 6 w - 30′ manual therapy and breathing ex + 30′ conventional auto-passive stretching - 2 × 30″/ex	**Global posture reeducation stretching** - 60′ × 2/w for 6 w - 30′ manual therapy and breathing ex + 30′ supervised muscle chain stretching - 2 postures: posterior and anterior chains (15′/posture)	**Pain:** - Pain intensity (VAS) **SF36-BP** (bodily pain items) ~baseline ~post-intervention (6 w) ~6 w follow-up	**Short-term effects (post-intervention):** VAS: - ↓ SI and NSI - ΔSI = ΔNSI SF36-BP: - ↑ SI and NSI - ΔSI = ΔNSI **Long-term effects (follow-up):** VAS: - ↓ SI and NSI - ΔSI = ΔNSI SF36-BP: - ↑ SI and NSI - ΔSI = ΔNSI

Abbreviations: ′, minute/s; ″, second/s; ↑, increased/higher; ↓, decreased/lower; =, no change; ♀, female subjects; EX, exercise; M, month/s; n, number of subjects; NSI, Non-specific intervention; REF, reference group; SI, specific intervention; VAS, visual analogical scale; W, week/s; Y, year/s.

3.4. Data Synthesis

3.4.1. Specific Strength vs. Non-Specific Aerobic Exercises

A total of 8 out of the 13 articles analyzed the effects of specific strength training compared to general aerobic exercises (Table 3).

- Acute effects

One article analyzed the acute effects of a single bout of exercise [26]: non-specific exercise, based on a generic aerobic program, caused an immediate post-exercise pain reduction. Specific strength training showed an immediate post-exercise pain increase during the first half of the training period that flattened near the end of the 10-week training program. Both pain increases and reductions leveled off 2 h after exercise.

- Short-term effects

Seven out of the 13 articles analyzed the short-term effects of physical exercise on pain behavior [21–26,32,33]. Both specific strength training and non-specific physical exercise programs of 10–12 weeks (20–30 min training, 2–3 days/week) resulted in a decrease in general pain [22,23,32,33], in pain during a repetitive task [24], and in the number of pain regions [33] compared to a reference intervention. However, in two articles, specific strength training for 20 min/day, 3 times/week was superior in reducing pain in general [26], pain at worst [26], and pain at rest [24] after 10 weeks of treatment in women with trapezius myalgia.

Two articles reported the effects of exercise on PPTs, reporting no differences between specific and non-specific training [21,25]. While Iversen et al. [21] found no changes after the exercise program, Nielsen et al. [25] reported that pain sensitivity at a pain-free reference muscle was decreased (i.e., higher PPTs) in response to both specific strength training (concentric and eccentric contractions) and non-specific fitness training (bicycle ergometer) after 10 weeks of exercise (20-min training, 3 days/week) in women with trapezius myalgia.

- Long-term effects

Two articles analyzed the effects of specific strength training vs. aerobic exercise 10 weeks after finishing the exercise program, with inconsistent results. Saeterbakken et al. [22] found that both exercise types (specific and non-specific) had a similar effect on pain reduction that lasted during follow-up compared with no effect in a reference group. Nevertheless, the study performed by Andersen et al. [26] reported that specific strength training resulted in significant pain reduction, in contrast to the non-specific aerobic exercise group, which consolidated in the further 10-week follow-up period.

In conclusion, there is low evidence that specific strengthening exercises and non-specific fitness training produce similar short-term effects regarding pain relief. There is only preliminary evidence that immediate acute response to exercise is more favorable for the non-specific exercise program. There is also very low evidence that the long-term effects are favored by specific strengthening exercises.

3.4.2. Specific Strength vs. Body Mind Exercises

A total of 4 out of the 13 articles analyzed the effects of specific strength training compared to body mind therapies (Table 4) [28–31].

- Short-term effects

All the mentioned articles reported positive short-term effects of exercise programs on pain behavior. There were no differences between specific strength training and NSE (body-mind exercises through body awareness and yoga), as both resulted in a decrease in the intensities of pain at motion [30], pain at present, pain at worst, and pain in general [28,29] after 9 or more weeks of treatment (3 days/week).

However, there were inconsistent results in two of the articles regarding three outcomes: specific strength training during 60 min/day, 3 times/week, reduced pain at worst after 10 weeks of treatment in women with trapezius myalgia compared to body-awareness exercises [28]. Yoga classes for 90 min/week reduced pain in general and bodily pain items from SF-36, after 9 weeks of practice, in patients with non-specific neck pain, compared to specific strength exercises [30].

Two articles reported the effects of exercise on PPTs [29,30]. Cramer et al. [30] demonstrated better results with non-specific interventions: yoga exercises, practiced with an instructor for 90 min/week for 9 weeks, decreased pressure sensitivity in non-specific neck pain patients compared to strength training for 10 min/day. The study of Waling et al. [29] found no differences between SE and NSE: pressure sensitivity significantly decreased at four myofascial trigger points of the trapezius muscle in both exercise regimens, compared to a reference group.

For pain drawings, no changes were seen in the extent of painful body area in any of the exercise groups (body awareness and specific strength) [29].

- Long-term effects

One article analyzed the effects of a 13-week specific-strength training (3 days/week) compared to relaxation training and a reference group, after 9 months follow-up, concluding that no difference was found in neck pain intensity in questions concerning neck pain disability between the three groups in a sample of 393 female office workers with chronic non-specific neck pain [31].

There is moderate evidence that exercises reduce pain in the short-term compared to a reference group and there seems to be no difference for different types of exercise. For the long-term, there is only preliminary evidence that there is no difference between exercise groups and the reference group.

3.4.3. Specific Stretch vs. General Stretch Exercises

- Short and long-term effects

One article investigated the effects, both short and long-term, of specific versus general stretches on pain reduction (Table 5) [27]. These authors suggest that conventional specific stretching and muscle chain stretching (30 min, 2 times/week), in association with manual therapy (30 min, 2 times/week), were equally effective in reducing the pain of female patients with chronic neck pain, both post-treatment and at six weeks after ending the treatment.

There is preliminary evidence that specific and non-specific stretching exercises are equally beneficial for pain reduction in female patients with chronic neck pain, although more studies are needed.

4. Discussion

This is the first systematic review specifically examining the effect of SE compared with NSE on pain in the rehabilitation of patients with CNSP.

The aim of this review was to evaluate the effect of SE, involving exercises focused on the neck and/or shoulder region, focused on CNSP patients, looking for pain reduction/increases compared to NSE.

There is considerable evidence of pain reduction after an exercise program, both specific and non-specific, in the short- and long-term [22,24,26,28,29,32,33]. For the short-term effects, 9 out of 13 articles did not favor a particular type of exercise [21–23,27–29,31–33], while 3 articles [24–26] found better effects on pain for specific training, and the other article favored non-specific training [30]. With regard to the long-term effects of exercise on pain, 3 out of 4 articles found that specific [26], or both exercise types independently (specific and non-specific) [22,27], had a lasting effect on pain reduction. The other article found that exercise had no long-term effects on pain [31]. Nevertheless, regarding the acute effect of single bouts of exercise, only one article assessed this aspect [26], reporting an immediate pain reduction after non-specific exercise in contrast to specific resistance exercises. Consequently, more research is needed, specifically about acute and long-term effects.

These results are in line with a Cochrane systematic review evaluating the use of motor control as a specific exercise strategy among a chronic non-specific neck pain population [8]. The study suggested that specific motor control exercises were not superior to more general exercise strategies. Furthermore, the review of Booth et al. [35] did not provide evidence for the superiority of one exercise type in chronic musculoskeletal pain conditions. Therefore, the type of exercise might be less important than the act of doing exercise. Sluka et al. [36] suggest that this lack of specificity of exercise type may be related to the multiple and widespread mechanisms by which exercise works to reduce pain.

Although this aspect is out of the scope of the present review, it is interesting to try to elucidate the mechanisms that could explain our findings. The reason that the research to date has not shown any specific exercise to be superior may be that psychological and/or neurophysiological factors that are common to all exercise approaches have the greatest mediating effects on pain [37]. If changes in pain and disability occur without changes in physical function, then specific modalities of exercise and their dosage seem to be less relevant in chronic musculoskeletal pain [35,38]. It is tempting to speculate that exercise can indeed desensitize the central nervous system. This hypothesis has recently been supported through a review of the current evidence on the central mechanisms underlying exercise-induced pain and analgesia [39].

Exercise is likely to be most effective if tailored to individual patients with spinal pain. As Falla and Hodges [40] stated, current exercise programs for spinal pain treatment often rely on a one-size-fits-all approach and usually fall short of success. These authors provide evidence supporting the hypothesis that the outcome of exercise interventions can be optimized when targeted to the *right* people and adapted to the individual's presentation. In the same line, tailoring exercise to individual patients has been recommended for chronic musculoskeletal pain [17,41], which requires an initial assessment to understand the biological, psychological, and social factors contributing to pain and disability [35]. The dominant pain mechanism must also be considered to optimize exercise prescription. Indeed, a recent systematic review concluded that global (non-specific) exercises are preferred in nociplastic pain conditions, while more SE should be emphasized in non-nociplastic conditions [42]. In the present review, however, all the included studies used standardized exercise programs and no prior assessment was made to determine the patient's profile.

The level of supervision is also an important aspect in promoting treatment adherence and patients' motivation [35]. Supervised exercise programs have been recommended for chronic musculoskeletal pain [17,43]. In the present review, all studies but one [23] included supervised exercise sessions. This could be the reason that the drop-out rate was relatively low in those studies.

Finally, ongoing self-monitoring can be helpful to identify barriers to [14] and facilitators of exercise participation, motivate positive exercise behavior and increase participation [44]. In the present review, only five articles out of 13 did not use diaries to register their adherence to the exercise programs [22,24–26,31], which could also explain the high participation rate.

Thus, supervised exercise, individualized therapy, and self-management techniques may help to promote a successful rehabilitation program [14]; however, the quality of trials assessing these interventions is low [43], and further research is warranted.

Limitations

First, the main weakness of this review is the risk of bias. Random sequence generation, accounted co-interventions, and concealment of allocation were often not attained. Therefore, a note of caution is due here. Most studies failed to achieve blinding of the patients. Furthermore, the majority of studies relied on self-reported measures, prohibiting blinding of the assessors as well. Although blinding participants and therapists in an exercise trial is difficult to implement and cannot obviate the risk of bias, future studies should endeavor to limit the potential bias with the appropriate blinding of at least the assessors. Keeping the patients and therapists naïve regarding the received treatment should be attempted, as specific expectations and beliefs could influence outcomes. Assuming naïve patients is only possible in the studies evaluating different exercise modalities. This should be considered in future studies. Second, the number of RCTs included was low. The limited number of studies published in this area also raises the possibility of publication bias. Third, patient activity between post-test and follow-up was not controlled in any study. Finally, only four articles analyzed the follow-up period [22,26,27,31]. In two of these, the follow-up was limited to less than three months, which seems to be insufficient, as CNSP can last for up to several years [26,27]. This aspect limits any comment on the maintenance of the effects of exercise. Ongoing research including acute and follow-up schemes over six months is required to further validate our findings and determine the long-term effects of the intervention.

Furthermore, there was a lack of uniformity in the obtained results regarding the differences in the benefits between specific and non-specific exercises. The term "specific exercise" has been used to describe different types of exercises, such as stabilization [45], strengthening [46], individualized [47], supervised [48], and even what appear to be general exercises [49]. Non-specific exercise protocols usually address general flexibility, strength, and/or endurance training, including all body regions. Such inconsistency, together with an incomplete description of exercise details regarding dosage [8], are a possible reason for the inconsistent results found in different chronic pain populations. Therefore, the working mechanisms and exact definition and dosage of the exercise therapy modalities need to be further elaborated.

5. Conclusions

This systematic review shows interesting findings for pain relief with regard to training effects using specific and/or non-specific exercise for CNSP. Both specific (neck and/or shoulder exercises) and NSE seem to be effective for short-term pain reduction in patients with CNSP.

Based on the acute effects, there is only preliminary evidence that a bout of non-specific exercise seems to be more tolerable for patients with CNSP, overcoming the exacerbation in the beginning. Regarding the long-term effects, SE seems to be the best option, although the evidence for this is very limited. As the evidence is still rather restricted, this review highlights the need for further RCTs comparing the effects of injury-focused (specific) exercises versus more general (non-specific) exercises, and a need to better understand the definition and dosage of exercise therapy modalities to improve clinical application.

Author Contributions: Conceptualization, M.M., L.V. and L.D.; methodology, M.M.; data collection and analysis, L.D., M.A.-R. and M.M.; writing—original draft preparation, L.D. and M.M.; writing—review and editing, M.A.-R., L.V., E.L., F.S., M.G.C.A.M.M. and K.D.M.; visualization, F.S. and M.G.C.A.M.M.; supervision, M.M. All authors have read and agreed to the published version of the manuscript.

Funding: This research received no external funding.

Institutional Review Board Statement: This is a systematic review of published data. We had no access to any individualized patient data. Therefore, no informed patient consent or ethical approval was needed for this study.

Informed Consent Statement: Not applicable.

Data Availability Statement: The data presented in this study are available from the corresponding author upon reasonable request.

Conflicts of Interest: The authors declare no conflict of interest.

References

1. Hakala, P.; Rimpelä, A.; Salminen, J.J.; Virtanen, S.M.; Rimpelä, M. Back, Neck, and Shoulder Pain in Finnish Adolescents: National Cross Sectional Surveys. *BMJ* **2002**, *325*, 743. [CrossRef] [PubMed]

2. Ihlebaek, C.; Brage, S.; Eriksen, H.R. Health Complaints and Sickness Absence in Norway, 1996–2003. *Occup. Med. Oxf. Engl.* **2007**, *57*, 43–49. [CrossRef] [PubMed]
3. Ferrari, R.; Russell, A.S. Regional Musculoskeletal Conditions: Neck Pain. *Best Pract. Res. Clin. Rheumatol.* **2003**, *17*, 57–70. [CrossRef]
4. Urwin, M.; Symmons, D.; Allison, T.; Brammah, T.; Busby, H.; Roxby, M.; Simmons, A.; Williams, G. Estimating the Burden of Musculoskeletal Disorders in the Community: The Comparative Prevalence of Symptoms at Different Anatomical Sites, and the Relation to Social Deprivation. *Ann. Rheum. Dis.* **1998**, *57*, 649–655. [CrossRef] [PubMed]
5. van der Windt, D.A.; Koes, B.W.; de Jong, B.A.; Bouter, L.M. Shoulder Disorders in General Practice: Incidence, Patient Characteristics, and Management. *Ann. Rheum. Dis.* **1995**, *54*, 959–964. [CrossRef] [PubMed]
6. Winters, J.C.; Sobel, J.S.; Groenier, K.H.; Arendzen, J.H.; Meyboom-de Jong, B. The Long-Term Course of Shoulder Complaints: A Prospective Study in General Practice. *Rheumatol. Oxf. Engl.* **1999**, *38*, 160–163. [CrossRef]
7. Linsell, L.; Dawson, J.; Zondervan, K.; Rose, P.; Randall, T.; Fitzpatrick, R.; Carr, A. Prevalence and Incidence of Adults Consulting for Shoulder Conditions in UK Primary Care; Patterns of Diagnosis and Referral. *Rheumatol. Oxf. Engl.* **2006**, *45*, 215–221. [CrossRef]
8. Gross, A.R.; Paquin, J.P.; Dupont, G.; Blanchette, S.; Lalonde, P.; Cristie, T.; Graham, N.; Kay, T.M.; Burnie, S.J.; Gelley, G.; et al. Exercises for Mechanical Neck Disorders: A Cochrane Review Update. *Man. Ther.* **2016**, *24*, 25–45. [CrossRef]
9. Teasell, R.W.; McClure, J.A.; Walton, D.; Pretty, J.; Salter, K.; Meyer, M.; Sequeira, K.; Death, B. A Research Synthesis of Therapeutic Interventions for Whiplash-Associated Disorder (WAD): Part 4-Noninvasive Interventions for Chronic WAD. *Pain Res. Manag.* **2010**, *15*, 313–322. [CrossRef]
10. Childs, J.D.; Cleland, J.A.; Elliott, J.M.; Teyhen, D.S.; Wainner, R.S.; Whitman, J.M.; Sopky, B.J.; Godges, J.J.; Flynn, T.W. American Physical Therapy Association Neck Pain: Clinical Practice Guidelines Linked to the International Classification of Functioning, Disability, and Health from the Orthopedic Section of the American Physical Therapy Association. *J. Orthop. Sports Phys. Ther.* **2008**, *38*, A1–A34. [CrossRef]
11. Stewart, M.J.; Maher, C.G.; Refshauge, K.M.; Herbert, R.D.; Bogduk, N.; Nicholas, M. Randomized Controlled Trial of Exercise for Chronic Whiplash-Associated Disorders. *Pain* **2007**, *128*, 59–68. [CrossRef]
12. Littlewood, C.; Bateman, M.; Brown, K.; Bury, J.; Mawson, S.; May, S.; Walters, S.J. A Self-Managed Single Exercise Programme versus Usual Physiotherapy Treatment for Rotator Cuff Tendinopathy: A Randomised Controlled Trial (the SELF Study). *Clin. Rehabil.* **2016**, *30*, 686–696. [CrossRef]
13. Lannersten, L.; Kosek, E. Dysfunction of Endogenous Pain Inhibition during Exercise with Painful Muscles in Patients with Shoulder Myalgia and Fibromyalgia. *Pain* **2010**, *151*, 77–86. [CrossRef]
14. Kroll, H.R. Exercise Therapy for Chronic Pain. *Phys. Med. Rehabil. Clin. N. Am.* **2015**, *26*, 263–281. [CrossRef]
15. Naugle, K.M.; Fillingim, R.B.; Riley, J.L. A Meta-Analytic Review of the Hypoalgesic Effects of Exercise. *J. Pain Off. J. Am. Pain Soc.* **2012**, *13*, 1139–1150. [CrossRef]
16. Nijs, J.; Kosek, E.; Van Oosterwijck, J.; Meeus, M. Dysfunctional Endogenous Analgesia during Exercise in Patients with Chronic Pain: To Exercise or Not to Exercise? *Pain Physician* **2012**, *15*, ES205–ES213. [CrossRef] [PubMed]
17. Meeus, M.; Nijs, J.; Van Wilgen, P.; Noten, S.; Goubert, D.; Huijnen, I. Moving on to Movement in Patients with Chronic Joint Pain. *Pain* **2016**, *1*, 23–35.
18. Moher, D.; Liberati, A.; Tetzlaff, J.; Altman, D.G. PRISMA Group Preferred Reporting Items for Systematic Reviews and Meta-Analyses: The PRISMA Statement. *PLoS Med.* **2009**, *6*, e1000097. [CrossRef]
19. Coghlan, J.A.; Buchbinder, R.; Green, S.; Johnston, R.V.; Bell, S.N. Surgery for Rotator Cuff Disease. *Cochrane Database Syst. Rev.* **2008**, *1*, CD005619. [CrossRef] [PubMed]
20. Balshem, H.; Helfand, M.; Schünemann, H.J.; Oxman, A.D.; Kunz, R.; Brozek, J.; Vist, G.E.; Falck-Ytter, Y.; Meerpohl, J.; Norris, S.; et al. GRADE Guidelines: 3. Rating the Quality of Evidence. *J. Clin. Epidemiol.* **2011**, *64*, 401–406. [CrossRef] [PubMed]
21. Iversen, V.M.; Vasseljen, O.; Mork, P.J.; Fimland, M.S. Resistance Training vs General Physical Exercise in Multidisciplinary Rehabilitation of Chronic Neck Pain: A Randomized Controlled Trial. *J. Rehabil. Med.* **2018**, *50*, 743–750. [CrossRef] [PubMed]
22. Saeterbakken, A.H.; Nordengen, S.; Andersen, V.; Fimland, M.S. Nordic Walking and Specific Strength Training for Neck- and Shoulder Pain in Office Workers: A Pilot-Study. *Eur. J. Phys. Rehabil. Med.* **2017**, *53*, 928–935. [CrossRef] [PubMed]
23. Rolving, N.; Christiansen, D.H.; Andersen, L.L.; Skotte, J.; Ylinen, J.; Jensen, O.K.; Nielsen, C.V.; Jensen, C. Effect of Strength Training in Addition to General Exercise in the Rehabilitation of Patients with Non-Specific Neck Pain. A Randomized Clinical Trial. *Eur. J. Phys. Rehabil. Med.* **2014**, *50*, 617–626.
24. Søgaard, K.; Blangsted, A.K.; Nielsen, P.K.; Hansen, L.; Andersen, L.L.; Vedsted, P.; Sjøgaard, G. Changed Activation, Oxygenation, and Pain Response of Chronically Painful Muscles to Repetitive Work after Training Interventions: A Randomized Controlled Trial. *Eur. J. Appl. Physiol.* **2012**, *112*, 173–181. [CrossRef] [PubMed]
25. Nielsen, P.K.; Andersen, L.L.; Olsen, H.B.; Rosendal, L.; Sjøgaard, G.; Søgaard, K. Effect of Physical Training on Pain Sensitivity and Trapezius Muscle Morphology. *Muscle Nerve* **2010**, *41*, 836–844. [CrossRef]
26. Andersen, L.L.; Kjaer, M.; Søgaard, K.; Hansen, L.; Kryger, A.I.; Sjøgaard, G. Effect of Two Contrasting Types of Physical Exercise on Chronic Neck Muscle Pain. *Arthritis Rheum.* **2008**, *59*, 84–91. [CrossRef]

27. Cunha, A.C.V.; Burke, T.N.; França, F.J.R.; Marques, A.P. Effect of Global Posture Reeducation and of Static Stretching on Pain, Range of Motion, and Quality of Life in Women with Chronic Neck Pain: A Randomized Clinical Trial. *Clin. Sao Paulo Braz.* **2008**, *63*, 763–770. [CrossRef] [PubMed]
28. Ahlgren, C.; Waling, K.; Kadi, F.; Djupsjöbacka, M.; Thornell, L.E.; Sundelin, G. Effects on Physical Performance and Pain from Three Dynamic Training Programs for Women with Work-Related Trapezius Myalgia. *J. Rehabil. Med.* **2001**, *33*, 162–169. [CrossRef]
29. Waling, K.; Sundelin, G.; Ahlgren, C.; Järvholm, B. Perceived Pain before and after Three Exercise Programs–a Controlled Clinical Trial of Women with Work-Related Trapezius Myalgia. *Pain* **2000**, *85*, 201–207. [CrossRef]
30. Cramer, H.; Lauche, R.; Hohmann, C.; Lüdtke, R.; Haller, H.; Michalsen, A.; Langhorst, J.; Dobos, G. Randomized-Controlled Trial Comparing Yoga and Home-Based Exercise for Chronic Neck Pain. *Clin. J. Pain* **2013**, *29*, 216–223. [CrossRef] [PubMed]
31. Viljanen, M.; Malmivaara, A.; Uitti, J.; Rinne, M.; Palmroos, P.; Laippala, P. Effectiveness of Dynamic Muscle Training, Relaxation Training, or Ordinary Activity for Chronic Neck Pain: Randomised Controlled Trial. *BMJ* **2003**, *327*, 475. [CrossRef]
32. Andersen, L.L.; Jørgensen, M.B.; Blangsted, A.K.; Pedersen, M.T.; Hansen, E.A.; Sjøgaard, G. A Randomized Controlled Intervention Trial to Relieve and Prevent Neck/Shoulder Pain. *Med. Sci. Sports Exerc.* **2008**, *40*, 983–990. [CrossRef]
33. Andersen, L.L.; Christensen, K.B.; Holtermann, A.; Poulsen, O.M.; Sjøgaard, G.; Pedersen, M.T.; Hansen, E.A. Effect of Physical Exercise Interventions on Musculoskeletal Pain in All Body Regions among Office Workers: A One-Year Randomized Controlled Trial. *Man. Ther.* **2010**, *15*, 100–104. [CrossRef]
34. *Review Manager (RevMan) The Cochrane Collaboration*; The Nordic Cochrane Centre: Copenhagen, Denmark, 2014.
35. Booth, J.; Moseley, G.L.; Schiltenwolf, M.; Cashin, A.; Davies, M.; Hübscher, M. Exercise for Chronic Musculoskeletal Pain: A Biopsychosocial Approach. *Musculoskelet. Care* **2017**, *15*, 413–421. [CrossRef]
36. Sluka, K.A.; Frey-Law, L.; Hoeger Bement, M. Exercise-Induced Pain and Analgesia? Underlying Mechanisms and Clinical Translation. *Pain* **2018**, *159* (Suppl. S1), S91–S97. [CrossRef]
37. Bialosky, J.E.; Beneciuk, J.M.; Bishop, M.D.; Coronado, R.A.; Penza, C.W.; Simon, C.B.; George, S.Z. Unraveling the Mechanisms of Manual Therapy: Modeling an Approach. *J. Orthop. Sports Phys. Ther.* **2018**, *48*, 8–18. [CrossRef] [PubMed]
38. Steiger, F.; Wirth, B.; de Bruin, E.D.; Mannion, A.F. Is a Positive Clinical Outcome after Exercise Therapy for Chronic Non-Specific Low Back Pain Contingent upon a Corresponding Improvement in the Targeted Aspect(s) of Performance? A Systematic Review. *Eur. Spine J. Off. Publ. Eur. Spine Soc. Eur. Spinal Deform. Soc. Eur. Sect. Cerv. Spine Res. Soc.* **2012**, *21*, 575–598. [CrossRef] [PubMed]
39. Lima, L.V.; Abner, T.S.S.; Sluka, K.A. Does Exercise Increase or Decrease Pain? Central Mechanisms Underlying These Two Phenomena. *J. Physiol.* **2017**, *595*, 4141–4150. [CrossRef] [PubMed]
40. Falla, D.; Hodges, P.W. Individualized Exercise Interventions for Spinal Pain. *Exerc. Sport Sci. Rev.* **2017**, *45*, 105–115. [CrossRef]
41. O'Riordan, C.; Clifford, A.; Van De Ven, P.; Nelson, J. Chronic Neck Pain and Exercise Interventions: Frequency, Intensity, Time, and Type Principle. *Arch. Phys. Med. Rehabil.* **2014**, *95*, 770–783. [CrossRef] [PubMed]
42. Ferro Moura Franco, K.; Lenoir, D.; Dos Santos Franco, Y.R.; Jandre Reis, F.J.; Nunes Cabral, C.M.; Meeus, M. Prescription of Exercises for the Treatment of Chronic Pain along the Continuum of Nociplastic Pain: A Systematic Review with Meta-Analysis. *Eur. J. Pain Lond. Engl.* **2021**, *25*, 51–70. [CrossRef]
43. Jordan, J.L.; Holden, M.A.; Mason, E.E.; Foster, N.E. Interventions to Improve Adherence to Exercise for Chronic Musculoskeletal Pain in Adults. *Cochrane Database Syst. Rev.* **2010**, *1*, CD005956. [CrossRef]
44. Moseley, G.L. Do Training Diaries Affect and Reflect Adherence to Home Programs? *Arthritis Rheum.* **2006**, *55*, 662–664. [CrossRef] [PubMed]
45. Ferreira, M.L.; Ferreira, P.H.; Latimer, J.; Herbert, R.D.; Hodges, P.W.; Jennings, M.D.; Maher, C.G.; Refshauge, K.M. Comparison of General Exercise, Motor Control Exercise and Spinal Manipulative Therapy for Chronic Low Back Pain: A Randomized Trial. *Pain* **2007**, *131*, 31–37. [CrossRef]
46. Holmgren, T.; Hallgren, H.B.; Öberg, B.; Adolfsson, L.; Johansson, K. Effect of Specific Exercise Strategy on Need for Surgery in Patients with Subacromial Impingement Syndrome: Randomised Controlled Study. *BMJ* **2012**, *344*, e787. [CrossRef] [PubMed]
47. Descarreaux, M.; Normand, M.C.; Laurencelle, L.; Dugas, C. Evaluation of a Specific Home Exercise Program for Low Back Pain. *J. Manip. Physiol. Ther.* **2002**, *25*, 497–503. [CrossRef]
48. Marshall, P.W.; Murphy, B.A. Muscle Activation Changes after Exercise Rehabilitation for Chronic Low Back Pain. *Arch. Phys. Med. Rehabil.* **2008**, *89*, 1305–1313. [CrossRef]
49. Hurwitz, E.L.; Morgenstern, H.; Chiao, C. Effects of Recreational Physical Activity and Back Exercises on Low Back Pain and Psychological Distress: Findings from the UCLA Low Back Pain Study. *Am. J. Public Health* **2005**, *95*, 1817–1824. [CrossRef] [PubMed]

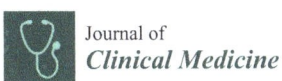

Review

Diet/Nutrition: Ready to Transition from a Cancer Recurrence/Prevention Strategy to a Chronic Pain Management Modality for Cancer Survivors?

Sevilay Tümkaya Yılmaz [1,2], Anneleen Malfliet [1,2,3,4], Ömer Elma [1,2], Tom Deliens [5], Jo Nijs [1,2,4,6], Peter Clarys [5], An De Groef [2,3,7,8] and Iris Coppieters [1,2,4,9,*]

[1] Pain in Motion Research Group (PAIN), Department of Physiotherapy, Human Physiology and Anatomy, Faculty of Physical Education and Physiotherapy, Vrije Universiteit Brussel, 1090 Brussels, Belgium; sevilay.tumkaya.yilmaz@vub.be (S.T.Y.); Anneleen.Malfliet@vub.be (A.M.); omer.elma@vub.ac.be (Ö.E.); Jo.Nijs@vub.be (J.N.)

[2] Pain in Motion International Research Group, 1090 Brussels, Belgium; an.degroef@kuleuven.be

[3] Research Foundation Flanders (FWO), 1000 Brussels, Belgium

[4] Department of Physical Medicine and Physiotherapy, University Hospital Brussels, 1090 Brussels, Belgium

[5] Department of Movement and Sport Sciences, Faculty of Physical Education and Physiotherapy, Vrije Universiteit Brussel, 1050 Brussels, Belgium; Tom.Deliens@vub.be (T.D.); Peter.Clarys@vub.be (P.C.)

[6] Institute of Neuroscience and Physiology, Unit of Physiotherapy, Department of Health & Rehabilitation, University of Gothenburg, 40530 Gothenburg, Sweden

[7] Department of Rehabilitation Sciences, Research Group for Rehabilitation in Internal Disorders, KU Leuven, 3000 Leuven, Belgium

[8] Department of Rehabilitation Sciences, MOVANT Research Group, University of Antwerp, 2000 Antwerp, Belgium

[9] Laboratory for Brain-Gut Axis Studies (LaBGAS), Translational Research Center for Gastrointestinal Disorders (TARGID), Department of Chronic Diseases, Metabolism, and Ageing, KU Leuven, 3000 Leuven, Belgium

* Correspondence: Iris.Coppieters@vub.be; Tel.: +32-(0)-2477-4326

Abstract: Evidence for the relationship between chronic pain and nutrition is mounting, and chronic pain following cancer is gaining recognition as a significant area for improving health care in the cancer survivorship population. This review explains why nutrition should be considered to be an important component in chronic pain management in cancer survivors by exploring relevant evidence from the literature and how to translate this knowledge into clinical practice. This review was built on relevant evidence from both human and pre-clinical studies identified in PubMed, Web of Science and Embase databases. Given the relationship between chronic pain, inflammation, and metabolism found in the literature, it is advised to look for a strategic dietary intervention in cancer survivors. Dietary interventions may result in weight loss, a healthy body weight, good diet quality, systemic inflammation, and immune system regulations, and a healthy gut microbiota environment, all of which may alter the pain-related pathways and mechanisms. In addition to being a cancer recurrence or prevention strategy, nutrition may become a chronic pain management modality for cancer survivors. Although additional research is needed before implementing nutrition as an evidence-based management modality for chronic pain in cancer survivors, it is already critical to counsel and inform this patient population about the importance of a healthy diet based on the data available so far.

Keywords: cancer survivors; chronic pain; pain management; nutrition; diet

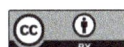

1. Introduction

The Survivorship Task Force describes cancer survivors as "all people who have been diagnosed with cancer, who have finalized primary cancer treatment (except the maintenance therapy, like immune and hormone therapy) and have no mark of active disease" [1]. With earlier diagnosis and improvements in treatment, cancer patients are more likely to survive the disease and therefore live longer [1,2], which is reflected in an increased prevalence of cancer survivors over the last 40 years [1]. Yet, although cancer survivors are considered disease-free, they often suffer from physical, social, and emotional problems that severely influence their quality of life [2].

In the cancer survivor population, the development of chronic pain ("pain that continues beyond the expected healing time" [3]) is one of the most often seen sequelae [4]. Pain is reported in 39.3% of survivors after curative treatment [5]. Severe chronic pain associated with a decrease in function is seen in 5 to 10% of survivors [6]. Moreover, pre-existing pain, repeated surgery, psychological vulnerability, radiation therapy, chemotherapy, sociodemographic and psychosocial (depression, anxiety, sleep disturbance, etc.) profiles, hormone therapy, body mass index (BMI) > 30 kg/m^2 are some of the "predisposing factors" for chronic pain in cancer survivors [4,7–9].

Besides chronic pain, cancer survivors often show significant nutritional deficiencies which crucially impact their quality of life [10]. Changed taste, anorexia, unintended weight loss, and, in certain cases, increased adiposity or obesity are all nutrition-related complications that may develop as a result of cancer and its treatment (i.e., chemo-radiotherapy etc.) since the systemic nature of cancer promotes metabolic dysregulation, increased catabolism, and even cachexia [11]. Significantly, an increase in body weight (or obesity) often occurs during cancer treatment and is related to a higher chance for comorbidities (including chronic pain) [12,13]. For that reason, besides a solution for pain, cancer survivors often look for information on nutrition and diet supplements to improve treatment outcome, quality of life and to increase their long-term survival rates [14].

Interest in the link between chronic pain and nutrition has increased tremendously in recent years. On the one hand, recent research indeed revealed that nutritional aspects can influence brain plasticity and function, and therefore may influence central nervous system health and disease (i.e., central sensitization) [15]. On the other hand, as shown by local and widespread pressure hypersensitivity and hyperalgesia, central sensitization occurs in survivors of breast [16], colon [17] and head and neck cancer [18].

Persistent pain in cancer survivors is often complex (neuropathic, nociplastic, and/or nociceptive) in nature [19], underrecognized, undertreated and less responsive to regular chronic pain management approaches (i.e., pharmacological treatments, rehabilitation, etc.) [7]. Additionally, in long-term survivors (in comparison to people without a history of cancer), it is known that the incidence and relative risk of chronic comorbidities is high [20], which result in significantly more functional limitations and pain intensity, making them less likely to respond to standard chronic pain treatment [21]. Despite crucial medical advances, multi-modal pain management approaches, and enhanced survival, the majority of cancer survivors with pain stated that their pain was only alleviated by 61% [22]. Patients and health care providers are frequently not aware of other possible rehabilitation approaches (like pain education, mind-body interventions) and their potential benefits in the pain management during and after cancer treatment [23]. Recently, the ability of daily diet to modulate pain onset and peripheral analgesic sensitivity has come to light as physicians are more attentive to the lifestyle of patients to better prevent side effects such as chronic pain onset, the main reason of medical intervention, healthcare costs, and outpatient counseling [24]. Nutritional medicine for treating persistent pain requires a comprehension of the disease process' pathogenesis that helps practitioners to prescribe ingredients with particular roles in alleviating the disease process, such as inflammation reduction, or with particular influences on other factors which contribute to pain (i.e., stress and insomnia) [25], or oxidative stress-modulating compounds and oxidative stress status [26].

Despite the increased awareness of the high prevalence, little research has been performed on chronic pain in the cancer population, leading to an important knowledge gap and a lack of clear management guidelines [22]. The most recent systematic review of the association between chronic pain and nutrition in cancer patients and survivors found no evidence in cancer survivors [27], which clearly identifies the knowledge gap and need to address this issue conceptually and scientifically. For all these reasons, this narrative review discusses the mechanisms involved in chronic pain and the critical interaction between these systems and survivors' diets. In addition, dietary interventions that might provide sustainable, long-term, self-manageable and cost-effective implications for chronic pain management in cancer survivors are proposed. It is shown that nutrition holds potential to become a chronic pain management modality for cancer survivors.

2. Methods

This narrative review was accomplished by looking for both pre-clinical and human studies in PubMed, Web of Science and Embase databases by combining the terms "chronic pain", "cancer survivors" and "nutrition" or "diet". English-language articles were accessed until September 2021. The reference lists from the articles that were retrieved were also carefully searched.

3. Pain and Nutrition in Cancer Survivors: An Update from Cancer and Chronic Pain Literature

Since both nutritional and chronic pain mechanisms and pathways are known for their complexity, it does not come as a surprise that research covering the link between both is complex, ambiguous and involves different explanatory components [24]. Dietary factors (like food preparation, food processing and dietary patterns) exert their impact by several pathways and mechanisms such as glucose-insulin homeostasis, blood lipids, blood pressure, functions of the endothelial, cardiac and adipocyte systems, the gut microbiome, systemic inflammation, and hunger and satiety [28]. Chronic pain and its treatment (like opioids), in turn, are known to have an interplay with the nervous systems and the immune system [29,30]. This narrative piece shines a light on the following different pathways and mechanisms to link diet/nutrition and (chronic) pain in cancer survivors (Figure 1): (1) through obesity; (2) through malnutrition, nutritional deficiency, and diet quality; (3) through the immune system and systemic inflammation; and (4) through gut microbiota.

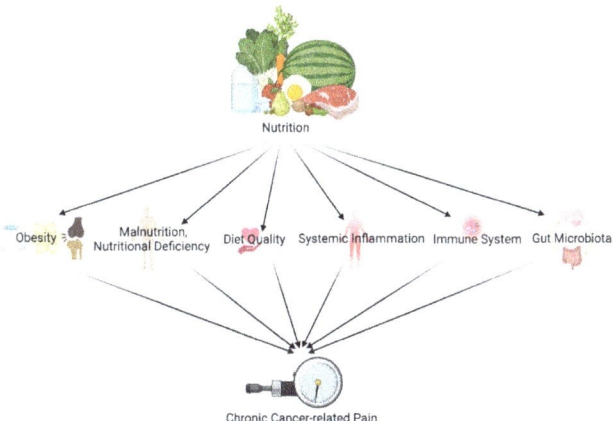

Figure 1. Different pathways and mechanisms to link diet/nutrition and (chronic) pain in cancer survivors (created with BioRender.com accessed on 23 December 2021).

3.1. Impact of Diet and Nutrition on Pain in Cancer Survivors through Obesity

Obesity continues to be a major public health concern, and it is especially frequent among cancer patients, thus determining its long-term impact on the expanding population of cancer survivors is critical [31]. Moreover, it has been known since the 1970s that women with breast cancer receiving adjuvant chemotherapy experience weight gain, commonly reported as 2–5 kg but with great variance [32]. Obesity, defined as a BMI of 30 kg/m^2

or higher, is also a common risk factor for poor health-related quality of life in cancer survivors, in particular colorectal, breast, and prostate cancer survivors [33].

Obesity can cause chronic pain through two primary processes: mechanical stress, which occurs when extra body weight puts stress on joints in the musculoskeletal system, and systemic proinflammatory state, which is linked to adipose tissue and can increase pain [34]. Obesity (particularly caused by excessive abdominal fat) is related to an increment in chronic systemic inflammation which can have a contribution to central sensitization [35]. According to Emery et al., a diet rich in anti-inflammatory foods, such as the consumption of seafood and plant protein, appears to be linked to the relationship between body fat and pain ratings in healthy adults so they advocated that diet can be addressed as part of pain treatment and evaluation, specifically among overweight and obese people [36]. Additionally, obesity has been linked to microbial homeostasis distortion, with a decrease in bacterial biodiversity and altered expression of bacterial genes, particularly those involved in dietary energy extraction [37]. The increased understanding of the interactions between the gut microbiota and the central nervous system, also known as the gut-brain axis, makes the hypothesis of the gut microbiota's possible effect on the pain processing and the pain perception reasonable [38], so does obesity. With good-to-moderate patient-centered evidence, the most recent review (n = 26) in taxane and platinum-treated cancer patients found a link between obesity and increased severity or occurrence of chemotherapy-induced peripheral neuropathy (CIPN) [39]. Additionally, weight gain (>5%) following breast cancer was found to be positively associated with above-average pain [40].

However, evidence on the relationship between obesity and (chronic) pain in cancer survivors remains very limited. One study found a correlation between a higher BMI and a lower physical quality of life in cancer survivors, including more pain even after taking into consideration age, race, education level, cancer type, and comorbidities [41]. Again, in a meta-analysis conducted by Leysen et al. [4], among other factors, a BMI of 30 kg/m^2 or higher was substantially linked with the development of chronic pain in breast cancer survivors. In another study, it has been suggested that cancer survivors with CIPN and co-occurring obesity may be more at risk of lower quality of life due to higher symptom severity and pain than non-obese survivors [33]. In parallel, among cancer survivors with CIPN who received platinum and/or taxane chemotherapeutic compounds, overweight and obese survivors experienced more severe pain and higher pain interference scores than normal-weight survivors [42]. Similar to that overweight or obese breast cancer survivors with weight loss of $\geq$ 5% showed improvement in their pain at 12 months, but these changes were not significantly different from those who lost < 5% [43]. Therefore, weight reduction techniques for obese cancer survivors suffering from chronic pain could be a key factor within pain management for this population. Moreover that studies examining whether dietary management results in pain relief in cancer patients receiving chemotherapy or in survivors after treatment (or in any other cancer treatment associated with pain) are urgently needed and represent an important research priority.

3.2. Impact of Diet and Nutrition on Pain in Cancer Survivors through Malnutrition, Nutritional Deficiency, and Diet Quality

Cancer patients suffer from a large catabolic imbalance which causes weight loss, the key indicator of cancer-associated malnutrition [44]. The prevalence of malnutrition is estimated to be between 50 and 80%, depending on the tools used and the populations studied [45], and can reach up to 85% of patients with certain cancers such as pancreatic [46]. According to many proposed mechanisms, which varying from signaling molecules included within the diet (such as oxidized lipids), vagus nerve activation, microbiota alterations, and oxidative stress to maladaptive neuroplasticity induced by hyper-palatable energy-dense foods, poor nutrition may also cause activation of the immune system, in particular by glial activation with increased inflammation and nervous system hypersensitivity as a consequence [47]. Available data clearly revealed that well-nourished breast cancer survivors had improved functions and less symptoms including pain in comparison to malnourished breast cancer survivors [48].

Additionally, nutritional reduction is frequently acknowledged as a component of the cancer course and treatment [49]. During chemotherapy, compared to women without cancer, breast cancer patients reported a significantly lower absolute protein, fat, and alcohol intake, but not carbohydrates and fiber. [50]. In Iranian breast cancer survivors, the average daily energy intake was lower than the estimated energy requirement as a reference value, with just 34% of participants meeting the estimated energy requirement, whereas the mean intakes of vitamin D, vitamin E, iron, and magnesium were insufficient to meet the Food and Nutrition Board's (1997–2001) guideline of dietary reference intakes [48].

In cancer patients, both at the time of diagnosis and during treatment, micronutrient deficits are common [11]. For instance, pancreatic cancer patients who have had their pancreas removed are at risk of many nutrition-related comorbidities, including an impact on gastrointestinal and hepatic function, glycaemic regulation, bone health, and the status of many micronutrients such as vitamin A, B12, D, E, iron, magnesium and zinc [51]. Similarly, one possible metabolic consequence after a gastrectomy after gastric cancer is vitamin B12 deficiency, which may lower cancer survivors' quality of life [52].

Importantly, low macro/micronutrient consumption, particularly omega-3 fatty acids, vitamins B1, B3, B6, B12, and D, magnesium, zinc, and -carotene, is associated with chronic neuropathic or inflammatory pain [53]. As seen in multiple systematic studies on various pain conditions, including aromatase inhibitor(AI)-related arthralgia in breast cancer [54], supplementing the diet with these specific nutrients helps to alleviate chronic pain [55]. For example, since estrogen increases vitamin D receptor activation, a low estrogen status could potentially reduce the available active vitamin D amount; 75 to 90% of women receiving AI therapy have a vitamin D deficiency [56], which might negatively contribute to a chronic pain state [57]. It is known that vitamin D deficiency causes a muscle and joint aches syndrome similar to Aromatase Inhibitor-Induced Arthralgias (AIA) [56]. As a result, it is suggested that vitamin D can have a crucial role in several cellular activities considered preventive against the development and modulation of chronic pain [57].

Interestingly, cancer and its treatment may increase the requirement for antioxidant nutrient intake such as vitamin C because of the increased free radicals [11]. Administrating some anti-cancer therapies has shown a significant reduction in patients' vitamin C concentrations and report of scurvy (vitamin C deficiency disease)-like symptoms so cancer patients are one of the many patient groups who have a high prevalence of hypovitaminosis C and vitamin C deficiency [58]. The mini-review that reviewed the few current trials exploring the impact of IV vitamin C on cancer- and chemotherapy-related quality of life discovered considerable reductions in pain following vitamin C administration [59].

Additionally, it is known that magnesium supplementation is used in a variety of neuropathic pain situations, including cancer-related neuropathic pain and chemotherapy-related neuropathy, as is shown in a recent review that looked for nutritional supplements for the treatment of neuropathic pain [60]. Still, evidence supporting magnesium supplementation for the treatment of (neuropathic pain) following cancer is lacking.

Similarly, short-chain fatty acids (SCFAs) are essential mediators of pain since they fundamentally modulate inflammation [24]. In a network meta-analysis with randomized controlled trials included in the six systematic reviews, Kim et al. [54] showed that omega-3 fatty acids are one of the treatment modalities which attained significant improvement in pain severity compared to wait list controls in breast cancer survivors with AIA. However, since the overall confidence level of each review was limited, no recommendations can be made at present to reduce pain in patients with AIA [54].

Apart from this, several studies have found a link between cancer survivors' health-related quality of life and their adherence to general non-cancer-specific dietary guidelines, such as the Healthy Eating Index and the Mediterranean diet [41,61]. Higher adherence to the traditional Mediterranean Diet (high consumption of plant-based foods (vegetables, fruit, whole grains, legumes, nuts, olive oil) and low or limited consumption of red meat, milk, and sweets) were linked to higher physical functioning and health status, as well as lower pain and insomnia symptoms, suggesting that this diet may play a role in the quality of life of recently diagnosed female breast cancer patients [62]. Likewise, Wayne et al. [63] claimed that women newly diagnosed with first primary breast cancer (in situ or stage I to IIIA disease) with excellent diet quality according to the Diet Quality Index received higher quality of life scores than women with poor diet quality, including physical health subscale category "bodily pain" with the highest scores.

Furthermore, cancer survivors are advised to follow some diet recommendations from the American Cancer Society (ACS) Guideline on Diet and Physical Activity for Cancer Prevention and the World Cancer Research Fund (WCRF)/American Institute for Cancer Research (AICR) Cancer Prevention (Table 1). Higher diet scores were associated with many aspects, including bodily pain among breast cancer survivors with stage II–III cancer, according to a cross-sectional study that looked at whether adherence to the American Cancer Society (ACS) guidelines was associated with health-related quality of life (HRQoL) among Korean breast cancer survivors [64]. A study of Chinese patients with breast cancer who followed the WCRF/AICR guidelines (BMI, physical activity, and diet) before and after their diagnosis found that following the BMI prescription resulted in reduced pain scores while adherence to dietary recommendations, on the other hand, was not linked to pain scores [65].

Table 1. Contents of the dietary recommendations/guidelines for cancer survivors.

Reference	The Dietary Recommendations

2020 American Cancer Society (ACS) Guideline on Diet and Physical Activity for Cancer Prevention [66]	1. Achieve and stay at a healthy weight throughout life.
	• Maintain a healthy body weight range throughout adulthood and avoid gaining weight.
	2. Engage in physical activity.
	• Adults should do 150–300 min of moderate-intensity physical activity each week, or 75–150 min of vigorous-intensity physical activity, or a combination of the two; reaching or beyond the upper limit of 300 min is ideal.
	• Every day, children and adolescents should do at least 1 h of moderate- to vigorous-intensity activity.
	• Limit sedentary behaviour such as sitting, lying down, and watching television or other screen-based entertainment.
	3. Keep a healthy eating habit during your life.
	• A healthy eating pattern comprises the following items:
	  ○ Foods rich in nutrients in amounts that aid reach and maintain healthy body weight;
	  ○ Various vegetables- dark green, red, and orange veggies, fibre-rich legumes (beans and peas), and others;
	  ○ Fruit, particularly entire fruit in various colours; and
	  ○ Whole grains.
	• A healthy eating pattern excludes or restricts:
	  ○ Meats, both red and processed;
	  ○ Sugar-sweetened drinks; or
	  ○ Refined grain products and highly processed foods.
	4. It is better not to consume alcohol.
	Those who choose to consume alcohol should limit their intake to one drink per day for women and two drinks per day for males. Recommendation for Community Action
	• At the national, state, and local levels, public, private, and community organizations should collaborate to develop, advocate for, and implement policy and environmental changes that increase access to affordable, nutritious foods; provide safe, enjoyable, and accessible opportunities for physical activity; and limit alcohol consumption for all people.

Table 1. *Cont.*

Reference	The Dietary Recommendations
World Cancer Research Fund (WCRF)/American Institute for Cancer Research (AICR) Diet, Nutrition, Physical Activity and Cancer: a Global Perspective (2018) [67]	1. Maintain a healthy body weight Maintain a healthy weight and prevent gaining weight in adult life. 2. Engage in physical activity Make physical activity a regular component of your everyday routine—walk more and sit less. 3. Include whole grains, vegetables, fruit and beans in your diet Make a major part of your usual daily diet from whole grains, vegetables, fruit, and pulses (legumes) such as beans and lentils. 4. Limit intake of 'fast foods'; and other processed foods that are high in fat, starches or sugars Limiting these foods can help you keep track of your calorie intake and maintain a healthy weight. 5. Limit red and processed meat consumption. Red meat, such as beef, pork, and lamb, should be consumed in moderation. Consume very little, if any, processed meat. 6. Limit sugar-sweetened drinks consumption Drink usually water and non-sweetened drinks. 7. Limit consumption of alcohol. It's best to not consume alcohol for preventing cancer. 8. Supplements should not be used to prevent cancer Aim to achieve nutritional needs solely through diet. 9. If you are a mother: if you are able, breastfeed your baby. Breastfeeding is beneficial to both mother and baby. 10. After recieving a cancer diagnosis: if you are able, follow our recommendations. 11. Consult your medical providers to determine what is right for you.

3.3. Impact of Diet and Nutrition on Pain in Cancer Survivors through the Immune System and Systemic Inflammation

Chronic pain frequently arises from a permanent pro-inflammatory state [55]. The proposed pathophysiology and mechanisms that maintain chronic pain emerge constantly, yet as part of the maladaptive synaptic plasticity related to chronic pain, proposing permanent low-grade inflammation (neuroinflammation) as a primary driver makes therapeutic approaches targeting immune activation to reduce the pro-inflammatory state important to consider for chronic pain management [47].

This pro-inflammatory state is also a characteristic of cancer. Independent of the increment in neural density noticed in the tumor environment, numerous pain modulating agents such as hydrogen ions, tumor necrosis factor-alpha (TNF-α), transforming growth factor-beta (TGF-β), prostaglandins, interleukin-1 (IL-1) and IL-6 are set free into the tumor vicinity, sensitizing and stimulating sensory fibers, possibly contributing to neuronal hyperexcitability and pain [1].

Dietary components have the potential to have substantial inflammatory or anti-inflammatory features [68]. Inflammation is linked to dietary consumption of omega-3 and omega-6 polyunsaturated fatty acids (PUFAs) in healthy populations, according to observational studies since higher omega-3 PUFAs are associated with lower levels of pro-inflammatory indicators such as interleukin (IL)-6, IL-1 receptor antagonist, TNF-α, and C-reactive protein (CRP), as well as higher levels of anti-inflammatory indicators such as IL-10 and transforming growth factor β [69]. Additionally, it is known that within the neurological system, certain combinations of omega-3 and micronutrients (like vitamin A and D) may show an even bigger synergistic effect on inhibiting microglial-mediated neuroinflammation [70]. Similarly, high consumption of dietary fibers is inversely related to the circulating inflammatory markers interleukin 6 (IL-6) and tumor necrosis factor α receptor 2 (TNF-α-R2) in postmenopausal women and C-reactive protein (CRP) in breast cancer survivors [71]. Moreover, a diet high in fruit, vegetables, whole grains, white meat, tomato, legumes, tea, and fruit juices is substantially and inversely related to indicators of systemic inflammation whereas consumption of refined cereals, red meat, butter, processed meat, high-fat dairy, sweets, desserts, pizza, potatoes, eggs, hydrogenated fats, and soft drinks, are found to be strongly and positively associated with systemic inflammation [72].

Looking at this matter from a dietary level rather than a nutritional level, the Mediterranean diet has a high anti-inflammatory micronutrients and phytochemical content such as n-3 fatty acids, flavonoids, carotenoids, and vitamins C and E [73]. Evidence shows that higher adherence to the Mediterranean diet is linked to a lower inflammatory status [74]. As a result, applying an intervention to increase the adherence to a Mediterranean diet pattern may have health benefits by reducing systemic inflammation [73]. In this regard, also more general, several studies have linked diet quality to inflammation. For example, breast cancer survivors with better postdiagnosis diet quality showed lower CRP levels (1.6 mg/L vs. 2.5 mg/L) and higher scores on the Healthy Eating Index (2005) [75]. Likewise, Orchard et al. observed that a higher HEI-2010 score was strongly associated with reduced IL-6 and TNFR-2 levels in breast cancer survivors [76].

Another approach to affect the nervous system's neuroimmune function is through metabolic alterations [47]. According to mounting evidence, oxidative stress can activate and maintain pain pathways via activating glutamatergic transmission and numerous inflammatory pathways (which are important for the development of peripheral and central sensitization), as well as directly influencing nociceptive centers in the brain [77]. Oxidative stress has been proven to be a significant contributor to the pain caused by chemotherapy-induced peripheral neuropathy (CIPN) [78]. The findings in mouse models showed that cisplatin-induced mechanical hypersensitivity is caused by peripheral oxidative stress sensitizing mechanical nociceptors, whereas paclitaxel-induced mechanical hypersensitivity is caused by central (spinal) oxidative stress maintaining central sensitization that abnormally produces pain in response to Aβ fiber inputs [78]. Furthermore, mitochondrial dysfunction caused by cancer cells (induced by the mitochondrial genome alterations, the associated oxidative stress etc.) [79] may play a role in chronic pain. Maintaining mitochondrial function has been proposed as a possible treatment technique for treating or preventing chronic pain [80]. For example, strategies that improve mitochondrial function have shown success in preventing and reversing CIPN in pre-clinical animal models and have begun to show some progress toward translation to the clinic [81]. Although dietary intake ultimately directs metabolism, only a few studies showed how metabolic pathways influenced by diet may have a role in the immune activation seen in chronic pain [82]. It is asserted that diets high in fruit and vegetable consumption can decrease oxidative stress [72]. For example, antioxidants produced from food, such as vitamin A, CoQ10, vitamin E, and vitamin C, have been demonstrated to play an important role in preventing oxidative stress, and several studies have found a link between the consumption of specific foods or food groups and plasma/serum antioxidant capacity [83]. In women who have had breast cancer, it has been demonstrated that drinking fresh carrot juice on a daily basis is a simple and effective way to increase plasma total carotenoids and, as a result, reduce oxidative stress, but not inflammatory markers [84].

Additionally, in vitro evidence demonstrated the role of nuclear factor-kappa B (NF-κB), which has a critical role in cancer development and progression [85], as well as in regulating inflammatory pain [86]. Evidence also found that tomato extracts inhibited TNFα induced NF-κB activity in the androgen-independent human-derived prostate cancer cells [87].

Taking into account the links between chronic pain, inflammation, and metabolic dysregulation, and there subsequent impact in cancer survivors, a strategic dietary intervention for this population that could modulate this pathophysiology is worth looking into [47]. However, specific evidence for these mechanisms in cancer survivors is yet to be generated and represent an important area for future research.

3.4. Impact of Diet and Nutrition on Pain in Cancer Survivors through Gut Microbiota

In cancer cohorts, cancer treatments, specifically chemotherapy, has been proven to have a negative impact on the gut microbiome [88]. In support of this, the gut microbiota has been linked to psychoneurological symptoms associated with cancer treatment including chemotherapy-induced peripheral neuropathy by generating pro- and anti-inflammatory cytokines or chemokines to be produced [89]. Recent research suggests that dysbiosis of the gut microbiome is also a critical factor in central sensitization, which leads to chronic pain and cancer-related pain [90].

An increasing body of research demonstrates the critical function of gut microbiota in acute and chronic pain (neuropathic, inflammatory, and viscera) modulation and has ushered into a new era in pain management [91,92]. Additionally, gut microbiota-derived mediators in the central nervous system may modulate induction and maintenance of central sensitization via regulating neuroinflammation, which involves the activation of blood–brain barrier cells, microglia, and infiltrating immune cells [91,93,94]. Animal models have shown that gut microbes can stimulate the vagus nerve, which controls brain and behavior, and that changes in gut microbial composition are linked to significant changes in mood, pain, and cognition behaviors [95]. Preclinical and clinical findings suggest that communication between the gut microbiome, inflammation and microglia is involved in the development of chronic pain, implying that manipulating the gut microbiome in chronic pain sufferers could be an effective way to improve pain outcomes [96].

Dietary composition and amount play a significant role in gut microbiota composition and function [37]. It has been shown that lesser gut microbial diversity is associated with poorer nutritional status, frailty, comorbidity, and inflammation indicators [97]. Based on animal and human studies, dietary intake is seen to be a main short-term and long-term regulator of the gut microbiota structure and function [98]. To illustrate; some findings point to a relationship between Vitamin D insufficiency and altered nociception, presumably through molecular processes affecting the endocannabinoid and associated mediator signaling systems [99]. Additionally, short-chain fatty acids (SCFAs), which are microbial metabolites, interact with vagal afferents, and impact inflammation and hormonal control may also affect the peripheral immune system to modulate brain function [100]. Hence, targeting gut microbiota by dietary intervention is one of the innovative and possibly productive options for chronic pain therapy [91].

In cancer survivors, there are a few studies examining the relationship between nutrition and gut microbiota. For example, volunteers with a prior history of colorectal cancer who received rice bran or bean powder had increased gut bacterial diversity and altered gut microbial composition after 28 days when compared to baseline [101]. In overweight breast cancer survivors, probiotics in addition to a Mediterranean diet (MD) enhance gut microbiota and metabolic and anthropometric parameters as compared to an MD alone [37]. Another evidence of positive associations between the abundances of Bifidobacterium among the gut microbiota and the levels of omega-3 PUFAs in the blood came from a cross-sectional study that looked at the relationship between PUFAs and the gut microbiota among breast cancer survivors [102].

Understanding the link between the gut microbiota, nutrition and chronic pain has practical implications for cancer survivors. Nutrients initially meet the gut microbiota before being absorbed as bioactive products; hence anything related to the link between diet and pain is closely associated with the gut microbiome [24]. Guo et al. [91] assert that gut microbiota modulates pain in the peripheral and central nervous systems, and that targeting gut microbiota through diet and pharmabiotic intervention could be a new therapeutic approach for chronic pain treatment including chemotherapy-induced peripheral neuropathy pain.

4. How Can We Implement This Knowledge in Clinical Practice?

Studies in cancer survivors showed differences in nutrient intake status (such as total energy intake, carbohydrates and vitamin B) before and after cancer diagnosis [103] and in comparison to cancer survivors with non-cancer individuals [104]. Moreover, studies displayed poor adherence to diet recommendations, reports, and guidelines [105–107].

Latest literature recommends that nutritional counseling focused on micro-/macronutrients (such as vitamins, minerals, saturated fat, proteins, etc.) does not end up with adequate development in eating behaviors and may also cause an unnecessary increase in supplements consumption [108]. Additionally, due to reduced dietary intake and changed metabolism and absorption, cancer survivors often do not respond well to nutritional supplements [11]. For that reason, dietary supplement use is common and controversial among cancer survivors; however, evidence on the amount of nutrients received through supplements is lacking [109]. Still, cancer survivors reported a higher prevalence and dose of dietary supplement use, but lower nutritional consumption from foods, than those who had not been diagnosed with cancer [110]. However, there is some evidence that shows supplementation could work in cancer patients. For example, diet supplementation with some particular nutrients such as omega-3 fatty acids, vitamins B1, B3, B6, B12 and D, magnesium, zinc and β-carotene contributes to the alleviating of chronic pain as seen in systematic reviews in different pain populations including aromatase inhibitor-related arthralgia in breast cancer [55].

Since the cancer survivors population grows, clinicians as well as the healthcare system will require adapting and learning new methods to support patients with persistent pain [111]. Biologic therapies such as diet targeting the underlying causes of pain as discussed above could potentially reduce costs associated with cancer-related pain in survivors. Additionally, cancer survivors are often curious about food choices, physical activity and dietary supplements since they would like to learn whether nutrition and physical activity may help them live longer or feel better [112]. As part of this, nearly half of cancer survivors used nutritional supplements on their own without contacting their health care provider, which could indicate a lack of communication between cancer survivors and their health care providers about supplement use [110]. According to a study, only 2% of 1081 cancer survivors received dietary supplement counseling from a licensed dietitian [113]. In addition, promoting a dietary pattern rather than a specific food or nutrient may offer more health advantages, but future treatments must develop techniques that allow people to change numerous dietary habits successfully [73].

Furthermore, moderate-certainty evidence has demonstrated that dietary interventions can also modify food and nutrient intakes and positively affect some anthropometric measurements (such as weight loss and body mass index) in cancer survivors, especially in women after breast cancer [114]. In addition to that as discussed, some evidence found those positive changes could improve pain in (breast) cancer survivors [43,115]. In the light of these considerations, cancer survivors should also be encouraged to follow the recommendations for body weight as has been reported in a recent systematic review [116].

In a recent review that addressed adult cancer survivors' perspectives on dietary advice following cancer treatment in the Australian context, cancer survivors reported a need for (a) individualized dietary strategies to address ongoing symptoms, (b) professional weight management support, and (c) practical skills for healthy eating [117]. Given that survivors are extremely motivated to improve their general health following a cancer diagnosis, healthy lifestyle recommendations from oncology providers can be a powerful motivator for survivors to embrace health behavior modifications [118]. A randomized controlled trial demonstrated that an education and culinary-based intervention in breast cancer survivors successfully increased adherence to a more anti-inflammatory dietary pattern by increasing consumption of anti-inflammatory foods, spices, and herbs while decreasing consumption of pro-inflammatory foods [73].

As a result, in order to make healthy lifestyle choices throughout survivorship, cancer survivors may benefit from additional advice and support [107]. However, cancer survivors receive a wide range of recommendations about what foods to consume or avoid, and what supplements to take, if any, from a variety of sources. Unfortunately, this advice is frequently inconsistent and unsupported by evidence [109]. However, even though more research is needed to completely integrate these approaches as management modality for chronic pain in cancer survivors, it is important to guide those people and inform them about the importance of healthy diet with so far accumulated evidence.

5. Conclusions

Obesity, malnutrition, nutritional deficiency, diet quality, immune system, systemic inflammation, and gut microbiota are some pathways/mechanisms associated with chronic pain in cancer survivors. As seen clearly, dietary interventions may provide weight reduction, a healthy body weight, good diet quality, regulations in systemic inflammation and immune system, and a healthy gut microbiota environment that could modify aforementioned pain-related pathways/mechanisms. For that reason, nutrition might have the potential to transition from being only prevention for cancer recurrence or cancer itself to a modality for chronic pain management for cancer survivors. In some available studies, nutrition has been already shown to improve survivors' pain and quality of life (including bodily pain), which provides some basis and rationale considering the role of nutrition in chronic pain management carefully.

In the future, more clinical studies that directly explore nutrition and chronic pain in cancer survivors should be done to better understand the particular mechanisms that connect nutrition to chronic pain. Exploring and implementing awareness, prevention and management approaches that recognize the links between these elements is crucial to providing pain relief to survivors.

Author Contributions: Conceptualization, all authors (S.T.Y., A.M., Ö.E., T.D., J.N., P.C., A.D.G. and I.C.); writing—original draft preparation, S.T.Y.; writing—review and editing, all authors. All authors have read and agreed to the published version of the manuscript.

Funding: This research received no external funding.

Institutional Review Board Statement: Not applicable.

Informed Consent Statement: Not applicable.

Acknowledgments: Sevilay Tümkaya Yılmaz and Ömer Elma are funded by the Ministry of National Education of the Turkish State as scholarship students for their Ph.D. research program. Anneleen Malfliet and An De Groef are postdoctoral research fellows funded by the Research Foundation Flanders (FWO), Belgium. Jo Nijs holds the Berekuyl Academy Chair in oncological rehabilitation, funded by the Berekuyl Academy, Hierden, The Netherlands. We thank Kelly Ickmans for creating Figure 1.

Conflicts of Interest: The authors declare no conflict of interest. The funders had no role in the design of the study; in the collection, analyses, or interpretation of data; in the writing of the manuscript, or in the decision to publish the results.

References

1. Brown, M.; Farquhar-Smith, P. Pain in cancer survivors; filling in the gaps. *Br. J. Anaesth.* **2017**, *119*, 723–736. [CrossRef] [PubMed]
2. Lu, W.; Rosenthal, D.S. Oncology Acupuncture for Chronic Pain in Cancer Survivors: A Reflection on the American Society of Clinical Oncology Chronic Pain Guideline. *Hematol. Oncol. Clin. N. Am.* **2018**, *32*, 519–533. [CrossRef] [PubMed]
3. Mailis, A.; Tepperman, P.S.; Hapidou, E.G. Chronic pain: Evolution of clinical definitions and implications for practice. *Psychol. Inj. Law* **2020**, *13*, 412–426. [CrossRef]
4. Leysen, L.; Beckwée, D.; Nijs, J.; Pas, R.; Bilterys, T.; Vermeir, S.; Adriaenssens, N. Risk factors of pain in breast cancer survivors: A systematic review and meta-analysis. *Support. Care Cancer* **2017**, *25*, 3607–3643. [CrossRef]
5. Van Den Beuken-Van, M.H.; Hochstenbach, L.M.; Joosten, E.A.; Tjan-Heijnen, V.C.; Janssen, D.J. Update on Prevalence of Pain in Patients With Cancer: Systematic Review and Meta-Analysis. *J. Pain Symptom Manag.* **2016**, *51*, 1070–1090.e9. [CrossRef]
6. Glare, P.A.; Davies, P.S.; Finlay, E.; Gulati, A.; Lemanne, D.; Moryl, N.; Oeffinger, K.C.; Paice, J.; Stubblefield, M.D.; Syrjala, K.L. Pain in Cancer Survivors. *J. Clin. Oncol.* **2014**, *32*, 1739–1747. [CrossRef]
7. Burton, A.W.; Fanciullo, G.J.; Beasley, R.D.; Fisch, M.J. Chronic Pain in the Cancer Survivor: A New Frontier. *Pain Med.* **2007**, *8*, 189–198. [CrossRef]
8. Azizoddin, D.R.; Schreiber, K.; Beck, M.R.; Enzinger, A.C.; Hruschak, V.; Darnall, B.D.; Edwards, R.R.; Allsop, M.J.; Tulsky, J.A.; Boyer, E.; et al. Chronic pain severity, impact, and opioid use among patients with cancer: An analysis of biopsychosocial factors using the CHOIR learning health care system. *Cancer* **2021**, *127*, 3254–3263. [CrossRef]
9. Habib, A.S.; Kertai, M.; Cooter, M.; Greenup, R.A.; Hwang, S. Risk factors for severe acute pain and persistent pain after surgery for breast cancer: A prospective observational study. *Reg. Anesth. Pain Med.* **2019**, *44*, 192–199. [CrossRef]
10. Virizuela, J.A.; Camblor-Álvarez, M.; Luengo-Pérez, L.M.; Grande, E.; Álvarez-Hernández, J.; Sendrós-Madroño, M.J.; Jiménez-Fonseca, P.; Peris, M.C.; Ocón-Bretón, M.J. Nutritional support and parenteral nutrition in cancer patients: An expert consensus report. *Clin. Transl. Oncol.* **2018**, *20*, 619–629. [CrossRef]
11. Inglis, J.E.; Lin, P.-J.; Kerns, S.L.; Kleckner, I.R.; Kleckner, A.S.; Castillo, A.D.; Mustian, K.M.; Peppone, L.J. Nutritional Interventions for Treating Cancer-Related Fatigue: A Qualitative Review. *Nutr. Cancer* **2019**, *71*, 21–40. [CrossRef] [PubMed]

12. Braakhuis, A.; Campion, P.; Bishop, K. The Effects of Dietary Nutrition Education on Weight and Health Biomarkers in Breast Cancer Survivors. *Med. Sci.* **2017**, *5*, 12. [CrossRef] [PubMed]
13. Rock, C.L.; Flatt, S.W.; Byers, T.E.; Colditz, G.A.; Demark-Wahnfried, W.; Ganz, P.A.; Wolin, K.Y.; Elias, A.; Krontiras, H.; Liu, J.; et al. Results of the Exercise and Nutrition to Enhance Recovery and Good Health for You (ENERGY) trial: A behavioral weight loss intervention in overweight or obese breast cancer survivors. *J. Clin. Oncol.* **2015**, *33*, 3169. [CrossRef]
14. Doyle, C.; Kushi, L.H.; Byers, T.; Courneya, K.S.; Demark-Wahnfried, W.; Grant, B.; McTiernan, A.; Rock, C.L.; Thompson, C.; Gansler, T.; et al. Nutrition and physical activity during and after cancer treatment: An American Cancer Society guide for informed choices. *CA Cancer J. Clin.* **2006**, *56*, 323–353. [CrossRef]
15. Gomez-Pinilla, F.; Gomez, A.G. The influence of dietary factors in central nervous system plasticity and injury recovery. *PM&R* **2011**, *3* (Suppl. S1), S111–S116.
16. Fernandez-Lao, C.; Cantarero-Villanueva, I.; Fernández-de-Las-Peñas, C.; Del-Moral-Avila, R.; Arendt-Nielsen, L.; Arroyo-Morales, M. Myofascial trigger points in neck and shoulder muscles and widespread pressure pain hypersensitivtiy in patients with postmastectomy pain: Evidence of peripheral and central sensitization. *Clin. J. Pain* **2010**, *26*, 798–806. [CrossRef]
17. Sánchez-Jiménez, A.; Cantarero-Villanueva, I.; Molina-Barea, R.; Fernández-Lao, C.; Galiano-Castillo, N.; Arroyo-Morales, M. Widespread Pressure Pain Hypersensitivity and Ultrasound Imaging Evaluation of Abdominal Area after Colon Cancer Treatment. *Pain Med.* **2014**, *15*, 233–240. [CrossRef] [PubMed]
18. Ortiz-Comino, L.; Fernández-Lao, C.; Castro-Martín, E.; Lozano-Lozano, M.; Cantarero-Villanueva, I.; Arroyo-Morales, M.; Martín-Martín, L. Myofascial pain, widespread pressure hypersensitivity, and hyperalgesia in the face, neck, and shoulder regions, in survivors of head and neck cancer. *Support. Care Cancer* **2019**, *28*, 2891–2898. [CrossRef]
19. Leysen, L.; Adriaenssens, N.; Nijs, J.; Pas, R.; Bilterys, T.; Vermeir, S.; Lahousse, A.; Beckwée, D. Chronic Pain in Breast Cancer Survivors: Nociceptive, Neuropathic, or Central Sensitization Pain? *Pain Pract.* **2018**, *19*, 183–195. [CrossRef]
20. Chao, C.; Bhatia, S.; Xu, L.; Cannavale, K.L.; Wong, F.L.; Huang, P.S.; Cooper, R.; Armenian, S.H. Chronic Comorbidities Among Survivors of Adolescent and Young Adult Cancer. *J. Clin. Oncol.* **2020**, *38*, 3161. [CrossRef]
21. Paice, J.A.; Portenoy, R.; Lacchetti, C.; Campbell, T.; Cheville, A.; Citron, M.; Constine, L.S.; Cooper, A.; Glare, P.; Keefe, F.; et al. Management of chronic pain in survivors of adult cancers: American Society of Clinical Oncology Clinical Practice Guideline. *J. Clin. Oncol.* **2016**, *34*, 3325–3345. [CrossRef] [PubMed]
22. Green, C.R.; Hart-Johnson, T.; Loeffler, D.R. Cancer-related chronic pain: Examining quality of life in diverse cancer survivors. *Cancer* **2011**, *117*, 1994–2003. [CrossRef] [PubMed]
23. De Groef, A.; Penen, F.; Dams, L.; Van der Gucht, E.; Nijs, J.; Meeus, M. Best-Evidence Rehabilitation for Chronic Pain Part 2: Pain during and after Cancer Treatment. *J. Clin. Med.* **2019**, *8*, 979. [CrossRef] [PubMed]
24. Bjørklund, G.; Aaseth, J.; Doşa, M.D.; Pivina, L.; Dadar, M.; Pen, J.J.; Chirumbolo, S. Does diet play a role in reducing nociception related to inflammation and chronic pain? *Nutrition* **2019**, *66*, 153–165. [CrossRef] [PubMed]
25. Audette, J.F.; Bailey, A. *Integrative Pain Medicine: The Science and Practice of Complementary and Alternative Medicine in Pain Management*; Springer Science & Business Media: Totowa, NJ, USA, 2008.
26. Hendrix, J.; Nijs, J.; Ickmans, K.; Godderis, L.; Ghosh, M.; Polli, A. The Interplay between Oxidative Stress, Exercise, and Pain in Health and Disease: Potential Role of Autonomic Regulation and Epigenetic Mechanisms. *Antioxidants* **2020**, *9*, 1166. [CrossRef]
27. Yilmaz, S.T.; Elma, Ö.; Deliens, T.; Coppieters, I.; Clarys, P.; Nijs, J.; Malfliet, A. Nutrition/Dietary Supplements and Chronic Pain in Patients with Cancer and Survivors of Cancer: A Systematic Review and Research Agenda. *Pain Physician* **2021**, *24*, 335–344.
28. Tapsell, L.C. Dietary behaviour changes to improve nutritional quality and health outcomes. *Chronic Dis. Transl. Med.* **2017**, *3*, 154–158. [CrossRef]
29. Ren, K.; Dubner, R. Interactions between the immune and nervous systems in pain. *Nat. Med.* **2010**, *16*, 1267–1276. [CrossRef]
30. Malafoglia, V.; Ilari, S.; Vitiello, L.; Tenti, M.; Balzani, E.; Muscoli, C.; Raffaeli, W.; Bonci, A. The Interplay between Chronic Pain, Opioids, and the Immune System. *Neuroscientist* **2021**, 10738584211030493. [CrossRef]
31. Parekh, N.; Chandran, U.; Bandera, E.V. Obesity in Cancer Survival. *Annu. Rev. Nutr.* **2012**, *32*, 311–342. [CrossRef]
32. Buch, K.; Gunmalm, V.; Andersson, M.; Schwarz, P.; Brøns, C. Effect of chemotherapy and aromatase inhibitors in the adjuvant treatment of breast cancer on glucose and insulin metabolism-A systematic review. *Cancer Med.* **2019**, *8*, 238–245. [CrossRef] [PubMed]
33. Cox-Martin, E.; Trahan, L.H.; Cox, M.G.; Dougherty, P.M.; Lai, E.A.; Novy, D.M. Disease burden and pain in obese cancer patients with chemotherapy-induced peripheral neuropathy. *Support. Care Cancer* **2017**, *25*, 1873–1879. [CrossRef] [PubMed]
34. Morelhão, P.K.; Tufik, S.; Andersen, M.L. The Interactions Between Obesity, Sleep Quality, and Chronic Pain. *J. Clin. Sleep Med.* **2018**, *14*, 1965–1966. [CrossRef] [PubMed]
35. Mínguez-Olaondo, A.; Martínez-Valbuena, I.; Romero, S.; Frühbeck, G.; Luquin, M.R.; Martínez-Vila, E.; Irimia, P. Excess abdominal fat is associated with cutaneous allodynia in individuals with migraine: A prospective cohort study. *J. Headache Pain* **2020**, *21*, 9. [CrossRef]
36. Emery, C.F.; Olson, K.L.; Bodine, A.; Lee, V.; Habash, D.L. Dietary intake mediates the relationship of body fat to pain. *Pain* **2017**, *158*, 273–277. [CrossRef]
37. Pellegrini, M.; Ippolito, M.; Monge, T.; Violi, R.; Cappello, P.; Ferrocino, I.; Cocolin, L.S.; De Francesco, A.; Bo, S.; Finocchiaro, C. Gut microbiota composition after diet and probiotics in overweight breast cancer survivors: A randomized open-label pilot intervention trial. *Nutrition* **2020**, *74*, 110749. [CrossRef]

38. Minerbi, A.; Gonzalez, E.; Brereton, N.J.; Anjarkouchian, A.; Dewar, K.; Fitzcharles, M.-A.; Chevalier, S.; Shir, Y. Altered microbiome composition in individuals with fibromyalgia. *Pain* **2019**, *160*, 2589–2602. [CrossRef]
39. Timmins, H.C.; Mizrahi, D.; Li, T.; Kiernan, M.C.; Goldstein, D.; Park, S.B. Metabolic and lifestyle risk factors for chemotherapy-induced peripheral neuropathy in taxane and platinum-treated patients: A systematic review. *J. Cancer Surviv.* **2021**, 1–15. [CrossRef]
40. Forsythe, L.P.; Alfano, C.M.; George, S.M.; McTiernan, A.; Baumgartner, K.B.; Bernstein, L.; Ballard-Barbash, R. Pain in long-term breast cancer survivors: The role of body mass index, physical activity, and sedentary behavior. *Breast Cancer Res. Treat.* **2013**, *137*, 617–630. [CrossRef]
41. Mosher, C.E.; Sloane, R.; Morey, M.C.; Snyder, D.C.; Cohen, H.J.; Miller, P.E.; Demark-Wahnefried, W. Associations between lifestyle factors and quality of life among older long-term breast, prostate, and colorectal cancer survivors. *Cancer Interdiscip. Int. J. Am. Cancer Soc.* **2009**, *115*, 4001–4009. [CrossRef]
42. Petrovchich, I.; Kober, K.M.; Wagner, L.; Paul, S.M.; Abrams, G.; Chesney, M.A.; Topp, K.; Smoot, B.; Schumacher, M.; Conley, Y.P. Deleterious effects of higher body mass index on subjective and objective measures of chemotherapy-induced peripheral neuropathy in cancer survivors. *J. Pain Symptom Manag.* **2019**, *58*, 252–263. [CrossRef] [PubMed]
43. Sheng, J.Y.; Santa-Maria, C.A.; Blackford, A.L.; Lim, D.; Carpenter, A.; Smith, K.L.; Cohen, G.I.; Coughlin, J.; Appel, L.J.; Stearns, V. The impact of weight loss on physical function and symptoms in overweight or obese breast cancer survivors: Results from POWER-remote. *J. Cancer Surviv.* **2021**. online ahead of print. [CrossRef] [PubMed]
44. Cederholm, T.; Jensen, G.L. To create a consensus on malnutrition diagnostic criteria: A report from the Global Leadership Initiative on Malnutrition (GLIM) meeting at the ESPEN Congress 2016. *J. Parenter. Enter. Nutr.* **2017**, *41*, 311–314. [CrossRef] [PubMed]
45. Prevost, V.; Joubert, C.; Heutte, N.; Babin, E. Assessment of nutritional status and quality of life in patients treated for head and neck cancer. *Eur. Ann. Otorhinolaryngol. Head Neck Dis.* **2014**, *131*, 113–120. [CrossRef]
46. Argiles, J.M. Cancer-associated malnutrition. *Eur. J. Oncol. Nurs.* **2005**, *9* (Suppl. S2), S39–S50. [CrossRef]
47. Field, R.; Pourkazemi, F.; Turton, J.; Rooney, K. Dietary Interventions Are Beneficial for Patients with Chronic Pain: A Systematic Review with Meta-Analysis. *Pain Med.* **2021**, *22*, 694–714. [CrossRef]
48. Mohammadi, S.; Sulaiman, S.; Koon, P.B.; Amani, R.; Hosseini, S.M. Association of Nutritional Status with Quality of Life in Breast Cancer Survivors. *Asian Pac. J. Cancer Prev.* **2013**, *14*, 7749–7755. [CrossRef]
49. Capra, S.; Ferguson, M.; Ried, K. Cancer: Impact of nutrition intervention outcome—Nutrition issues for patients. *Nutrition* **2001**, *17*, 769–772. [CrossRef]
50. De Vries, Y.; Van Den Berg, M.; De Vries, J.; Boesveldt, S.; de Kruif, J.T.C.; Buist, N.; Haringhuizen, A.; Los, M.; Sommeijer, D.; Timmer-Bonte, J. Differences in dietary intake during chemotherapy in breast cancer patients compared to women without cancer. *Supportive Care Cancer* **2017**, *25*, 2581–2591. [CrossRef]
51. Petzel, M.Q.B.; Hoffman, L. Nutrition Implications for Long-Term Survivors of Pancreatic Cancer Surgery. *Nutr. Clin. Pract.* **2017**, *32*, 588–598. [CrossRef]
52. Hu, Y.; Kim, H.-I.; Hyung, W.J.; Song, K.J.; Lee, J.H.; Kim, Y.M.; Noh, S.H. Vitamin B12 deficiency after gastrectomy for gastric cancer: An analysis of clinical patterns and risk factors. *Ann. Surg.* **2013**, *258*, 970–975. [CrossRef] [PubMed]
53. Philpot, U.; Johnson, M. Diet therapy in the management of chronic pain: Better diet less pain? *Pain Manag.* **2019**, *9*, 335–338. [CrossRef] [PubMed]
54. Kim, T.-H.; Kang, J.W.; Lee, T.H. Therapeutic options for aromatase inhibitor-associated arthralgia in breast cancer survivors: A systematic review of systematic reviews, evidence mapping, and network meta-analysis. *Maturitas* **2018**, *118*, 29–37. [CrossRef] [PubMed]
55. Dragan, S.; Serban, M.-C.; Damian, G.; Buleu, F.; Valcovici, M.; Christodorescu, R. Dietary Patterns and Interventions to Alleviate Chronic Pain. *Nutrients* **2020**, *12*, 2510. [CrossRef]
56. Niravath, P.; Chen, B.; Chapman, J.-A.W.; Agarwal, S.K.; Welschhans, R.L.; Bongartz, T.; Kalari, K.R.; Shepherd, L.E.; Bartlett, J.; Pritchard, K. Vitamin D levels, vitamin D receptor polymorphisms, and inflammatory cytokines in aromatase inhibitor-induced Arthralgias: An analysis of CCTG MA. 27. *Clin. Breast Cancer* **2018**, *18*, 78–87. [CrossRef]
57. Martin, K.R.; Reid, D.M. Is there a role for vitamin D in the treatment of chronic pain? *Ther. Adv. Musculoskelet. Dis.* **2017**, *9*, 131–135. [CrossRef]
58. Carr, A.C.; McCall, C. The role of vitamin C in the treatment of pain: New insights. *J. Transl. Med.* **2017**, *15*, 77. [CrossRef]
59. Carr, A.C.; Vissers, M.C.M.; Cook, J.S. The Effect of Intravenous Vitamin C on Cancer- and Chemotherapy-Related Fatigue and Quality of Life. *Front. Oncol.* **2014**, *4*, 283. [CrossRef]
60. Abdelrahman, K.; Hackshaw, K. Nutritional Supplements for the Treatment of Neuropathic Pain. *Biomedicines* **2021**, *9*, 674. [CrossRef]
61. Schlesinger, S.; Walter, J.; Hampe, J.; von Schönfels, W.; Hinz, S.; Küchler, T.; Jacobs, G.; Schafmayer, C.; Nöthlings, U. Lifestyle factors and health-related quality of life in colorectal cancer survivors. *Cancer Causes Control.* **2014**, *25*, 99–110. [CrossRef]
62. Porciello, G.; Montagnese, C.; Crispo, A.; Grimaldi, M.; Libra, M.; Vitale, S.; Palumbo, E.; Pica, R.; Calabrese, I.; Cubisino, S. Mediterranean diet and quality of life in women treated for breast cancer: A baseline analysis of DEDiCa multicentre trial. *PLoS ONE* **2020**, *15*, e0239803. [CrossRef] [PubMed]
63. Wayne, S.J.; Baumgartner, K.; Baumgartner, R.N.; Bernstein, L.; Bowen, D.J.; Ballard-Barbash, R. Diet quality is directly associated with quality of life in breast cancer survivors. *Breast Cancer Res. Treat.* **2006**, *96*, 227–232. [CrossRef] [PubMed]
64. Koh, D.; Song, S.; Moon, S.-E.; Jung, S.-Y.; Lee, E.S.; Kim, Z.; Youn, H.J.; Cho, J.; Yoo, Y.B.; Lee, S.K. Adherence to the American Cancer Society guidelines for cancer survivors and health-related quality of life among breast cancer survivors. *Nutrients* **2019**, *11*, 2924. [CrossRef]

65. Lei, Y.-Y.; Ho, S.C.; Cheng, A.; Kwok, C.; Lee, C.-K.I.; Cheung, K.L.; Lee, R.; Loong, H.H.; He, Y.-Q.; Yeo, W. Adherence to the World Cancer Research Fund/American Institute for Cancer Research Guideline is associated with better health-related quality of life among Chinese patients with breast cancer. *J. Natl. Compr. Cancer Netw.* **2018**, *16*, 275–285. [CrossRef]
66. Rock, C.L.; Thomson, C.; Gansler, T.; Gapstur, S.M.; McCullough, M.L.; Patel, A.V.; Andrews, K.S.; Bandera, E.V.; Spees, C.K.; Robien, K. American Cancer Society guideline for diet and physical activity for cancer prevention. *CA Cancer J. Clin.* **2020**, *70*, 245–271. [CrossRef] [PubMed]
67. World Cancer Research Fund/American Institute for Cancer Research. *Diet, Nutrition, Physical Activity and Cancer: A Global Perspective*; Continuous Update Project Expert Report; World Cancer Research Fund: London, UK, 2018.
68. Christensen, M.A.; Smoak, P.; Lisano, J.K.; Hayward, R.; Coronado, C.; Kage, K.; Shackelford, D.; Stewart, L.K. Cardiorespiratory fitness, visceral fat, and body fat, but not dietary inflammatory index, are related to C-reactive protein in cancer survivors. *Nutr. Health* **2019**, *25*, 195–202. [CrossRef]
69. Alfano, C.M.; Imayama, I.; Neuhouser, M.L.; Kiecolt-Glaser, J.K.; Smith, A.W.; Meeske, K.; McTiernan, A.; Bernstein, L.; Baumgartner, K.B.; Ulrich, C.M. Fatigue, inflammation, and ω-3 and ω-6 fatty acid intake among breast cancer survivors. *J. Clin. Oncol.* **2012**, *30*, 1280. [CrossRef]
70. Kurtys, E.; Eisel, U.; Verkuyl, J.; Broersen, L.; Dierckx, R.; de Vries, E. The combination of vitamins and omega-3 fatty acids has an enhanced anti-inflammatory effect on microglia. *Neurochem. Int.* **2016**, *99*, 206–214. [CrossRef]
71. Guest, D.D.; Evans, E.M.; Rogers, L.Q. Diet components associated with perceived fatigue in breast cancer survivors. *Eur. J. Cancer Care* **2013**, *22*, 51–59. [CrossRef]
72. Lowry, E.; Marley, J.; McVeigh, J.G.; McSorley, E.; Allsopp, P.; Kerr, D. Dietary Interventions in the Management of Fibromyalgia: A Systematic Review and Best-Evidence Synthesis. *Nutrients* **2020**, *12*, 2664. [CrossRef]
73. Zuniga, K.E.; Parma, D.L.; Muñoz, E.; Spaniol, M.; Wargovich, M.; Ramirez, A.G. Dietary intervention among breast cancer survivors increased adherence to a Mediterranean-style, anti-inflammatory dietary pattern: The Rx for Better Breast Health Randomized Controlled Trial. *Breast Cancer Res. Treat.* **2019**, *173*, 145–154. [CrossRef] [PubMed]
74. Esposito, K.; Marfella, R.; Ciotola, M.; Di Palo, C.; Giugliano, F.; Giugliano, G.; D'Armiento, M.; D'Andrea, F.; Giugliano, D. Effect of a Mediterranean-style diet on endothelial dysfunction and markers of vascular inflammation in the metabolic syndrome: A randomized trial. *JAMA* **2004**, *292*, 1440–1446. [CrossRef] [PubMed]
75. George, S.M.; Neuhouser, M.L.; Mayne, S.T.; Irwin, M.L.; Albanes, D.; Gail, M.H.; Alfano, C.M.; Bernstein, L.; McTiernan, A.; Reedy, J. Postdiagnosis diet quality is inversely related to a biomarker of inflammation among breast cancer survivors. *Cancer Epidemiol. Prev. Biomark.* **2010**, *19*, 2220–2228. [CrossRef] [PubMed]
76. Orchard, T.S.; Andridge, R.R.; Yee, L.D.; Lustberg, M.B. Diet quality, inflammation, and quality of life in breast cancer survivors: A cross-sectional analysis of pilot study data. *J. Acad. Nutr. Diet.* **2018**, *118*, 578–588.e1. [CrossRef]
77. Nashed, M.G.; Balenko, M.D.; Singh, G. Cancer-induced oxidative stress and pain. *Current Pain Headache Reports* **2014**, *18*, 384. [CrossRef]
78. Shim, H.S.; Bae, C.; Wang, J.; Lee, K.-H.; Hankerd, K.M.; Kim, H.K.; Chung, J.M.; La, J.-H. Peripheral and central oxidative stress in chemotherapy-induced neuropathic pain. *Mol. Pain* **2019**, *15*, 1744806919840098. [CrossRef]
79. Luo, Y.; Ma, J.; Lu, W. The Significance of Mitochondrial Dysfunction in Cancer. *Int. J. Mol. Sci.* **2020**, *21*, 5598. [CrossRef]
80. Sui, B.-D.; Xu, T.-Q.; Liu, J.-W.; Wei, W.; Zheng, C.-X.; Guo, B.-L.; Wang, Y.-Y.; Yang, Y.-L. Understanding the role of mitochondria in the pathogenesis of chronic pain. *Postgrad. Med. J.* **2013**, *89*, 709–714. [CrossRef]
81. Doyle, T.M.; Salvemini, D. Mini-Review: Mitochondrial dysfunction and chemotherapy-induced neuropathic pain. *Neurosci. Lett.* **2021**, *760*, 136087. [CrossRef]
82. Totsch, S.K.; Waite, M.E.; Sorge, R.E. Dietary influence on pain via the immune system. *Prog. Mol. Biol. Transl. Sci.* **2015**, *131*, 435–469.
83. Skouroliakou, M.; Grosomanidis, D.; Massara, P.; Kostara, C.; Papandreou, P.; Ntountaniotis, D.; Xepapadakis, G. Serum antioxidant capacity, biochemical profile and body composition of breast cancer survivors in a randomized Mediterranean dietary intervention study. *Eur. J. Nutr.* **2018**, *57*, 2133–2145. [CrossRef] [PubMed]
84. Butalla, A.C.; Crane, T.E.; Patil, B.; Wertheim, B.C.; Thompson, P.; Thomson, C.A. Effects of a Carrot Juice Intervention on Plasma Carotenoids, Oxidative Stress, and Inflammation in Overweight Breast Cancer Survivors. *Nutr. Cancer* **2012**, *64*, 331–341. [CrossRef] [PubMed]
85. Schatz, A.A.; Oliver, T.K.; Swarm, R.A.; Paice, J.A.; Darbari, D.S.; Dowell, D.; Meghani, S.H.; Winckworth-Prejsnar, K.; Bruera, E.; Plovnick, R.M.; et al. Bridging the Gap Among Clinical Practice Guidelines for Pain Management in Cancer and Sickle Cell Disease. *J. Natl. Compr. Cancer Netw.* **2020**, *18*, 392–399. [CrossRef]
86. Hartung, J.E.; Eskew, O.; Wong, T.; Tchivileva, I.E.; Oladosu, F.A.; O'Buckley, S.C.; Nackley, A.G. Nuclear factor-kappa B regulates pain and COMT expression in a rodent model of inflammation. *Brain Behav. Immun.* **2015**, *50*, 196–202. [CrossRef] [PubMed]
87. Kolberg, M.; Pedersen, S.; Bastani, N.E.; Carlsen, H.; Blomhoff, R.; Paur, I. Tomato paste alters NF-κB and cancer-related mRNA expression in prostate cancer cells, xenografts, and xenograft microenvironment. *Nutr. Cancer* **2015**, *67*, 305–315. [CrossRef] [PubMed]
88. Deleemans, J.M.; Chleilat, F.; Reimer, R.A.; Henning, J.-W.; Baydoun, M.; Piedalue, K.-A.; McLennan, A.; Carlson, L.E. The chemo-gut study: Investigating the long-term effects of chemotherapy on gut microbiota, metabolic, immune, psychological and cognitive parameters in young adult Cancer survivors; study protocol. *BMC Cancer* **2019**, *19*, 1243. [CrossRef]

89. Song, B.C.; Bai, J. Microbiome-gut-brain axis in cancer treatment-related psychoneurological toxicities and symptoms: A systematic review. *Supportive Care Cancer* **2021**, *29*, 605–617. [CrossRef]
90. Kelly, D.L.; Lyon, D.E.; Yoon, S.L.; Horgas, A.L. The microbiome and cancer: Implications for oncology nursing science. *Cancer Nurs.* **2016**, *39*, E56–E62. [CrossRef]
91. Guo, R.; Chen, L.-H.; Xing, C.; Liu, T. Pain regulation by gut microbiota: Molecular mechanisms and therapeutic potential. *Br. J. Anaesth.* **2019**, *123*, 637–654. [CrossRef]
92. Santoni, M.; Miccini, F.; Battelli, N. Gutmicrobiota, immunity and pain. *Immunol. Lett.* **2021**, *229*, 44–47. [CrossRef]
93. Nijs, J.; Yilmaz, S.T.; Elma, O.; Tatta, J.; Mullie, P.; Vanderweeen, L.; Clarys, P.; Deliens, T.; Coppieters, I.; Weltens, N.; et al. Nutritional intervention in chronic pain: An innovative way of targeting central nervous system sensitization? *Expert Opin. Ther. Targets* **2020**, *24*, 793–803. [CrossRef] [PubMed]
94. Nijs, J.; Elma, Ö.; Yilmaz, S.T.; Mullie, P.; Vanderweeën, L.; Clarys, P.; Deliens, T.; Coppieters, I.; Weltens, N.; Van Oudenhove, L. Nutritional neurobiology and central nervous system sensitisation: Missing link in a comprehensive treatment for chronic pain? *Br. J. Anaesth.* **2019**, *123*, 539–543. [CrossRef] [PubMed]
95. Forsythe, P.; Kunze, W.A.; Bienenstock, J. On communication between gut microbes and the brain. *Curr. Opin. Gastroenterol.* **2012**, *28*, 557–562. [CrossRef]
96. Dworsky-Fried, Z.; Kerr, B.J.; Taylor, A.M. Microbes, microglia, and pain. *Neurobiol. Pain* **2020**, *7*, 100045. [CrossRef] [PubMed]
97. Croisier, E.; Brown, T.; Bauer, J. The Efficacy of Dietary Fiber in Managing Gastrointestinal Toxicity Symptoms in Patients with Gynecologic Cancers undergoing Pelvic Radiotherapy: A Systematic Review. *J. Acad. Nutr. Diet.* **2021**, *121*, 261–277.e2. [CrossRef]
98. Lynch, S.V.; Pedersen, O. The Human Intestinal Microbiome in Health and Disease. *N. Engl. J. Med.* **2016**, *375*, 2369–2379. [CrossRef]
99. Guida, F.; Boccella, S.; Belardo, C.; Iannotta, M.; Piscitelli, F.; De Filippis, F.; Paino, S.; Ricciardi, F.; Siniscalco, D.; Marabese, I. Altered gut microbiota and endocannabinoid system tone in vitamin D deficiency-mediated chronic pain. *Brain Behav. Immun.* **2020**, *85*, 128–141. [CrossRef]
100. Dalile, B.; Van Oudenhove, L.; Vervliet, B.; Verbeke, K. The role of short-chain fatty acids in microbiota–gut–brain communication. *Nat. Rev. Gastroenterol. Hepatol.* **2019**, *16*, 461–478. [CrossRef]
101. Sheflin, A.M.; Borresen, E.C.; Kirkwood, J.S.; Boot, C.M.; Whitney, A.K.; Lu, S.; Brown, R.J.; Broeckling, C.D.; Ryan, E.P.; Weir, T.L. Dietary supplementation with rice bran or navy bean alters gut bacterial metabolism in colorectal cancer survivors. *Mol. Nutr. Food Res.* **2017**, *61*, 1500905. [CrossRef]
102. Horigome, A.; Okubo, R.; Hamazaki, K.; Kinoshita, T.; Katsumata, N.; Uezono, Y.; Xiao, J.; Matsuoka, Y. Association between blood omega-3 polyunsaturated fatty acids and the gut microbiota among breast cancer survivors. *Benef. Microbes* **2019**, *10*, 751–758. [CrossRef]
103. Fassier, P.; Zelek, L.; Lécuyer, L.; Bachmann, P.; Touillaud, M.; Druesne-Pecollo, N.; Galan, P.; Cohen, P.; Hoarau, H.; Latino-Martel, P. Modifications in dietary and alcohol intakes between before and after cancer diagnosis: Results from the prospective population-based NutriNet-Santé cohort. *Int. J. Cancer* **2017**, *141*, 457–470. [CrossRef] [PubMed]
104. Park, B.; Lee, J.; Kim, J. Imbalanced nutrient intake in cancer survivors from the examination from the nationwide health examination center-based cohort. *Nutrients* **2018**, *10*, 212. [CrossRef]
105. Zhang, F.F.; Liu, S.; John, E.M.; Must, A.; Demark-Wahnefried, W. Diet quality of cancer survivors and noncancer individuals: Results from a national survey. *Cancer* **2015**, *121*, 4212–4221. [CrossRef] [PubMed]
106. Zhang, F.F.; Ojha, R.P.; Krull, K.R.; Gibson, T.M.; Lu, L.; Lanctot, J.; Chemaitilly, W.; Robison, L.L.; Hudson, M.M. Adult Survivors of Childhood Cancer Have Poor Adherence to Dietary Guidelines. *J. Nutr.* **2016**, *146*, 2497–2505. [CrossRef]
107. Tollosa, D.N.; Holliday, E.; Hure, A.; Tavener, M.; James, E.L. A 15-year follow-up study on long-term adherence to health behaviour recommendations in women diagnosed with breast cancer. *Breast Cancer Res. Treat.* **2020**, *182*, 727–738. [CrossRef] [PubMed]
108. Polak, R.; Dacey, M.; Phillips, E.M. Time for food—Training physiatrists in nutritional prescription. *J. Rehabil. Med.* **2017**, *49*, 106–112. [CrossRef]
109. Song, S.; Youn, J.; Lee, Y.J.; Kang, M.; Hyun, T.; Song, Y.; Lee, J.E. Dietary supplement use among cancer survivors and the general population: A nation-wide cross-sectional study. *BMC Cancer* **2017**, *17*, 891. [CrossRef]
110. Du, M.; Luo, H.; Blumberg, J.B.; Rogers, G.; Chen, F.; Ruan, M.; Shan, Z.; Biever, E.; Zhang, F.F. Dietary supplement use among adult cancer survivors in the United States. *J. Nutr.* **2020**, *150*, 1499–1508. [CrossRef]
111. Boland, E.; Ahmedzai, S. Persistent pain in cancer survivors. *Curr. Opin. Support. Palliat. Care* **2017**, *11*, 181–190. [CrossRef]
112. Rock, C.L.; Doyle, C.; Demark-Wahnefried, W.; Meyerhardt, J.; Courneya, K.S.; Schwartz, A.L.; Bandera, E.V.; Hamilton, K.K.; Grant, B.; McCullough, M.; et al. Nutrition and physical activity guidelines for cancer survivors. *CA Cancer J. Clin.* **2012**, *62*, 275–276. [CrossRef]
113. Pouchieu, C.; Fassier, P.; Druesne-Pecollo, N.; Zelek, L.; Bachmann, P.; Touillaud, M.; Bairati, I.; Hercberg, S.; Galan, P.; Cohen, P. Dietary supplement use among cancer survivors of the NutriNet-Sante cohort study. *Br. J. Nutr.* **2015**, *113*, 1319–1329. [CrossRef] [PubMed]
114. Burden, S.; Jones, D.J.; Sremanakova, J.; Sowerbutts, A.M.; Lal, S.; Pilling, M.; Todd, C. Dietary interventions for adult cancer survivors. *Cochrane Database Syst. Rev.* **2019**, *2019*, CD011287. [CrossRef] [PubMed]
115. Befort, C.A.; Klemp, J.R.; Austin, H.L.; Perri, M.G.; Schmitz, K.H.; Sullivan, D.K.; Fabian, C.J. Outcomes of a weight loss intervention among rural breast cancer survivors. *Breast Cancer Res. Treat.* **2012**, *132*, 631–639. [CrossRef]

116. Tjon-A-Joe, S.; Pannekoek, S.; Kampman, E.; Hoedjes, M. Adherence to diet and body weight recommendations among cancer survivors after completion of initial cancer treatment: A systematic review of the literature. *Nutr. Cancer* **2019**, *71*, 367–374. [CrossRef] [PubMed]
117. Barlow, K.H.; van der Pols, J.C.; Ekberg, S.; Johnston, E.A. Cancer survivors' perspectives of dietary information provision after cancer treatment: A scoping review of the Australian context. *Health Promot. J. Aust.* **2021**, *33*, 232–244. [CrossRef]
118. Vijayvergia, N.; Denlinger, C.S. Lifestyle factors in cancer survivorship: Where we are and where we are headed. *J. Pers. Med.* **2015**, *5*, 243–263. [CrossRef] [PubMed]

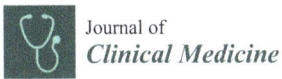

Article

Individual Patterns and Temporal Trajectories of Changes in Fear and Pain during Exposure In Vivo: A Multiple Single-Case Experimental Design in Patients with Chronic Pain

Jente Bontinck [1,2], Marlies den Hollander [3,4], Amanda L. Kaas [5], Jeroen R. De Jong [3,6] and Inge Timmers [2,3,*]

[1] Department of Rehabilitation Sciences and Physiotherapy, Ghent University, 9000 Ghent, Belgium; jente.bontinck@ugent.be
[2] Pain in Motion International Research Group, Department of Physiotherapy, Human Physiology and Anatomy, Faculty of Physical Education & Physiotherapy, Vrije Universiteit Brussel, 1090 Brussels, Belgium
[3] Department of Rehabilitation Medicine, Maastricht University, 6211 LK Maastricht, The Netherlands; m.hollander@adelante-zorggroep.nl (M.d.H.); jeroen.dejong@integrin.nl (J.R.D.J.)
[4] Adelante Centre of Expertise in Rehabilitation and Audiology, 6430 AB Hoensbroek, The Netherlands
[5] Department of Cognitive Neuroscience, Maastricht University, 6229 EV Maastricht, The Netherlands; a.kaas@maastrichtuniversity.nl
[6] Intergrin Academy for Specialized Healthcare, 6167 AC Geleen, The Netherlands
* Correspondence: inge.timmers@maastrichtuniversity.nl

Abstract: Exposure in vivo (EXP) is an effective treatment to reduce pain-related fear and disability in chronic pain populations. Yet, it remains unclear how reductions in fear and pain relate to each other. This single-case experimental design study attempted to identify patterns in the individual responses to EXP and to unravel temporal trajectories of fear and pain. Daily diaries were completed before, during and after EXP. Multilevel modelling analyses were performed to evaluate the overall effect. Temporal effects were scrutinized by individual regression analyses and determination of the time to reach a minimal clinically important difference. Furthermore, individual graphs were visually inspected for potential patterns. Twenty patients with chronic low back pain and complex regional pain syndrome type I were included. On a group level, both fear and pain were reduced following EXP. Individually, fear was significantly reduced in 65% of the patients, while pain in only 20%. A decrease in fear was seen mostly in the first weeks, while pain levels reduced later or remained unchanged. Daily measurements provided rich data on temporal trajectories of reductions in fear and pain. Overall, reductions in fear preceded pain relief and seemed to be essential to achieve pain reductions.

Keywords: chronic pain; exposure in vivo; pain-related fear; rehabilitation; chronic low back pain; complex regional pain syndrome

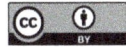

1. Introduction

Chronic pain is characterized by a complex interaction between physical and psychosocial factors, and therefore remains a therapeutic challenge [1]. Psychosocial factors have been recognised as important contributors to the development and maintenance of chronic pain and related disability. A major role is played by pain-related fear [2]. After an acute injury, it is a beneficial protection mechanism to fear and avoid activities that are associated with pain and potential further damage. Yet, this behaviour becomes maladaptive when it persists into the chronic stage [3]. Avoidance of daily activities results in functional deterioration, contributes to more pain and increases the fear of (re)injury [4]. This vicious circle is described as the fear-avoidance model [2].

Pain-related fear has been considered an important contributing factor in chronic musculoskeletal pain populations [2,5,6]. For instance, in patients with chronic low back pain (cLBP), fear contributes more to disability than pain intensity [7] and is associated with poorer recovery [8,9]. Furthermore, the recovery of patients with complex regional pain syndrome type I (CRPS-I) is adversely influenced by pain-related fear [10,11]. In fact, both populations showcase high similarities in fear and its association with disability [12].

Consequently, it is important to address pain-related fear in the rehabilitation of patients with chronic pain. Exposure in vivo (EXP) is a cognitive-behavioural treatment that stimulates patients to perform threatening movements and activities, in order to modify their expectations about movement and injury, and to reduce their avoidance behaviour [13]. Combining exposure with pain education teaches patients that their disability is self-manageable and their pain is not necessarily a reliable indicator of injury [14]. EXP has been demonstrated to be effective in patients with cLBP [15–17], CRPS [18,19], and other pain types [20,21]. Although EXP decreases fear and disability in most patients, approximately 40–60% does not respond with clinically relevant changes in pain experiences [17,22]. Importantly, this treatment does not explicitly target pain levels. The primary intention is to lower pain-related fear and consequently disability, as they show a strong association unaffected by pain intensity [4]. Conversely, fear does mediate the associations between pain and disability [9]. Fear influences the report of pain [23], but is also identified as a consequence rather than a precipitating factor of pain [24]. These findings suggest an unique but also complicated relationship between fear and pain. It has been anecdotally reported that during EXP fear is reduced first and then followed by reductions in pain, but this has not been formally investigated. It also remains unclear whether reductions in fear are a prerequisite for pain relief.

Therefore, the primary aim of this study was to examine the temporal relationship between changes in pain-related fear and pain intensity during EXP in patients with chronic pain. Daily diaries were used to scrutinise the chronology of treatment effects and to identify individual patterns. These insights could help clinicians to improve patient-tailored treatment approaches. Our hypothesis was that decreases in fear during EXP would precede pain relief.

2. Materials and Methods

2.1. Study Design

A sequential single-case experimental design (SCED) was used in this study, in which several outcomes per participant were repeatedly assessed throughout different phases [25]. Participants completed daily repeated measures during a baseline period (phase A), an intervention phase (phase B), and an immediate post-intervention period (phase C). In addition to the diaries, online questionnaires were completed at baseline and post-treatment.

2.2. Procedures

This SCED study is part of a larger study investigating effects of EXP on chronic pain, "BrainEXPain". BrainEXPain was approved by the Medical Ethical Committee of Maastricht University Hospital/Maastricht University (MUMC+/UM). The protocol is registered at ClinicalTrials.gov [NCT02347579]. Previous papers of the "BrainEXPain" project focused on fMRI [22,26], in relation to pain-related questionnaires. The results of the diaries have not been described yet.

Patients were recruited via the department of Rehabilitation Medicine at MUMC+/ Adelante Rehabilitation Centre, between January 2015 and August 2017. They were referred by a physiatrist to a multidisciplinary screening procedure and were requested to fill out an online screening questionnaire (Qualtrics, Provo, UT, USA). Eligible patients, for whom pain-related fear was suspected to be a major contributing factor, were briefed on the study procedure, daily diaries, and treatment approach, and were asked to sign the informed consent. If both the multidisciplinary team and the patient gave a green light, information about EXP and an introduction to pain education was provided. Prior to the first study visit in which an MRI scan was performed, patients were requested to fill out online questionnaires and to start with filling out daily diaries (Qualtrics, Provo, UT, USA) for five consecutive days or more, which resulted in a pseudo-randomized baseline period. Three days prior to the first treatment session, patients were requested to start completing daily diaries again and to continue throughout the whole treatment period. Daily diaries were consistently sent out at 9:00 am. The online questionnaires were repeated post-treatment and the patients were asked to continue filling out the diaries for another two weeks (Figure 1).

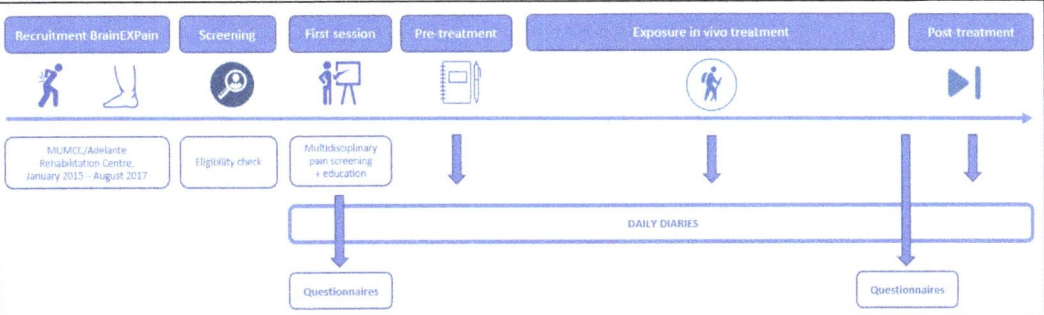

Figure 1. Timeline study procedure.

2.3. Participants

The study included patients with cLBP as well as patients with CRPS, between 18 and 65 years old. To be included, patients had to experience non-specific LBP for at least 6 months or to be diagnosed with complex regional pain syndrome type-I (CRPS-I) based on the Budapest criteria [27]. Patients were referred for EXP if irrational cognitions and pain-related fear was deemed to be a maintaining factor for pain-related disability, by an experienced rehabilitation team (including a physiatrist, a physical therapist, a psychologist, and an occupational therapist). Exclusion criteria were other diagnoses that could explain the symptoms, pregnancy, and serious psychopathology diagnosed with the Symptom Checklist (SCL-90) [28].

2.4. Exposure In Vivo Treatment

Exposure in vivo (EXP) is standard care for patients with chronic pain and elevated pain-related fear at MUMC+/Adelante. This treatment exposes patients to feared movements and activities, in order to challenge and adjust their exaggerated expectations related to harm and (re-)injury. EXP aims to modify fear-avoidance beliefs by increasing knowledge about pain, encouraging to perform threatening activities, and challenging patient's expectations about consequences of movement. A detailed description of the EXP-protocol can be found in Vlaeyen et al. [29]. First, individual threatening activities were identified by using the photograph series of daily activities (PHODA) [30]. Treatment started subsequently with pain education, in which was explained that pain is not an indicator of harm and may persist in a vicious fear-avoidance circle. In the EXP sessions, threatening activities selected from the patient's completed PHODA were performed to challenge their expectancies and were encouraged to repeatedly perform relevant threatening activities until they no longer intended to avoid them. EXP typically consist of 16 sessions, but the number could be adapted based on clinicians' and patient's decision.

2.5. Outcomes

2.5.1. Daily Measures

Daily levels of pain intensity and self-reported fear of three personally relevant daily-life movements/activities were assessed using electronic diaries. These individually tailored activities were selected based on a ranking of movements/activities (PHODA) by the participant as being threatening and personally relevant. Participants received a daily reminder to complete a brief questionnaire. Participants were requested to complete the daily assessments from baseline until two weeks after the end of treatment. Due to variations in scheduling, the baseline period differed for each participant and hence was pseudo-randomized. All items were rated on a visual analogue scale (VAS) ranging from 0 to 100. The daily questions are described in Table 1. Diaries have been shown to be sensitive to capture the effect of exposure in vivo treatment [11,18,31].

Table 1. Diary questions.

Topic	Question	Scale
Pain-related fear	"How threatening would it be for you to perform this activity at this moment?" (one question for each of the three tailored activities)	0 = not at all–100 = very
Pain intensity	"How intense is your pain at this moment?" "How intense was your most intense pain during the last 24 h?" "How intense was your least intense pain during the last 24 h?"	0 = not at all–100 = worst imaginable

2.5.2. Non-Daily Questionnaires

Online questionnaires were filled out at baseline and post-treatment. The following standardised questionnaires were included: Pain Disability Index [32], photograph series of daily activities (PHODA) for low back [33], upper [34], or lower extremities [35], Tampa Scale of Kinesiophobia (TSK) [36], Pain Catastrophizing Scale (PCS) [37], Hospital Anxiety and Depression Scale (HADS) [38], Pain Vigilance and Awareness Questionnaire (PVAQ), Short-Form McGill Pain Questionnaire (SFMPQ) [39], and the Resilience Scale (RS) [40]. Participants were also asked to score their pain on a standard 11-point numeric rating scale from 0 ("no pain") to 10 ("most pain imaginable") [41]. An average pain score was calculated; combining the current pain, pain from the night before and the worst, the best, and average pain in the last week.

2.6. Statistical Analyses

Initially, descriptive statistics of baseline characteristics, including the average fear and pain levels, were examined. Our statistical analyses of daily diary data were conducted with the MultiSCED app (http://34.251.13.245/MultiSCED/; 1 October 2021). MultiSCED has been developed in R to provide the possibility to investigate intervention effects at the individual level and to combine SCED data across cases through multilevel modelling [42]. By creating a multilevel model, the strong internal validity of monitoring a single case can be extended to estimate overall treatment effects [43]. To evaluate the overall changes in pain-related fear and pain intensity, the pre- and post-treatment daily data were compared on a group level. The significance level was set at $\alpha = 0.05$, 95% CI. Missing data was handled according to the randomized-marker method, in which all days the diary was not completed were displayed as "NA" (not applicable) [44,45].

Subsequently, individual data were examined to identify individual patterns and to unravel interactions between pain-related fear and pain intensity. Individual regression analyses were performed, comparing baseline (phase A) and post-intervention results (phase C) to examine the effect of EXP per individual.

In order to investigate when treatment effects occur during the intervention:

(1) Different phases were created to be used in a sliding window approach. We started comparing baseline data (phase A) with all intervention and post-intervention data (Phase B + C). Afterwards, we systematically added one week to phase A to obtain a timeline for treatment effects (e.g., Phase A + 1w), until phase B consists of less than five measurements.

(2) The time to reach the minimal clinically important difference (MCID) was scrutinized. To unravel the relevance of EXP to patient care, it is useful to not only focus on statistically significant changes, but also on clinically important differences. Even if the statistical result is not significant, the patient might still feel meaningful pain

relief or physical improvement due to treatment. A reduction of 30% in pain intensity on a 11-point numeric rating scale has been considered as a MCID in chronic pain populations [46,47]. Therefore, the 30% cut-off value, starting from the baseline average, for pain intensity and for pain-related fear was calculated for each patient. The moment the patient scored lower than this value for at least three consecutive days, was considered as the point of MCID.

(3) Individual visual graphs and descriptive values were explored to divide the patients into clusters based on their response to EXP. Patterns in temporal changes were analysed within these clusters and compared to the results of the sliding window approach, the time to reach the MCID and the differences between baseline and post-intervention questionnaires.

Pre- and post-intervention questionnaires were analysed using SPSS (version 27). First, normality was checked with the Shapiro-Wilk test. Treatment effects of normally distributed variables were analysed with the paired Student's *t*-test and the paired Wilcoxon-test was used for non-normally distributed variables.

At last, moderator variables for treatment effectiveness were also exploratively scrutinized, by including them one by one in the pre–post multilevel model (e.g., gender, age, population, and the baseline results of the non-daily questionnaires).

3. Results

3.1. Participant Characteristics

The recruitment period resulted in 38 included patients in BrainEXPain, of which 23 initiated and completed EXP. Based on the completeness of the daily diaries (minimal duration of treatment of five weeks with at least 40% of the daily diaries completed), 20 patients were analysed as single-cases in this study (Figure 2), including thirteen patients with cLBP and seven with CRPS. The baseline demographic characteristics and most relevant reported outcomes can be found in Table 2. Detailed information on baseline scores for all questionnaires can be accessed in Supplementary materials.

Table 2. Baseline patient characteristics.

Case	Population	Age	Sex (% M)	BMI	Duration Complaints (Total = Median)	Average Pain Score	PDI	PHODA
C01	CRPS LE	43	M	27.47	3–6 m	6.4	34	45.00
C02	CLBP	55	F	26.29	>5 y	5	28	49.43
C03	CLBP	41	F	25.71	2–5 y	6.8	50	61.30
C04	CRPS UE	28	M	24.22	1–2 y	7.6	57	73.00
C05	CLBP	35	M	28.40	2–5 y	3.4	7	18.28
C06	CLBP	36	M	28.70	6–12 m	7	48	43.38
C07	CLBP	28	F	25.00	2–5 y	3.8	41	40.25
C08	CLBP	23	M	22.64	>5 y	7.6	45	71.15
C09	CLBP	37	M	20.28	2–5 y	4	19	28.20
C10	CLBP	53	M	26.85	2–5 y	5.8	39	65.35
C11	CLBP	32	M	29.39	1–2 y	5.6	38	35.38
C12	CLBP	57	M	25.00	2–5 y	4.6	49	71.28
C13	CLBP	52	M	30.76	1–2 y	5.2	35	40.55
C14	CLBP	40	M	29.39	>5 y	3.6	19	54.00
C15	CRPS LE	33	F	27.76	6–12 m	6.2	42	47.95
C16	CLBP	44	M	27.93	>5 y	0	57	70.40
C17	CRPS LE	62	F	31.99	>5 y	6.4	44	83.88
C18	CRPS LE	27	F	24.81	2–5 y	3.6	35	7.28
C19	CRPS UE	34	F	44.63	3–6 m	8.4	49	72.17
C20	CRPS LE	29	F	37.11	1–2 y	8	29	25.25
Mean CLBP	13	41	77%	27	2–5 y	5	37	50
Mean CRPS	7	37	29%	31	1–2 y	7	41	51
Overall mean	20	39	60%	28	2–5 y	5	38	50

CLBP = chronic low back pain; CRPS = complex regional pain syndrome type I; F = female; LE = lower extremities; M = male; PDI = Pain Disability Index (0–70); UE = upper extremities.

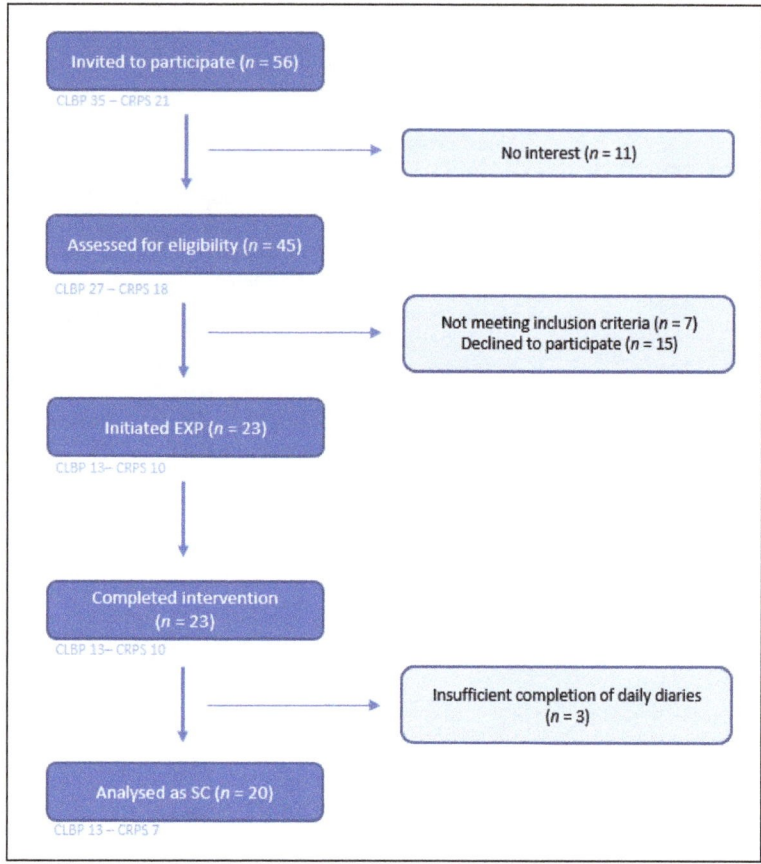

Figure 2. Flow chart of recruitment process. CLBP = chronic low back pain; CRPS = complex regional pain syndrome type I; Exp = exposure in vivo treatment; SC = single case subject.

3.2. Treatment Characteristics

Patients initially received two sessions per week, which was reduced to one session per week in the generalisation phase. Total treatment duration ranged from 5 to 14 weeks, with an average of 9 weeks, which was determined by a common decision between the therapist and the patient (Table 3).

Table 3. Completeness of daily measurements.

Case	Duration Baseline		Duration EXP		Duration Post-Intervention	
	Duration (Days)	Measurements	Duration (Days (Weeks))	Completion (%)	Duration (Days)	Completion (%)
C01	23	12	94 (14)	100	19	100
C02	9	9	72 (11)	90	12	61
C03	34	9	47 (7)	64	17	56
C04	33	10	66 (10)	41	19	61
C05	7	7	30 (5)	67	0	-
C06	33	10	29 (5)	79	9	89
C07	26	5	59 (9)	66	0	-
C08	35	6	43 (7)	53	0	-

Table 3. Cont.

Case	Duration Baseline		Duration EXP		Duration Post-Intervention	
	Duration (Days)	Measurements	Duration (Days (Weeks))	Completion (%)	Duration (Days)	Completion (%)
C09	27	11	37 (6)	97	7	89
C10	34	11	66 (10)	55	4	56
C11	47	11	45 (7)	56	0	-
C12	42	11	51 (8)	64	0	-
C13	93	10	57 (9)	88	7	86
C14	31	5	52 (8)	88	0	-
C15	9	9	96 (14)	81	0	-
C16	41	5	57 (9)	81	0	-
C17	52	3	92 (14)	89	12	100
C18	29	9	57 (9)	81	0	-
C19	113	10	52 (8)	51	0	-
C20	65	9	57 (9)	59	0	-
Average	39.15	8.60	57.95 (8.95)	72.50	5.30	77.55

3.3. Diary Completion

An overview of the diary completion per patient and period can be found in Table 3. Baseline data contained 3 to 12 measures scattered throughout the five months prior to treatment, of which at least the three days right before the start of treatment were acquired. Completion during treatment had an average of 72.5%. Post-intervention data varied between 0 and 19 measures. Unfortunately, eleven patients did not complete the diaries after finishing treatment. When no follow up data was available, the last seven measurements during treatment were utilized for further analyses.

3.4. Multi-Level Modelling of Daily Diary Outcomes

Multi-level analyses of pre- and post-intervention diaries were performed to evaluate overall treatment effects (Table S1). Comparison of the daily measurements in phase A versus phase C showed significant improvements in pain related fear (MD = −29.44; SD = 7.30; t = −4.03; $p \leq 0.001$) and pain intensity (MD = −9.28; SD = 2.61; t = −3.55; $p = 0.002$) (both outcomes were scored on a scale from 0 to 100).

3.5. Descriptive and One-Level Analyses of Daily Diary Outcomes

The evolution of individual daily measurements of pain-related fear and pain intensity across all participants is shown in Figure 3. Visual inspection of these graphs reveals reduction of pain-related fear in almost all patients. Some showed an immediate response to EXP, while others display a delayed reaction. When observing pain intensity, only about half of the patients showed a decrease between baseline and post-intervention. Various patterns can be identified, emphasising that not all patients respond similarly to EXP and strong conclusions based on visual inspection are challenging.

Therefore, a schematic overview of the one-level analyses is presented in Figures 4 and 5, and detailed statistical information can be found in Tables S2 and S3. First, all daily measurements during baseline phase A were compared with those during the post-intervention phase C. This comparison showcases the effectiveness of EXP for the relevant outcomes. For pain-related fear, the effect of treatment manifests itself in significant reductions in 13 out of 20 patients (65%). By contrast, only four showed a significant reduction for pain between the baseline and post-intervention phase (20%).

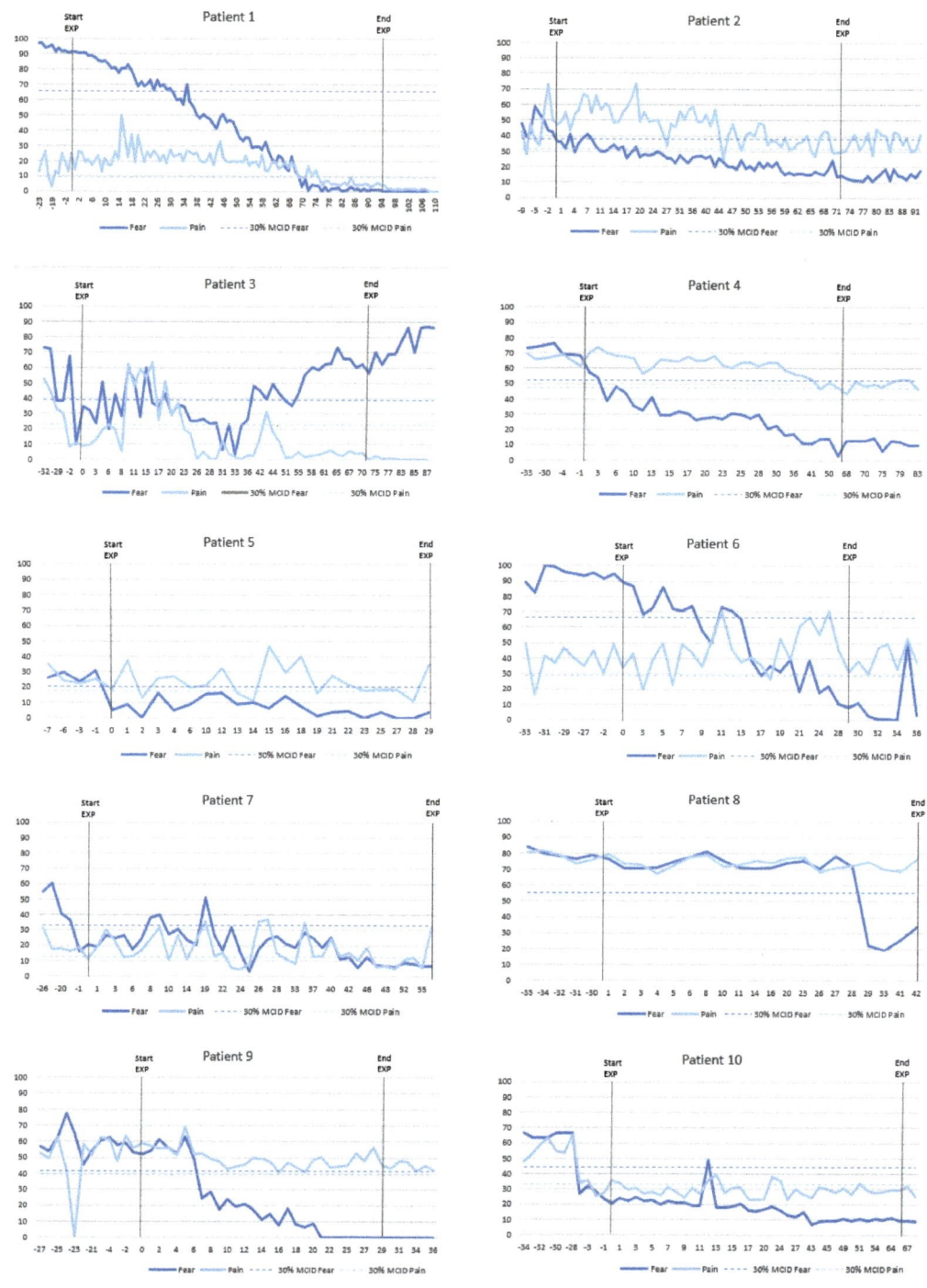

Figure 3. *Cont.*

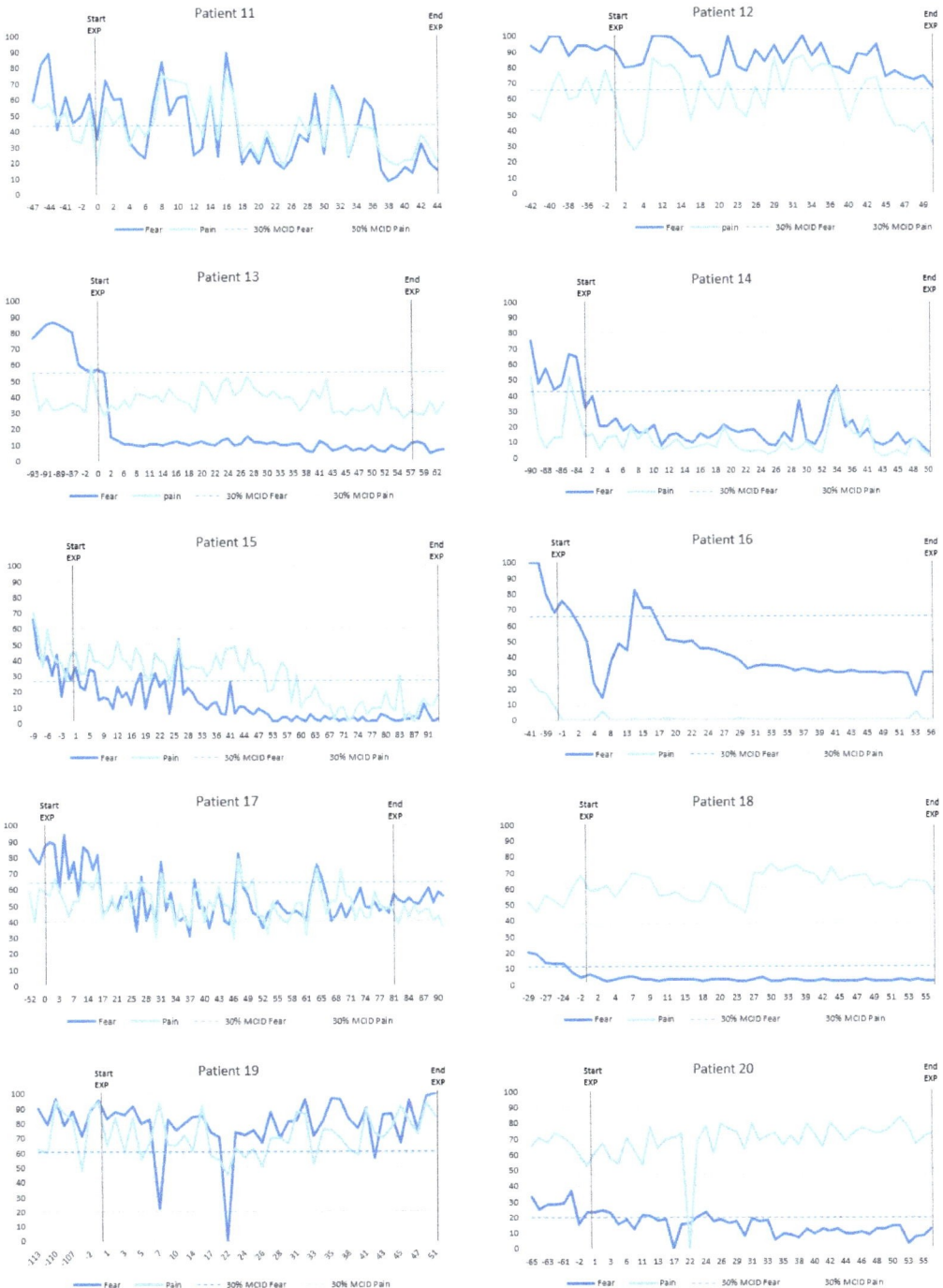

Figure 3. Graphs of daily measurements of pain-related fear and pain intensity.

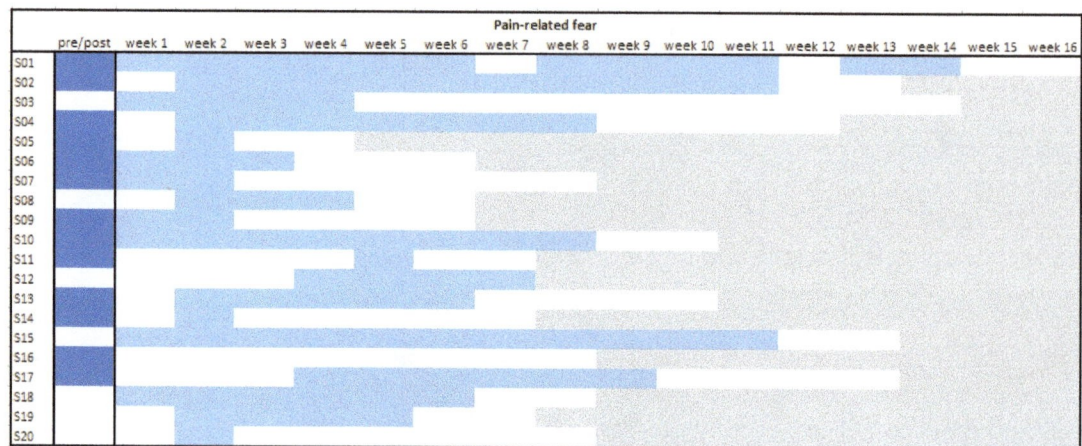

Figure 4. Overview of individual significant reductions per phase for pain-related fear. ▇ pre–post effect ($p < 0.05$); ▭ change in trend ($p < 0.05$); ▭ non-significant change; ▭ end of EXP. Note. A light blue box means the trend of scores before that specific week was significantly different than the trend of scores after this point. A white box after a light blue box means that that week no big changes occurred anymore.

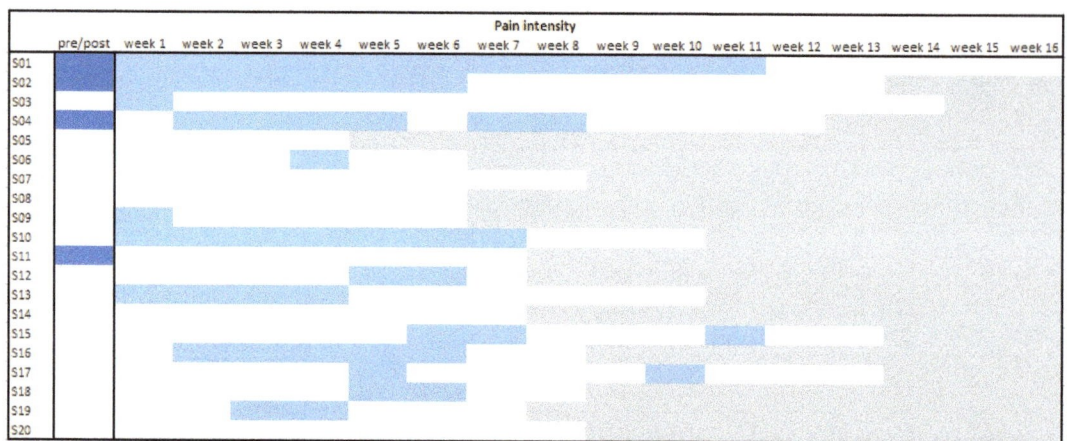

Figure 5. Overview of individual significant reductions per phase for pain intensity. ▇ pre-post effect ($p < 0.05$); ▭ change in trend ($p < 0.05$); ▭ non-significant change; ▭ end of EXP. Note. A light blue box means the trend of scores before that specific week was significantly different than the trend of scores after this point. A white box after a light blue box means that that week no big changes occurred anymore.

Consequently, it was analysed during which week a significant change in trend appeared by comparing all data before the respective week with all further data (i.e., sliding window approach). These results were rather variable, but visual inspection of Figures 4 and 5 shows that patients had earlier and more continuous changes in pain-related fear than in pain intensity. After two weeks, the scores for fear were significantly influenced in 16 of the patients (80%), and for pain, only, in 8 of the patients (40%). Only one patient did not experience a significant change in fear at any point during treatment (even though the overall pre–post comparison did yield a significant difference), while for pain six patients did not show a change in trend at any point.

3.6. Time to Reach the Minimal Clinically Important Differences (MCID)

An overview of these findings is given in Figure 6. The earlier the clinically meaningful effect occurred, the darker blue the box is coloured. Inspection of this figure quickly shows that the cut-off values for fear were more often and sooner reached than for pain intensity. The fear scores reached the cut-off in all but two patients, while the pain scores reached the MCID in only half of the patients. Of those who reached a MCID for pain, it preceded an MCID in fear in only one patient (10%). The others showed a MCID in fear before or during the same week as an MCID in pain. The range in which the MCID was reached was week 1 to 7 for fear and week 1 to 11 for pain. Additionally, during the first four weeks 15 of the 20 patients reached the MCID for fear, compared to only five for pain.

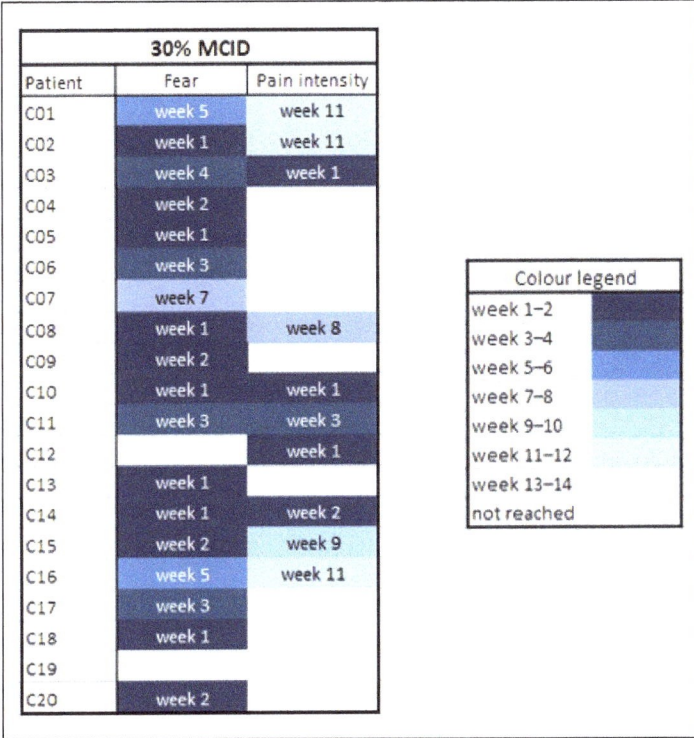

Figure 6. Time to reach the minimal clinically important difference per patient. MCID = minimal clinically important difference, fixed at 30% of the mean baseline score.

3.7. Visual Inspection of Clusters in Single Cases

Closer inspection of the individual graphs in Figure 3 shows that each patient responded differently to EXP. However, different patterns can be recognized and enables us to divide the patients into clusters. Based on the temporal effect on pain-related fear and pain intensity, four clusters could be identified (Figure 7).

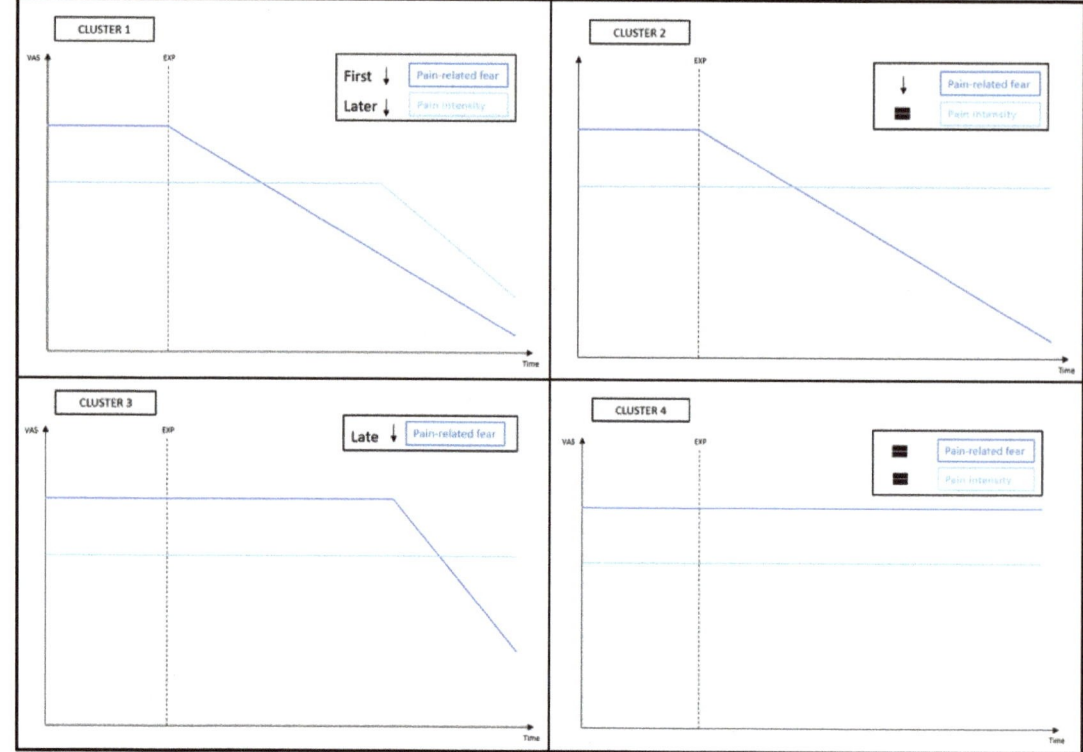

Figure 7. Overview of the clusters.

Cluster 1: Quick decrease in fear, pain follows

Patients in this cluster showed a decrease in pain-related fear quickly after the start of EXP, while a decrease in pain intensity only occurs later. Seven patients (i.e., 1, 2, 4, 7, 10, 14, and 15) showcase this pattern in greater or lesser extent.

Cluster 2: Decrease in fear, pain unaffected

This pattern is characterized by a decrease in pain-related fear, while the pain remained unchanged. This phenomenon is recognisable in the graphs of five patients (i.e., 5, 6, 9, 13, and 17).

Cluster 3: Late effect in fear

Three patients (i.e., 8, 11, and 16) showed a rather late decrease in pain-related fear, reflecting that they needed multiple treatment sessions and repeated exposure before the effect occurred. While patient 8 has a sudden drop in fear after four weeks, patient 11 had enormous fluctuations until far in treatment, and patient 16 had an initial early drop but relapsed before improvements slowly occurred again. Patient 8 showed no change in pain intensity, while the pain of patient 11 followed the same pattern of the fear and patient 16 described no pain throughout the whole treatment period.

Cluster 4: No clear effect

Based on visual inspection of the graphs, five patients (i.e., 3, 12, 18, 19, and 20) showed little to no change in pain-related fear or pain intensity.

3.8. Non-Daily Questionnaires

Before and after treatment the patients filled out online questionnaires. All results can be found in Table S4A,B. All variables were normally distributed. Comparisons of pre- and post-EXP data of all patients showed significant improvements in average pain score (-1.64 ± 2.16; $p = 0.003$), pain-related disability (PDI; -27.4 ± 15.36 SD; $p < 0.001$), pain-related fear (PHODA; -33.33 ± 22.69 SD; $p < 0.001$), fear of movement (TSK; -10.65 ± 7.39 SD; $p < 0.001$), pain catastrophizing (PCS; -12.4 ± 13.08 SD; $p < 0.001$), pain vigilance (PVAQ; -13.75 ± 16.57 SD; $p = 0.001$), pain rating (SFMPQ; -5.4 ± 6.48 SD; $p = 0.001$), and resilience (RS; -7.1 ± 7.45 SD; $p < 0.001$), but not on anxiety and depression (HADS; -2.35 ± 7.17; $p = 0.16$).

Based on the distribution into the four clusters, differences can also be exploratively inspected in questionnaires results. Baseline average pain scores were the highest in cluster 4 compared to the other clusters, while the gain by EXP was the lowest. Baseline PDI scores were higher in cluster 3 and 4, while cluster 2 and 4 showed smaller improvement in disability after treatment. No differences between the clusters were seen in baseline PHODA and RS scores, yet cluster 4 showed again the least improvement in these questionnaires. Other between clusters results were comparable.

3.9. Moderating Factors of Treatment Efficacy

In order to evaluate which characteristics influenced the effect of EXP on the outcomes, the baseline scores were included as moderator variables in the pre–post multilevel model (Table S5). Treatment effect on pain-related fear was significantly moderated by gender ($p = 0.001$), showing a lower reduction of fear in women compared to men, but not by age, population, or any of the questionnaire results. None of the baseline characteristics significantly moderated the effect of EXP on pain intensity.

The text continues here. Proofs must be formatted as follows.

4. Discussion

The primary aim of this SCED study was to disentangle individual patterns in the temporal effect of EXP on pain-related fear and pain intensity. SCEDs have proven to be valid for demonstrating intervention effectiveness at an individual level and to observe these changes over time [43]. The strong internal validity of monitoring one participant has also been extended by creating a multilevel model, allowing to estimate overall effects across cases. Multilevel analyses revealed that daily fear and pain scores were lower after than before treatment, showing that—overall—EXP had a positive impact on both outcomes. The findings of this study are consistent with previous SCED studies that concluded that EXP had a positive effect on fear and intensity in patients with CRPS-I [18] and cLBP [48]. In addition to the positive group-level effects, individual subject analyses demonstrated that the majority of patients (65%) responded with a reduction in fear, while the effect on pain was more limited (20%). Both the sliding window approach and the time to reach MCID showcased that fear reductions occurred sooner or in absence of pain reductions.

When considering the temporal trajectories by the sliding window approach, it is remarkable that none of the patients showed an improvement in pain without an improvement in fear. This suggests that it is necessary to lower fear to obtain an effect on pain. This fits the idea to predominantly treat fear, as it is more disabling than pain itself [7] and contributes to the maintenance of chronic disability [49]. Disability was reduced by EXP, but it could have been useful to investigate when this effect occurs to understand its relationship with fear and pain. It might be that first new expectations are formed and subsequently fear reduces. Hence, individuals restart to perform formerly threatening activities and eventually their functionality increases. The reduction in pain subsequent to the reduction of fear could be explained by the fact that they share common brain networks [50,51]. Fear of pain involves similar neural circuits as pain perception, including the amygdala, limbic structures, anterior insula, and the adrenomedullary system [52–54]. Pain-related fear also recruits distinguishable networks, compared to non-pain related fears [55]. Previous neuroimaging analyses of this project established the involvement of cortico-limbic connectivity in the effect of EXP on pain intensity [22]. In particular, larger decreases in resting-state connectivity between the hippocampus and the posterior medial cortex were associated with larger pain relief and mediated the relationship between catastrophizing and pain. Furthermore, EXP had a positive impact on the medial prefrontal cortex and the right posterior insula, which play a fundamental role in the pain experience [56,57]. The description of pain as an unpleasant sensory and emotional experience [58] and the classification of chronic primary pain [59], highlight the neural and conceptual link between pain and emotion [60]. Pain is inextricably linked with biological, psychological, and socio-cultural factors. Fear, as a strong emotion, can influence pain experiences and reductions in fear can consequentially lead to pain reduction.

Scrutinizing daily assessments showed that each patient responded differently. However, based on the chronology of treatment effects, four patterns could be identified. The pattern of the first cluster—*quick decrease in fear, pain follows*—underscores our hypothesis. The sliding window approach showed that the patients in this cluster benefited already in the first two weeks concerning fear. This pattern is in accordance with the objective of EXP: to target fear and not pain itself. It is also in line with anecdotal reports of clinicians that many patients experience an early eye-opener, after which they manage to "flip the switch". This group also showed the largest improvement in disability. Their questionnaires results support the daily diaries, which showcases that SCEDs are appropriate to capture individual effects. Concerning the goal of EXP to lower fear, patients in cluster two—*decrease in fear, pain unaffected*—still responded well. Clusters one and two demonstrate an effect in the early phase, what may suggest that pain education and limited exposure sessions already affect fear. Patients in cluster three—*late effect in fear*—needed more EXP sessions before their fear levels distinctly decreased. Remarkable is that this cluster had the highest initial disability and fear. This group may have needed more persuasion before they let go of their avoidance and/or safety behaviours. The difference with cluster one could lay in what they are afraid of. For instance, fear of what can happen during threatening activities could be quickly reduced by EXP, while fear of not being able to handle the pain could be more persistent. However, this remains speculative and would need to be further investigated. Based on the diaries, patients of cluster four—*no clear effect*—did not respond positively. However, questionnaire scores still improved remarkably. Various explanations of why they did not respond as strongly as the others could be considered. First, it cannot be ruled out that their treatment period was too short or delayed treatment effects were not captured within the follow-up period. Delayed effects on pain-related fear have also been seen in youth with chronic pain [61]. Contradictory, short-term EXP might have better results than long-term [17]. Second, while a variety of activities were performed during treatment, only fear of three activities were daily questioned. These may not have been representative enough, given that the complete PHODA showed positive results. Third, it is noticeable that the baseline average pain was higher, while they did not score higher on fear. It may be that patients with higher initial pain benefited less from EXP than patients with higher fear. The presence of pain may not always be a reason to rise fear and to avoid activities. Morley et al. (2005) showed that fear is more common when the meaning attached to pain is negative and the individual considers their future self to be conditional on the presence of pain. These patients may have been more stubborn in their maladaptive thoughts and behaviour, or were unable to reflect their cognitions due to underlying psychiatric comorbidities. Therefore, it could be possible that for this heterogenic group EXP is not sufficient and these patients require a more extensive or different treatment approach [62,63].

No moderating factors were revealed, except for gender. Men's fear levels benefited more from EXP than women's. Noteworthy, they had higher baseline fear. This is in contrast with the fact that women are more likely to have higher fear levels [64], but it could be ascribed to the small sample size. Patients with higher fear levels were assumed to benefit more from EXP, but no moderator could not demonstrate that. However, it is worth mentioning that all patients already had elevated levels as they were referred to EXP based on the presence of pain-related fear and worries. In addition, no differences between patients with CRPS-I and cLBP were found. This suggests that they did not respond differently to EXP, and conclusions could be applicable for both populations. It has been stated that both populations have similar levels of fear, pain, and disability [12]. Previous research found fast improvement of fear by EXP in patients with cLBP emphasizing insight learning [65], but more gradual progression by trial-and-error learning in patients with CRPS-I [18]. However, our study did not reveal differences in response to EXP based on population.

It is noteworthy that the Body Mass Index of these patients was rather high. Obesity can interact with disability, whether as cause or result [66]. This could have an impact on treatment effects. The fact that exercise programs are able to reduce pain in patients with cLBP and overweight [67] raises the question whether increased activity could explain at least part of the effects. Furthermore, this factor may explain why some patients do not benefit from EXP alone, as obesity requires specific treatment as well [68].

Strengths and Limitations

One of the strengths of this SCED study is the high number of examined cases. Twenty patients filled out daily diaries with a total of 1136 observations, while previous research established that most SCED studies have an average of three to four cases [69]. Daily diaries were not only interpreted by visual graphs, but also by individual analyses, MCID calculations and multilevel modelling. However, this study also has some limitations. First, the baseline period was mostly short and unstable and not fully randomized (rather the practical context resulted in pseudo-randomization). Second, this study did not include long-term data. Therefore, we cannot evaluate long-term effects. Third, although at least 20 observations per case were collected to prevent biased intervention effects [43], diary completion was rather low. Fourth, interpretation of the MCID should be approached with caution. The cut-off value was determined by three successive measurements, but because of enormous fluctuations later increases are possible. Fifth and last, although the internal validity of SCED studies is strong [43], conclusions should be generalized to the total population with cautiousness. Future research should synthesize information obtained from multiple SCED studies and multiple variables to increase the external validity, especially for identifying treatment moderators.

5. Conclusions

The overall findings of this SCED study indicate that EXP reduced pain-related fear as well as pain intensity in patients with cLBP and CRPS-I. However, not all patients responded similarly and different patterns of treatment responses were identified. On an individual level, a reduction in fear was seen in most cases, prior to or in absence of a reduction in pain. For most patients, fear reduced already in the early stage of EXP, and it seemed that fear reductions are necessary to achieve pain relief. The idea that reductions in fear might be necessary to lower pain should encourage clinicians to target fear during rehabilitation. Future research should examine long term effects and should further unravel the benefits of patient clustering for screening and treatment approaches.

Supplementary Materials: The following supporting information can be downloaded at: https://www.mdpi.com/article/10.3390/jcm11051360/s1, Table S1: Multilevel modelling results of the pre-post EXP comparison; Table S2: Individual regression results per week for pain-related fear; Table S3: Individual regression results per week for pain intensity; Table S4A–C: results of non-daily questionnaires; Table S5: Moderating factors in multilevel pre-post model.

Author Contributions: Conceptualization, I.T., M.d.H., J.R.D.J., A.L.K. and J.B.; methodology, I.T., M.d.H., J.R.D.J. and A.L.K.; software, J.B. and M.d.H.; validation, I.T., M.d.H., J.R.D.J., A.L.K. and J.B.; formal analysis, J.B.; investigation, I.T.; resources, I.T., A.L.K. and J.R.D.J.; data curation, M.d.H., I.T. and J.B.; writing—original draft preparation, J.B.; writing—review and editing I.T., M.d.H., A.L.K.

and J.R.D.J.; visualization, J.B.; supervision, I.T., M.d.H., A.L.K. and J.R.D.J.; project administration, I.T., A.L.K. and J.R.D.J.; funding acquisition, I.T., A.L.K. and J.R.D.J. All authors have read and agreed to the published version of the manuscript.

Funding: This work was financially supported by the Health Foundation Limburg (Stichting Sint Annadal, Maastricht, to J.R.D.J., A.L.K.), Board of Directors of Maastricht University Medical Center (MUMC+, to J.R.D.J., A.L.K., I.T.), and Esperance Foundation (Stichting Esperance, to J.R.D.J.). Jente Bontinck was funded by the Special Research Fund of Ghent University (BOF01962334).

Institutional Review Board Statement: The study was approved by the Medical Ethical Committee of Maastricht University.

Informed Consent Statement: Informed consent was obtained from all subjects involved in the study.

Data Availability Statement: The datasets generated for this study are available on reasonable request to the responding author.

Acknowledgments: We would like to thank all participants for their time and effort. We also thank the staff of the department of Rehabilitation Medicine at MUMC+/Adelante Rehabilitation Centre and Patrick Onghena and Wim Van De Noortgate for their helpful advice concerning the MULTISCED app. Our beloved colleague, Amanda Kaas, passed away in September 2021. Her contributions to the project prior to her passing were significant and of incredible value.

Conflicts of Interest: The authors declare no conflict of interest. The funding sources had no role in the study design, collection, analysis, or interpretation of the data. One of the co-authors, Jeroen R. de Jong, currently works at Intergrin as a psychologist. Intergrin Academy for Specialized Healthcare is one of the affiliations that de Jong had when important parts of the work (i.e., the analyses, interpretation and writing) were carried out.

References

1. Miller, R.M.; Kaiser, R.S. Psychological Characteristics of Chronic Pain: A Review of Current Evidence and Assessment Tools to Enhance Treatment. *Curr. Pain Headache Rep.* **2018**, *22*, 22. [CrossRef] [PubMed]
2. Vlaeyen, J.W.S.; Linton, S.J. Fear-avoidance and its consequences in chronic musculoskeletal pain: A state of the art. *Pain* **2000**, *85*, 317–332. [CrossRef]
3. Crombez, G.; Eccleston, C.; Van Damme, S.; Vlaeyen, J.W.; Karoly, P. Fear-avoidance model of chronic pain: The next generation. *Clin. J. Pain* **2012**, *28*, 475–483. [CrossRef] [PubMed]
4. Zale, E.L.; Lange, K.L.; Fields, S.A.; Ditre, J.W. The relation between pain-related fear and disability: A meta-analysis. *J. Pain* **2013**, *14*, 1019–1030. [CrossRef]
5. Martinez-Calderon, J.; Flores-Cortes, M.; Morales-Asencio, J.M.; Luque-Suarez, A. Pain-Related Fear, Pain Intensity and Function in Individuals With Chronic Musculoskeletal Pain: A Systematic Review and Meta-Analysis. *J. Pain* **2019**, *20*, 1394–1415. [CrossRef]
6. Luque-Suarez, A.; Martinez-Calderon, J.; Falla, D. Role of kinesiophobia on pain, disability and quality of life in people suffering from chronic musculoskeletal pain: A systematic review. *Br. J. Sports Med.* **2019**, *53*, 554–559. [CrossRef]
7. Crombez, G.; Vlaeyen, J.W.; Heuts, P.H.; Lysens, R. Pain-related fear is more disabling than pain itself: Evidence on the role of pain-related fear in chronic back pain disability. *Pain* **1999**, *80*, 329–339. [CrossRef]
8. Wertli, M.M.; Rasmussen-Barr, E.; Weiser, S.; Bachmann, L.M.; Brunner, F. The role of fear avoidance beliefs as a prognostic factor for outcome in patients with nonspecific low back pain: A systematic review. *Spine J.* **2014**, *14*, 816–836. [CrossRef]
9. Marshall, P.W.M.; Schabrun, S.; Knox, M.F. Physical activity and the mediating effect of fear, depression, anxiety, and catastrophizing on pain related disability in people with chronic low back pain. *PLoS ONE* **2017**, *12*, e0180788. [CrossRef]
10. Bean, D.J.; Johnson, M.H.; Heiss-Dunlop, W.; Lee, A.C.; Kydd, R.R. Do psychological factors influence recovery from complex regional pain syndrome type 1? A prospective study. *Pain* **2015**, *156*, 2310–2318. [CrossRef]
11. De Jong, J.R.; Vlaeyen, J.W.; de Gelder, J.M.; Patijn, J. Pain-related fear, perceived harmfulness of activities, and functional limitations in complex regional pain syndrome type I. *J. Pain* **2011**, *12*, 1209–1218. [CrossRef] [PubMed]
12. Bean, D.J.; Johnson, M.H.; Kydd, R.R. Relationships between psychological factors, pain, and disability in complex regional pain syndrome and low back pain. *Clin. J. Pain* **2014**, *30*, 647–653. [CrossRef] [PubMed]
13. Vlaeyen, J.W.; Morley, S.; Linton, S.J.; Boersma, K.; de Jong, J. *Pain-Related Fear: Exposure-Based Treatment of Chronic Pain*; IASP Press: Malaga, Spain, 2012.
14. Vlaeyen, J.W.S.; Crombez, G. Behavioral Conceptualization and Treatment of Chronic Pain. *Annu. Rev. Clin. Psychol.* **2020**, *16*, 187–212. [CrossRef] [PubMed]
15. Woods, M.P.; Asmundson, G.J.G. Evaluating the efficacy of graded in vivo exposure for the treatment of fear in patients with chronic back pain: A randomized controlled clinical trial. *Pain* **2008**, *136*, 271–280. [CrossRef] [PubMed]

16. Leeuw, M.; Goossens, M.; van Breukelen, G.J.P.; de Jong, J.R.; Heuts, P.; Smeets, R.; Köke, A.J.A.; Vlaeyen, J.W.S. Exposure in vivo versus operant graded activity in chronic low back pain patients: Results of a randomized controlled trial. *Pain* **2008**, *138*, 192–207. [CrossRef]
17. Glombiewski, J.A.; Holzapfel, S.; Riecke, J.; Vlaeyen, J.W.S.; de Jong, J.; Lemmer, G.; Rief, W. Exposure and CBT for chronic back pain: An RCT on differential efficacy and optimal length of treatment. *J. Consult. Clin. Psychol.* **2018**, *86*, 533–545. [CrossRef]
18. De Jong, J.R.; Vlaeyen, J.W.S.; Onghena, P.; Cuypers, C.; den Hollander, M.; Ruijgrok, J. Reduction of pain-related fear in complex regional pain syndrome type I: The application of graded exposure In Vivo. *Pain* **2005**, *116*, 264–275. [CrossRef]
19. Den Hollander, M.; Goossens, M.; de Jong, J.; Ruijgrok, J.; Oosterhof, J.; Onghena, P.; Smeets, R.; Vlaeyen, J.W.S. Expose or protect? A randomized controlled trial of exposure in vivo vs pain-contingent treatment as usual in patients with complex regional pain syndrome type 1. *Pain* **2016**, *157*, 2318–2329. [CrossRef]
20. De Jong, J.R.; Vlaeyen, J.W.S.; van Eijsden, M.; Loo, C.; Onghena, P. Reduction of pain-related fear and increased function and participation in work-related upper extremity pain (WRUEP): Effects of exposure In Vivo. *Pain* **2012**, *153*, 2109–2118. [CrossRef]
21. Dekker, C.; Goossens, M.; Winkens, B.; Remerie, S.; Bastiaenen, C.; Verbunt, J. Functional Disability in Adolescents with Chronic Pain: Comparing an Interdisciplinary Exposure Program to Usual Care. *Children* **2020**, *7*, 288. [CrossRef]
22. Timmers, I.; van de Ven, V.; Vlaeyen, J.W.S.; Smeets, R.J.; Verbunt, J.A.; de Jong, J.R.; Kaas, A.L. Cortico-Limbic Circuitry in Chronic Pain Tracks Pain Intensity Relief Following Exposure In Vivo. *Biol. Psychiatry Glob. Open Sci.* **2021**, *1*, 28–36. [CrossRef]
23. Labrenz, F.; Icenhour, A.; Schlamann, M.; Forsting, M.; Bingel, U.; Elsenbruch, S. From Pavlov to pain: How predictability affects the anticipation and processing of visceral pain in a fear conditioning paradigm. *NeuroImage* **2016**, *130*, 104–114. [CrossRef] [PubMed]
24. Gheldof, E.L.; Crombez, G.; Van den Bussche, E.; Vinck, J.; Van Nieuwenhuyse, A.; Moens, G.; Mairiaux, P.; Vlaeyen, J.W. Pain-related fear predicts disability, but not pain severity: A path analytic approach of the fear-avoidance model. *Eur. J. Pain* **2010**, *14*, e871–e879. [CrossRef]
25. Onghena, P.; Edgington, E.S. Customization of pain treatments: Single-case design and analysis. *Clin. J. Pain* **2005**, *21*, 56–68. [CrossRef] [PubMed]
26. Timmers, I.; de Jong, J.R.; Goossens, M.; Verbunt, J.A.; Smeets, R.J.; Kaas, A.L. Exposure in vivo Induced Changes in Neural Circuitry for Pain-Related Fear: A Longitudinal fMRI Study in Chronic Low Back Pain. *Front. Neurosci.* **2019**, *13*, 970. [CrossRef] [PubMed]
27. Harden, N.R.; Bruehl, S.; Perez, R.S.G.M.; Birklein, F.; Marinus, J.; Maihofner, C.; Lubenow, T.; Buvanendran, A.; Mackey, S.; Graciosa, J.; et al. Validation of proposed diagnostic criteria (the "Budapest Criteria") for Complex Regional Pain Syndrome. *Pain* **2010**, *150*, 268–274. [CrossRef]
28. Derogatis, L.R.; Unger, R. Symptom checklist-90-revised. *Corsini Encycl. Psychol.* **2010**, 1–2. [CrossRef]
29. Vlaeyen, J.W.S.; den Hollander, M.; de Jong, J.; Simons, L. Exposure In Vivo for pain-related fear. In *Psychological Approaches to Pain Management*, 3rd ed.; Turk, D., Gatchel, R., Eds.; Guilford Press: New York, NY, USA, 2018.
30. Trost, Z.; France, C.R.; Thomas, J.S. Examination of the photograph series of daily activities (PHODA) scale in chronic low back pain patients with high and low kinesiophobia. *Pain* **2009**, *141*, 276–282. [CrossRef]
31. Hollander, M.D.; de Jong, J.; Onghena, P.; Vlaeyen, J.W.S. Generalization of exposure in vivo in Complex Regional Pain Syndrome type I. *Behav. Res.* **2020**, *124*, 103511. [CrossRef]
32. Tait, R.C.; Pollard, C.A.; Margolis, R.B.; Duckro, P.N.; Krause, S.J. The Pain Disability Index: Psychometric and validity data. *Arch. Phys. Med. Rehabil.* **1987**, *68*, 438–441.
33. Leeuw, M.; Goossens, M.E.; van Breukelen, G.J.; Boersma, K.; Vlaeyen, J.W. Measuring perceived harmfulness of physical activities in patients with chronic low back pain: The Photograph Series of Daily Activities-short electronic version. *J. Pain* **2007**, *8*, 840–849. [CrossRef] [PubMed]
34. Dubbers, A.T.; Vikström, M.H.; Jong, J.D. *The Photograph Series of Daily Activities (PHODA-UE): Cervical Spine and Shoulder, CD-Rom Version 1.2*; Zuyd University, Institute for Rehabilitation Research (iRv), Maastricht University: Heerlen/Maastricht, The Netherlands, 2003.
35. Jelinek, S.; Germes, D.; Leyckes, N.; de Jong, J.R. *The Photograph Series of Daily Activities (PHODA-LE): Lower Extremities, CD-Rom Version 1.2*; Zuyd University, Institute for Rehabilitation Research (iRv), Maastricht University: Heerlen/Maastricht, The Netherlands, 2003.
36. Miller, R.; Kori, S.; Todd, D. The tampa scale for kinisophobia. *Clin. J. Pain* **1991**, *7*, 51. [CrossRef]
37. Van Damme, S.; Crombez, G.; Bijttebier, P.; Goubert, L.; Van Houdenhove, B. A confirmatory factor analysis of the Pain Catastrophizing Scale: Invariant factor structure across clinical and non-clinical populations. *Pain* **2002**, *96*, 319–324. [CrossRef]
38. Snaith, R.P. The Hospital Anxiety And Depression Scale. *Health Qual. Life Outcomes* **2003**, *1*, 29. [CrossRef]
39. Melzack, R. The short-form McGill Pain Questionnaire. *Pain* **1987**, *30*, 191–197. [CrossRef]
40. Smith, B.W.; Dalen, J.; Wiggins, K.; Tooley, E.; Christopher, P.; Bernard, J. The brief resilience scale: Assessing the ability to bounce back. *Int. J. Behav. Med.* **2008**, *15*, 194–200. [CrossRef]
41. Hjermstad, M.J.; Fayers, P.M.; Haugen, D.F.; Caraceni, A.; Hanks, G.W.; Loge, J.H.; Fainsinger, R.; Aass, N.; Kaasa, S. Studies comparing Numerical Rating Scales, Verbal Rating Scales, and Visual Analogue Scales for assessment of pain intensity in adults: A systematic literature review. *J. Pain Symptom. Manag.* **2011**, *41*, 1073–1093. [CrossRef]

42. Declercq, L.; Cools, W.; Beretvas, S.N.; Moeyaert, M.; Ferron, J.M.; Van den Noortgate, W. MultiSCED: A tool for (meta-)analyzing single-case experimental data with multilevel modeling. *Behav. Res. Methods* **2020**, *52*, 177–192. [CrossRef]
43. Moeyaert, M.; Manolov, R.; Rodabaugh, E. Meta-Analysis of Single-Case Research via Multilevel Models: Fundamental Concepts and Methodological Considerations. *Behav. Modif.* **2020**, *44*, 265–295. [CrossRef]
44. De, T.K.; Michiels, B.; Tanious, R.; Onghena, P. Handling missing data in randomization tests for single-case experiments: A simulation study. *Behav. Res. Methods* **2020**, *52*, 1355–1370. [CrossRef]
45. Edgington, E.; Onghena, P. *Randomization Tests*; CRC Press: Boca Raton, FL, USA, 2007.
46. Rowbotham, M.C. What is a "clinically meaningful" reduction in pain? *Pain* **2001**, *94*, 131–132. [CrossRef]
47. Farrar, J.T.; Young, J.P., Jr.; LaMoreaux, L.; Werth, J.L.; Poole, R.M. Clinical importance of changes in chronic pain intensity measured on an 11-point numerical pain rating scale. *Pain* **2001**, *94*, 149–158. [CrossRef]
48. Vlaeyen, J.W.; de Jong, J.; Geilen, M.; Heuts, P.H.; van Breukelen, G. Graded exposure in vivo in the treatment of pain-related fear: A replicated single-case experimental design in four patients with chronic low back pain. *Behav. Res.* **2001**, *39*, 151–166. [CrossRef]
49. Volders, S.; Boddez, Y.; De Peuter, S.; Meulders, A.; Vlaeyen, J.W.S. Avoidance behavior in chronic pain research: A cold case revisited. *Behav. Res.* **2015**, *64*, 31–37. [CrossRef] [PubMed]
50. Hayes, D.J.; Northoff, G. Common brain activations for painful and non-painful aversive stimuli. *BMC Neurosci.* **2012**, *13*, 60. [CrossRef]
51. Vogt, B.A. Pain and emotion interactions in subregions of the cingulate gyrus. *Nat. Rev. Neurosci.* **2005**, *6*, 533–544. [CrossRef]
52. Elman, I.; Borsook, D. Threat Response System: Parallel Brain Processes in Pain vis-à-vis Fear and Anxiety. *Front. Psychiatry* **2018**, *9*, 29. [CrossRef]
53. Ochsner, K.N.; Ludlow, D.H.; Knierim, K.; Hanelin, J.; Ramachandran, T.; Glover, G.C.; Mackey, S.C. Neural correlates of individual differences in pain-related fear and anxiety. *Pain* **2006**, *120*, 69–77. [CrossRef]
54. Sambuco, N.; Costa, V.D.; Lang, P.J.; Bradley, M.M. Assessing the role of the amygdala in fear of pain: Neural activation under threat of shock. *J. Affect. Disord.* **2020**, *276*, 1142–1148. [CrossRef]
55. Biggs, E.E.; Timmers, I.; Meulders, A.; Vlaeyen, J.W.S.; Goebel, R.; Kaas, A.L. The neural correlates of pain-related fear: A meta-analysis comparing fear conditioning studies using painful and non-painful stimuli. *Neurosci. Biobehav. Rev.* **2020**, *119*, 52–65. [CrossRef]
56. Uddin, L.Q.; Nomi, J.S.; Hébert-Seropian, B.; Ghaziri, J.; Boucher, O. Structure and Function of the Human Insula. *J. Clin. Neurophysiol.* **2017**, *34*, 300–306. [CrossRef] [PubMed]
57. Ong, W.-Y.; Stohler, C.S.; Herr, D.R. Role of the Prefrontal Cortex in Pain Processing. *Mol. Neurobiol.* **2019**, *56*, 1137–1166. [CrossRef] [PubMed]
58. Merskey, H.; Bogduk, N. Part III pain terms, a current list with definitions and notes on usage. In *Classification of Chronic Pain*, 2nd ed.; IASP Press: Seattle, DC, USA, 1994; pp. 207–214.
59. Nicholas, M.; Vlaeyen, J.W.S.; Rief, W.; Barke, A.; Aziz, Q.; Benoliel, R.; Cohen, M.; Evers, S.; Giamberardino, M.A.; Goebel, A.; et al. The IASP classification of chronic pain for ICD-11: Chronic primary pain. *Pain* **2019**, *160*, 28–37. [CrossRef] [PubMed]
60. Gilam, G.; Gross, J.J.; Wager, T.D.; Keefe, F.J.; Mackey, S.C. What Is the Relationship between Pain and Emotion? Bridging Constructs and Communities. *Neuron* **2020**, *107*, 17–21. [CrossRef]
61. Simons, L.E.; Vlaeyen, J.W.S.; Declercq, L.; Smith, A.M.; Beebe, J.; Hogan, M.; Li, E.; Kronman, C.A.; Mahmud, F.; Corey, J.R.; et al. Avoid or engage? Outcomes of graded exposure in youth with chronic pain using a sequential replicated single-case randomized design. *Pain* **2020**, *161*, 520–531. [CrossRef] [PubMed]
62. Wood, L.; Hendrick, P.A. A systematic review and meta-analysis of pain neuroscience education for chronic low back pain: Short-and long-term outcomes of pain and disability. *Eur. J. Pain* **2019**, *23*, 234–249. [CrossRef]
63. Watson, J.A.; Ryan, C.G.; Cooper, L.; Ellington, D.; Whittle, R.; Lavender, M.; Dixon, J.; Atkinson, G.; Cooper, K.; Martin, D.J. Pain Neuroscience Education for Adults with Chronic Musculoskeletal Pain: A Mixed-Methods Systematic Review and Meta-Analysis. *J. Pain* **2019**, *20*, 1140.e1–1140.e22. [CrossRef]
64. Marques, A.A.; Bevilaqua, M.C.d.N.; da Fonseca, A.M.P.; Nardi, A.E.; Thuret, S.; Dias, G.P. Gender Differences in the Neurobiology of Anxiety: Focus on Adult Hippocampal Neurogenesis. *Neural Plast.* **2016**, *2016*, 5026713. [CrossRef]
65. Vlaeyen, J.W.S.; de Jong, J.; Geilen, M.; Heuts, P.H.T.G.; van Breukelen, G. The Treatment of Fear of Movement/(Re)injury in Chronic Low Back Pain: Further Evidence on the Effectiveness of Exposure In Vivo. *Clin. J. Pain* **2002**, *18*, 251–261. [CrossRef]
66. Ells, L.J.; Lang, R.; Shield, J.P.; Wilkinson, J.R.; Lidstone, J.S.; Coulton, S.; Summerbell, C.D. Obesity and disability-a short review. *Obes. Rev.* **2006**, *7*, 341–345. [CrossRef]
67. Wasser, J.G.; Vasilopoulos, T.; Zdziarski, L.A.; Vincent, H.K. Exercise Benefits for Chronic Low Back Pain in Overweight and Obese Individuals. *PM R* **2017**, *9*, 181–192. [CrossRef] [PubMed]
68. Narouze, S.; Souzdalnitski, D. Obesity and chronic pain: Systematic review of prevalence and implications for pain practice. *Reg. Anesth. Pain Med.* **2015**, *40*, 91–111. [CrossRef] [PubMed]
69. Shadish, W.R.; Sullivan, K.J. Characteristics of single-case designs used to assess intervention effects in 2008. *Behav. Res. Methods* **2011**, *43*, 971–980. [CrossRef] [PubMed]

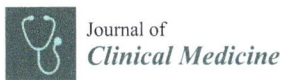

Article

Association between Dietary Protein Intake, Regular Exercise, and Low Back Pain among Middle-Aged and Older Korean Adults without Osteoarthritis of the Lumbar Spine

Hye-Mi Noh [1], Yi Hwa Choi [2,*], Soo Kyung Lee [2], Hong Ji Song [1], Yong Soon Park [3], Namhyun Kim [2] and Jeonghoon Cho [2]

[1] Department of Family Medicine, Hallym University Sacred Heart Hospital, College of Medicine, Hallym University, Anyang 14068, Korea; hyeminoh@hallym.or.kr (H.-M.N.); hongji@hallym.or.kr (H.J.S.)

[2] Department of Anesthesiology and Pain Medicine, Hallym University Sacred Heart Hospital, College of Medicine, Hallym University, Anyang 14068, Korea; agneta@hallym.or.kr (S.K.L.); alisia94@hallym.or.kr (N.K.); chojh137@hallym.or.kr (J.C.)

[3] Department of Family Medicine, Chuncheon Sacred Heart Hospital, College of Medicine, Hallym University, Chuncheon 24253, Korea; pyongs@hallym.or.kr

* Correspondence: pcyhchoi@hallym.or.kr; Tel.: +82-31-380-3943

Citation: Noh, H.-M.; Choi, Y.H.; Lee, S.K.; Song, H.J.; Park, Y.S.; Kim, N.; Cho, J. Association between Dietary Protein Intake, Regular Exercise, and Low Back Pain among Middle-Aged and Older Korean Adults without Osteoarthritis of the Lumbar Spine. *J. Clin. Med.* **2022**, *11*, 1220. https://doi.org/10.3390/jcm11051220

Academic Editors: Jo Nijs and Felipe J J Reis

Received: 22 December 2021
Accepted: 22 February 2022
Published: 24 February 2022

Publisher's Note: MDPI stays neutral with regard to jurisdictional claims in published maps and institutional affiliations.

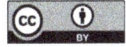

Copyright: © 2022 by the authors. Licensee MDPI, Basel, Switzerland. This article is an open access article distributed under the terms and conditions of the Creative Commons Attribution (CC BY) license (https://creativecommons.org/licenses/by/4.0/).

Abstract: This study aimed to evaluate the effect of dietary protein intake and regular exercise on low back pain (LBP) using data from the Korea National Health and Nutrition Examination Survey. A total of 2367 middle-aged and older adults (≥50 years) who underwent dual-energy X-ray absorptiometry and plain radiography of the lumbar spine were included. LBP was defined using a questionnaire to determine the presence of LBP lasting more than 30 days in the preceding three months. Twenty-four-hour dietary recall data were used to estimate protein intake, and regular exercise was assessed using the International Physical Activity Questionnaire. Multivariable logistic regression analysis revealed that men who did not perform regular exercise had a high probability of LBP (odds ratio [OR] 2.34; 95% confidence interval [CI] 1.24–4.44). Low protein intake (<0.8 g/kg/day) was associated with high odds for LBP in women (OR 1.83; 95% CI 1.12–2.99). Low protein intake and lack of regular exercise were also associated with a higher probability of LBP in women (OR 2.91; 95% CI 1.48–5.72). We recommend that women over 50 years of age consume the recommended daily amount of protein to prevent LBP and engage in regular exercise.

Keywords: exercise; low back pain; older adults; protein intake; physical activity; KNHANES

1. Introduction

Low back pain (LBP) is a common condition with a reported prevalence of 1.0% to 58.1% [1]. The medical costs attributable to LBP are estimated to be USD 26 billion, and the additional cost of productivity lost because of LBP is estimated to be USD 23.5 billion [2]. Chronic pain in older adults, which is commonly associated with musculoskeletal disorders, results in adverse health outcomes, including disability, falls, depression, insomnia, and social isolation [3].

LBP is also associated with a sedentary lifestyle. A recent systematic review and meta-analysis reported that strengthening by stretching or aerobic exercises helped to prevent LBP in both the general and working populations [4]. Exercise therapy was found to be effective in reducing pain and improving functionality in patients with non-specific LBP in the absence of specific pathology [5,6]. However, older patients encounter difficulty when trying to incorporate exercise into their daily lives in the real world due to frailty and poor performance caused by low muscle strength, comorbidities, and progressive degenerative changes in multiple joints.

Dietary protein intake can sustain muscle mass and physical function and prolong independent living in the older population [7,8]. Intake of sufficient dietary protein enables preservation or an increase in muscle mass resulting from a positive balance between synthesis and breakdown of muscle protein in older adults [9,10]. Many patients with LBP and their caregivers have questions concerning nutritional requirements and supplements in clinical practice. However, considering the level of interest among affected individuals, few studies have focused on daily dietary intake in patients with chronic LBP [11,12]. To date, the association between dietary protein intake and regular exercise in older patients with chronic LBP has been unclear.

Lifestyle factors, such as physical activity and nutrition, may be associated with LBP in the aging population. However, there is limited relevant literature in the Asian context. This study aimed to evaluate the association between dietary protein intake, regular exercise, and LBP in the absence of osteoarthritis of the lumbar spine, using a nationally representative sample of middle-aged and older Korean adults.

2. Materials and Methods

2.1. Study Population

Data from the Fifth Korea National Health and Nutrition Examination Survey (KNHANES V-1 and V-2) collected in 2010–2011 by the Korea Centers for Disease Control and Prevention (KCDC) were analyzed in this study. The KNHANES is a nationwide cross-sectional survey that has been conducted since 1998 by the KCDC. The KCDC selected 21,527 individuals using a complex, stratified, multistage probability sampling design. A total of 17,476 study participants completed the survey, giving a response rate of 81.2%. The present study included 3988 participants (aged $\geq$50 years) who underwent dual-energy X-ray absorptiometry (DEXA) and plain radiography of the lumbar spine. We excluded subjects who had a specific pathology causing LBP, namely those with radiographic evidence of osteoarthritis (OA) on a lumbar radiograph (n = 1327) and those with a history of vertebral fracture (n = 15). Participants with no response to questionnaire items on LBP (n = 34) or missing data for dietary protein intake (n = 244) or body weight (n = 1) were also excluded. Finally, data for 2367 subjects were included in the study. The 2010 and 2011 KNHANES were approved by the Institutional Review Board of the Korea Centers for Disease Control and Prevention (2010-02CON-21-C and 2011-02CON-06-C, respectively). Written informed consent was obtained from all study participants.

2.2. Data Collection and Measurements

Face-to-face interviews and standardized health examinations were conducted. The questionnaire included age, sex, educational attainment, occupation, household income, disease status, and lifestyle risk factors. Smoking status was classified into three categories: current smoker (more than five packs of cigarettes during lifetime and currently smokes every day), ex-smoker (smoked a month ago but has now quit), and never-smoker. Alcohol consumption was defined as consuming alcohol at least once every month over the past year. Physical activity was evaluated using the International Physical Activity Questionnaire [13]. We defined regular exercise as follows: aerobic exercise/weight training/stretching exercise on at least two days in a week or walking as a physical activity for at least 30 min on five days in a week. Aerobic exercise included swimming, doubles tennis, volleyball, badminton, table tennis, and occupational or sports activities, such as carrying objects, except for walking. Weight training consisted of push-ups, sit-ups, lifting dumbbells or barbells, and pull-up bars. Stretching exercise included back stretching, relaxation exercises, and calisthenics. Past medical history, including chronic diseases and vertebral fractures, was assessed using a self-report questionnaire. Chronic diseases included hypertension, diabetes mellitus, liver cirrhosis, chronic kidney disease, cancer, rheumatoid arthritis, and major depressive disorder.

2.3. Low Back Pain

We defined study participants as having LBP if they answered "yes" to the question "Have you suffered LBP for more than 30 days during the past three months?"

2.4. Radiographic Examination and Body Composition Measurements

Plain radiographs (anteroposterior and lateral views) of the lumbar spine were obtained using an SD 3000 Synchro Stand (Accele Ray SYFM Co., Seoul, Korea). Two musculoskeletal radiologists independently evaluated the severity of OA in all facet joints using the Kellgren–Lawrence grading system. The radiologic grade was classified using the method devised by Yoshimura et al. [14]: 0, normal (no abnormalities including slight osteophytes); 1, suspicious (clear osteophytes); and 2, abnormal (stenosis, osteosclerosis, and large osteophytes). If there was a difference in the radiologists' grades, the higher grade was selected. The inter-rater agreement was 92.8% [15]. Body composition and bone mineral density were measured by DEXA (DISCOVERY-W, Hologic Inc., Marlborough, MA, USA). Muscle mass was calculated as the difference between lean body mass and bone mineral content, and appendicular skeletal muscle mass (ASM) was defined as the sum of the values recorded for the upper and lower extremities bilaterally. The ASM index was calculated as ASM/(height $[m])^2$. Low skeletal muscle mass was defined according to the 2019 Asian Working Group for Sarcopenia consensus statement; the cut-off value for diagnosis of low muscle mass as sarcopenia is <7.0 kg/m^2 in men and <5.4 kg/m^2 in women [16]. According to the World Health Organization criteria, bone mineral density of the lumbar spine is defined as normal (T-score ≥ -1.0), osteopenia ($-2.5 <$ T-score < -1.0), or osteoporosis (T-score ≤ -2.5) [17].

2.5. Assessment of Dietary Intake

The frequency of dietary intake and amount of each food item were evaluated using a semi-quantitative food frequency questionnaire, with verified validity for 112 food items. Dietary intake was assessed using a 24 h dietary recall to determine the average intake frequency and average daily intake per serving during the preceding year. Trained dietitians helped participants recall their dietary information, such as consumed food, amount, and recipes. The total energy of the dietary intake and each nutrient was calculated using the National Standard Food Composition Table developed by the Rural Development Administration [18]. The daily intake of energy and nutrients for each individual was calculated based on the sum of all the items consumed. Protein intake was classified according to the recommended daily allowance (RDA) for dietary protein (0.8 g/kg/day) as low (<0.8 g/kg/day) or good ($\geq$0.8 g/kg/day) [19].

2.6. Statistical Analysis

Complex sample analysis was performed for all the statistical analyses. Continuous variables are presented as the mean ± standard error and compared between groups using the Student's *t*-test. Categorical data are shown as the estimated percentage (standard error) and compared using the chi-squared test. We performed multivariable logistic regression analysis to estimate the associations between protein intake, regular exercise, and LBP. We divided the subjects into four groups according to protein intake (low, <0.8 g/kg/day; good, $\geq$0.8 g/kg/day) and regular exercise status (specified exercises or walking for physical activity) as follows: low protein intake with exercise, good protein intake with exercise, low protein intake without exercise, and good protein intake without exercise. The good protein intake with exercise group was defined as the reference group; crude odds ratios (ORs) for LBP were calculated for the other three groups. Age and sex were adjusted in model 1. Body mass index, factors associated with socioeconomic status (household income, occupation, and education level), and lifestyle factors (smoking status and alcohol consumption) were additionally included in model 2. Bone mineral density of the lumbar spine (normal, osteopenia, and osteoporosis), Kellgren–Lawrence grading of the lumbar spine (normal or grade 1), comorbidities, and total energy intake were added to the final model (model 3). All statistical analyses were performed using SPSS software (version 20.0; IBM Corp., Armonk, NY, USA). A *p*-value < 0.05 was considered statistically significant.

3. Results

The study sample consisted of 1047 men and 1320 women. The mean age (standard error) was 59.4 years (0.34) in men and 59.7 years (0.30) in women. Table 1 shows the demographic and clinical characteristics of the study participants according to sex. Smoking and alcohol consumption were significantly more common in men than in women (both $p < 0.001$). Furthermore, 34.5% (2.0) of men and 15.3% (1.2) of women were engaged in regular exercise; the difference was statistically significant ($p < 0.001$). However, there was no significant difference in the frequency of walking for physical activity between men and women (40.4% vs. 40.2%). Regarding body composition and bone mineral density measured by DEXA, the ASM index was higher in men than in women, but there was no difference in the prevalence of low skeletal muscle mass between the sexes. Osteopenia and osteoporosis of the lumbar spine were more common in women than in men ($p < 0.001$). Daily protein intake (g/kg/day) was lower in women than in men. Furthermore, low protein intake and LBP were significantly more common in women than in men (41.6% vs. 24.1% and 29.7% vs. 12.6%, respectively, both $p < 0.001$).

Table 1. Characteristics of study participants by sex.

Variable	Men (n = 1047)	Women (n = 1320)	p-Value
Age (years)	59.4 (0.34)	59.7 (0.30)	0.620
Body mass index (kg/m^2)	23.9 (0.12)	24.3 (0.11)	0.031
Educational level			<0.001
≤Elementary school	28.9% (2.1)	53.3% (2.1)	
Middle and high school	52.2% (2.1)	40.3% (1.9)	
≥College	18.9% (1.8)	6.3% (0.9)	
Occupation			<0.001
Office work	12.4% (1.2)	3.4% (0.5)	
Sales and services	11.0% (1.3)	13.9% (1.2)	
Agriculture, forestry, and fisheries	20.7% (2.5)	11.9% (1.7)	
Machine fitting and simple labor	28.2% (1.9)	15.9% (1.2)	
Unemployed	27.7% (1.5)	55.0% (1.9)	
Household income			0.192
Low	26.6% (1.9)	24.1% (1.6)	
Lower middle	26.7% (1.7)	24.4% (1.7)	
Upper middle	24.9% (1.6)	28.5% (1.5)	
High	21.8% (1.6)	23.0% (1.7)	
Smoking status			<0.001
Ex-smoker	50.4% (2.0)	2.8% (0.7)	
Current smoker	35.7% (1.8)	3.6% (0.7)	
Alcohol consumption	71.5% (1.8)	30.5% (1.6)	<0.001
Muscle strengthening exercise [a]	34.5% (2.0)	15.3% (1.2)	<0.001
Walking for physical activity [b]	40.4% (1.8)	40.2% (1.7)	0.935
DEXA			
Trunk lean mass (kg)	24.69 (0.15)	18.50 (0.09)	<0.001
Appendicular skeletal muscle mass/height^2	7.48 (0.04)	5.86 (0.03)	<0.001
Low skeletal muscle mass [c]	28.8% (2.1)	25.4% (1.8)	0.146
Lumbar spine BMD			<0.001
Normal	59.0% (1.9%)	28.1% (1.7%)	
Osteopenia	35.6% (1.8%)	45.9% (2.0%)	
Osteoporosis	5.4% (0.8%)	26.0% (1.8%)	
Protein intake (g/day)	81.0 (1.41)	55.8 (1.12)	<0.001
Protein intake (g/kg/day)	1.22 (0.02)	0.98 (0.02)	<0.001
Low protein intake < 0.8 g/kg/day	24.1% (1.6)	41.6% (1.7)	<0.001
Total energy intake (kcal/day)	2320.1 (34.54)	1643.5 (28.74)	<0.001

Table 1. *Cont.*

Variable	Men (n = 1047)	Women (n = 1320)	p-Value
Comorbidity [d]			0.176
None	45.8% (2.3)	41.4% (1.9)	
1–2	36.6% (2.0)	39.0% (1.5)	
≥3	17.6% (1.6)	19.7% (1.5)	
Lumbar spine osteoarthritis			0.120
Normal	24.3% (1.9)	28.0% (1.8)	
Grade 1	75.7% (1.9)	72.0% (1.8)	
Low back pain	12.6% (1.6)	29.7% (1.9)	<0.001

Values are presented as the mean ± standard error or estimated percentage (standard error). [a] Muscle strengthening exercises (push-ups, sit-ups, and lifting dumbbells or weights) for at least two days a week; [b] walking for at least 30 min for five days a week; [c] low skeletal muscle mass (the 2019 Asian Working Group for Sarcopenia consensus statement defines the cut-off values for a diagnosis of low muscle mass as sarcopenia is <7.0 kg/m^2 in men and <5.4 kg/m^2 in women by DEXA); [d] comorbidity (hypertension, diabetes mellitus, chronic kidney disease, rheumatoid arthritis, cancer, liver cirrhosis, and depression). BMD, bone mineral density; DEXA, dual-energy X-ray absorptiometry.

Table 2 shows the factors associated with LBP in men. Men with LBP were significantly older (p = 0.006) and more likely to smoke (p = 0.018) and have a lower body mass index (p < 0.001) and educational level (p = 0.002) than men without LBP. Men without LBP tended to engage in exercise more often than men with LBP (p = 0.001). Men without LBP also had a significantly higher ASM index (p = 0.003); however, there was no significant difference in the frequency of low skeletal muscle mass between those with and without LBP. Daily protein intake (g/kg/day) and the proportion with low protein intake were similar between the groups. OA in the lumbar spine was significantly more common in men with LBP than in those without LBP (p = 0.039).

Table 2. Factors associated with low back pain in men.

Variable	Low Back Pain		p-Value
	Yes (n = 127)	No (n = 920)	
Age (years)	61.6 (0.90)	59.1 (0.33)	0.006
Body mass index (kg/m^2)	23.0 (0.23)	24.0 (0.13)	<0.001
Educational level			0.002
≤Elementary school	45.3% (6.0)	26.5% (2.1)	
Middle and high school	35.8% (5.7)	54.6% (2.0)	
≥College	18.9% (4.6)	18.9% (1.9)	
Occupation			0.202
Office work	13.7% (4.0)	15.2% (1.6)	
Sales and services	6.9% (3.5)	13.3% (1.9)	
Agriculture, forestry, and fisheries	24.9% (6.1)	16.5% (2.5)	
Machine fitting and simple labor	24.7% (5.3)	31.4% (2.5)	
Unemployed	29.8% (4.9)	23.6% (1.8)	
Household income			0.313
Low	30.5% (5.2)	26.0% (2.0)	
Lower middle	29.9% (5.6)	26.3% (1.8)	
Upper middle	16.8% (4.0)	26.0% (1.8)	
High	22.8% (3.7)	21.7% (1.7)	
Smoking status			0.018
Ex-smoker	57.9% (5.7)	49.3% (2.2)	
Current smoker	38.2% (5.7)	35.4% (2.0)	
Alcohol consumption	72.9% (4.5)	71.3% (2.0)	0.742
Muscle strengthening exercise [a]	19.3% (3.9)	36.7% (2.2)	0.001
Walking for physical activity [b]	42.0% (5.1)	40.2% (2.0)	0.743

Table 2. Cont.

Variable	Low Back Pain		p-Value
	Yes (n = 127)	No (n = 920)	
DEXA			
Trunk lean mass (kg)	23.97 (0.32)	24.79 (0.16)	0.015
Appendicular skeletal muscle mass/height^2	7.26 (0.08)	7.51 (0.04)	0.003
Low skeletal muscle mass ^{c}	30.6% (5.1)	28.5% (2.1)	0.695
Lumbar spine BMD			0.078
Normal	48.4% (5.5)	60.5% (1.9)	
Osteopenia	44.8% (5.5)	34.3% (1.8)	
Osteoporosis	6.8% (2.5)	5.2% (0.8)	
Protein intake (g/day)	75.2 (3.55)	81.8 (1.50)	0.083
Protein intake (g/kg/day)	1.17 (0.06)	1.23 (0.02)	0.382
Low protein intake < 0.8 g/kg/day	27.9% (3.6)	23.6% (1.7)	0.267
Total energy intake (kcal/day)	2126.5 (65.47)	2348.0 (37.55)	0.003
Comorbidity ^{d}			0.717
None	48.8% (6.1)	45.3% (2.4)	
1–2	32.8% (4.4)	37.2% (2.2)	
≥3	18.4% (4.2)	17.5% (1.6)	
Lumbar spine osteoarthritis			0.039
Normal	15.2% (3.9)	25.6% (2.1)	
Grade 1	84.8% (3.9)	74.4% (2.1)	

Values are presented as the mean ± standard error or as the estimated percentage (standard error). ^{a} Muscle strengthening exercises (push-ups, sit-ups, and lifting dumbbells or weights) for at least two days a week; ^{b} walking for at least 30 min for five days a week; ^{c} low skeletal muscle mass (the 2019 Asian Working Group for Sarcopenia consensus statement states the cut-off value for a diagnosis of low muscle mass as sarcopenia is <7.0 kg/m^2 in men by DEXA); ^{d} comorbidity (hypertension, diabetes mellitus, chronic kidney disease, rheumatoid arthritis, cancer, liver cirrhosis, and depression). BMD, body mass index; DEXA, dual-energy X-ray absorptiometry.

Table 3 shows the factors associated with LBP in women. Women with LBP were significantly older ($p < 0.001$) and had a significantly lower educational level ($p < 0.001$) and lower household income ($p = 0.024$). Women with LBP were more likely to work in agriculture, forestry, fisheries, machine fitting, or simple labor ($p = 0.004$). Women without LBP tended to engage in exercise more often than women with LBP ($p = 0.045$). There was no significant difference in the mean ASM index value or the proportion with low skeletal muscle mass between those with and without LBP. Both daily protein intake (g/kg/day) and the proportion with low protein intake were significantly lower in women with LBP than in those without LBP ($p = 0.011$ and $p = 0.008$, respectively). Women with LBP had a higher prevalence of multiple comorbidities ($p = 0.014$) and OA in the lumbar spine than those without LBP ($p < 0.001$).

The results of multivariable logistic regression analysis of the association between protein intake, regular exercise, and LBP are presented in Table 4. In the subgroup analysis according to sex, the association between muscle strengthening exercise and LBP was significant in men (OR 2.34; 95% CI 1.24–4.44) but not in women (OR 0.89; 95% CI 0.51–1.55). Low protein intake (<0.8 g/kg/day) was associated with high odds for LBP only in women (OR 1.83; 95% CI 1.12–2.99).

Table 5 shows the association between combined protein intake, regular exercise, and LBP. After designating the participants having good protein intake in the exercise group as the reference group, it was found that the risk of LBP was higher in participants with a low protein intake and no exercise (OR 2.00; 95% CI 1.20–3.33) than in the reference group. The risk of LBP in the low protein intake with exercise group and good protein intake without exercise group was not significantly different from that in the reference group. When subgroup analysis was performed according to sex, women with low protein intake and no exercise had a higher risk of LBP (OR 2.91; 95% CI 1.48–5.72) than women in the reference group. However, the association was not significant in men (OR 1.55; 95% C, 0.72–3.34).

Table 3. Factors associated with low back pain in women.

Variable	Low Back Pain		p-Value
	Yes (n = 380)	No (n = 940)	
Age (years)	61.6 (0.63)	58.8 (0.32)	<0.001
BMI (kg/m^2)	24.5 (0.23)	24.2 (0.12)	0.222
Educational level			<0.001
≤Elementary school	67.2% (3.3)	47.5% (2.6)	
Middle and high school	29.3% (3.0)	45.0% (2.4)	
≥College	3.5% (1.1)	7.5% (1.2)	
Occupation			0.004
Office work	1.5% (0.6)	5.7% (0.9)	
Sales and services	17.3% (2.4)	17.5% (1.8)	
Agriculture, forestry, and fisheries	15.4% (2.8)	9.3% (2.5)	
Machine fitting and simple labor	19.3% (2.9)	15.8% (1.6)	
Unemployed	46.4% (3.5)	51.7% (2.5)	
Household income			0.024
Low	29.9% (2.9)	21.6% (1.8)	
Lower middle	23.7% (2.9)	24.7% (2.2)	
Upper middle	29.1% (2.8)	28.3% (1.9)	
High	17.2% (2.4)	25.4% (2.2)	
Smoking status			0.802
Ex-smoker	2.5% (0.9)	2.9% (0.8)	
Current smoker	4.1% (1.4)	3.4% (0.7)	
Alcohol consumption	26.9% (3.0)	32.1% (1.9)	0.149
Muscle strengthening exercise [a]	11.4% (1.9)	16.9% (1.6)	0.045
Walking for physical activity [b]	36.6% (3.1)	41.7% (2.2)	0.212
DEXA			
Trunk lean mass (kg)	18.54 (0.16)	18.49 (0.10)	0.753
Appendicular skeletal muscle mass/height^2	5.92 (0.05)	6.32 (0.09)	0.107
Low skeletal muscle mass [c]	22.2% (2.4)	26.7% (2.1)	0.123
Lumbar spine BMD			0.097
Normal	24.9% (2.9)	29.5% (2.0)	
Osteopenia	44.0% (3.5)	46.7% (2.3)	
Osteoporosis	31.1% (2.0)	23.8% (2.2)	
Protein intake (g/day)	51.9 (1.76)	53.9 (2.38)	0.015
Protein intake (g/kg/day)	0.91 (0.03)	0.93 (0.04)	0.011
Low protein intake < 0.8 g/kg/day	49.1% (3.5)	38.5% (1.8)	0.008
Total energy intake (kcal/day)	1605.6 (46.94)	1659.6 (30.82)	0.269
Comorbidity [d]			0.014
None	34.4% (2.4)	44.3% (2.3)	
1–2	40.6% (2.9)	38.3% (2.0)	
≥3	25.0% (2.9)	17.4% (1.6)	
Lumbar spine osteoarthritis			<0.001
Normal	17.6% (2.6)	32.4% (2.3)	
Grade 1	82.4% (2.6)	67.6% (2.3)	

Values are presented as the mean ± standard error or as the estimated percentage (standard error). [a] Muscle strengthening exercises (push-ups, sit-ups, and lifting dumbbells or weights) for at least two days a week; [b] walking for at least 30 min for five days a week; [c] low skeletal muscle mass (the 2019 Asian Working Group for Sarcopenia consensus statement states the cut-off value for a diagnosis of low muscle mass as sarcopenia is <5.4 kg/m^2 in women by DEXA); [d] comorbidity (hypertension, diabetes mellitus, chronic kidney disease, rheumatoid arthritis, cancer, liver cirrhosis, and depression). BMD, body mass index; DEXA, dual-energy X-ray absorptiometry.

Table 4. Association between protein intake, regular exercise, and low back pain.

	Crude OR	95% CI	Model 1 [a] OR	95% CI	Model 2 [b] OR	95% CI	Model 3 OR	95% CI
Total study population								
Protein intake < 0.8 g/kg/day	1.88	(1.42–2.49)	1.46	(1.09–1.95)	1.44	(1.05–1.96)	1.32 [c]	(0.90–1.92)
Protein intake ≥ 0.8 g/kg/day	1		1		1		1	
Muscle strengthening exercise (-)	2.38	(1.60–3.53)	1.69	(1.15–2.48)	1.48	(1.01–2.17)	1.43 [d]	(0.95–2.16)
Muscle strengthening exercise (+)	1		1		1		1	
Walking for physical activity (-)	1.13	(0.84–1.51)	1.16	(0.85–1.58)	1.16	(0.84–1.60)	1.18 [e]	(0.84–1.66)
Walking for physical activity (+)	1		1		1		1	
Men								
Protein intake < 0.8 g/kg/day	1.33	(0.87–2.01)	1.24	(0.80–1.90)	1.32	(0.82–2.11)	1.07 [c]	(0.59–1.96)
Protein intake ≥ 0.8 g/kg/day	1		1		1		1	
Muscle strengthening exercise (-)	2.57	(1.43–4.59)	2.45	(1.35–4.55)	2.29	(1.23–4.24)	2.34 [d]	(1.24–4.44)
Muscle strengthening exercise (+)	1		1		1		1	
Walking for physical activity (-)	0.92	(0.55–1.53)	0.95	(0.57–1.61)	0.93	(0.54–1.60)	0.76 [e]	(0.42–1.39)
Walking for physical activity (+)	1		1		1		1	
Women								
Protein intake < 0.8 g/kg/day	1.68	(1.16–2.43)	1.59	(1.08–2.32)	1.57	(1.04–2.36)	1.83 [c]	(1.12–2.99)
Protein intake ≥ 0.8 g/kg/day	1		1		1		1	
Muscle strengthening exercise (-)	1.24	(0.74–2.10)	1.16	(0.70–1.93)	0.95	(0.58–1.54)	0.89 [d]	(0.51–1.55)
Muscle strengthening exercise (+)	1		1		1		1	
Walking for physical activity (-)	1.26	(0.87–1.85)	1.29	(0.89–1.88)	1.32	(0.89–1.95)	1.53 [e]	(0.99–2.35)
Walking for physical activity (+)	1		1		1		1	

[a] Model 1: age, sex; [b] Model 2: age, sex, BMI, smoking, alcohol consumption, education, occupation, household income; [c] Model 3: age, sex, BMI, smoking, alcohol consumption, education, occupation, household income, osteoporosis of the lumbar spine, severity of lumbar osteoarthritis, comorbidity, total energy intake, muscle strengthening exercise, walking for physical activity; [d] Model 3: age, sex, BMI, smoking, alcohol consumption, education, occupation, household income, osteoporosis of the lumbar spine, severity of lumbar osteoarthritis, comorbidity, protein intake, total energy intake, walking for physical activity; [e] Model 3: age, sex, BMI, smoking, alcohol consumption, education, occupation, household income, osteoporosis of the lumbar spine, severity of lumbar osteoarthritis, comorbidity, protein intake, total energy intake, muscle strengthening exercise. BMI, body mass index; CI, confidence interval; OR, odds ratio.

Table 5. Association between combined protein intake, regular exercise, and low back pain.

	Crude OR	95% CI	Model 1 [b] OR	95% CI	Model 2 [c] OR	95% CI	Model 3 [d] OR	95% CI
Total study population								
Low protein intake and exercise [a] (-)	2.62	(1.84–3.74)	1.86	(1.29–2.67)	1.99	(1.27–3.11)	2.00	(1.20–3.33)
Low protein intake and exercise (+)	1.35	(0.93–1.96)	1.01	(0.69–1.50)	1.11	(0.72–1.72)	0.97	(0.58–1.63)
Good protein intake and exercise (-)	1.38	(1.004–1.91)	1.26	(0.92–1.74)	1.19	(0.82–1.73)	1.17	(0.78–1.75)
Good protein intake and exercise (+)	1		1		1		1	
Men								
Low protein intake and exercise (-)	2.08	(1.23–3.50)	1.83	(1.06–3.15)	1.93	(1.04–3.59)	1.55	(0.72–3.34)
Low protein intake and exercise (+)	0.92	(0.43–1.96)	0.83	(0.38–1.82)	1.06	(0.44–2.54)	0.89	(0.35–2.26)
Good protein intake and exercise (-)	1.32	(0.77–2.26)	1.37	(0.80–2.34)	1.27	(0.66–2.46)	1.18	(0.63–2.24)
Good protein intake and exercise (+)	1		1		1		1	
Women								
Low protein intake and exercise (-)	2.08	(1.32–3.28)	1.87	(1.17–2.96)	2.06	(1.15–3.67)	2.91	(1.48–5.72)
Low protein intake and exercise (+)	1.23	(0.80–1.88)	1.09	(0.69–1.70)	1.24	(0.74–2.08)	1.36	(0.72–2.54)
Good protein intake and exercise (-)	1.24	(0.84–1.84)	1.21	(0.82–1.78)	1.16	(0.73–1.86)	1.21	(0.70–2.08)
Good protein intake and exercise (+)	1		1		1		1	

[a] Low protein intake, <0.8 g/kg/day; good protein intake, ≥0.8 g/kg/day; exercise, muscle-strengthening exercise or walking for physical activity. [b] Model 1: age, sex; [c] Model 2: age, sex, BMI, smoking, alcohol consumption, education, occupation, household income; [d] Model 3: age, sex, BMI, smoking, alcohol consumption, education, occupation, household income, lumbar spine osteoporosis, the severity of lumbar OA, comorbidity, total energy intake. BMI, body mass index; OR, odds ratio; 95% CI, 95% confidence interval; OA, osteoarthritis.

4. Discussion

This study evaluated the relationship between daily dietary protein intake, regular exercise, and LBP using nationally representative data from the KNHANES. Not performing muscle-strengthening exercise was associated with a higher risk of LBP in men, and low protein intake was associated with a higher risk of LBP in women.

Multiple factors can cause LBP, including structural changes in the lumbar spine and lifestyle, psychological, and social factors. Aerobic exercise plays a crucial role in relieving LBP by increasing blood flow and providing nutrients to the soft tissues in the lumbar structures, thereby improving the healing process in the damaged tissues and reducing stiffness [20]. In addition, physical activity, which can increase aerobic capacity and muscle strength, especially of the lumbar extensor muscles, assists patients with LBP in undertaking everyday activities [21]. Several studies have evaluated the effect of exercise in the aging population with LBP. Liu et al. and Jou et al. found that Tai Chi and core stabilization exercises reduced pain and protected neuromuscular function in the lower limbs in aging individuals (aged 50 years old or older) with LBP [22,23]. Our present findings are in line with the previous reports, i.e., regular exercise or walking is an important lifestyle factor that can prevent LBP in middle-aged and older adults.

In clinical practice, many older adults are vulnerable to LBP because of their inability to exercise enough to achieve the required clinical outcome. Age-related endocrine and metabolic alterations lead to changes in body composition, including progressive loss of muscle and bone mass and acquisition of fat mass [24]. Moreover, older adults have degenerative changes in the spine or multiple joints. The reduced walking speed is insufficient to rebuild muscles that undergo atrophy because of frailty, malnutrition, and anabolic resistance [25]. Protein intake has been shown to preserve muscle mass, prevent loss of physical function and prolong independent living in older adults [7,26]. However, in the real world, 7–41% of older adults are reported to have a daily protein intake lower than the RDA [27]. Over half of Korean adults over 60 years of age have a dietary protein intake that is lower than the RDA [28].

In our study, the probability of LBP was higher in women who had low protein intake and did not exercise than in their counterparts who had a good protein intake and exercised. Furthermore, 41.6% of women and 24.1% of men had a protein intake below the RDA (<0.8 g/kg/day). The marked association between protein intake and LBP in women may reflect their lower skeletal muscle mass relative to men. Although the impact of protein intake on LBP remains unclear, there are several plausible mechanisms. First, a prospective Women's Health Initiative study that analyzed the data of 24,417 women found that a higher protein intake was associated with better preservation of muscle strength [29]. Low muscle strength is associated with an increased risk of LBP [30,31]. Second, protein intake may play a significant role in alleviating pain via muscle recovery. It was reported that the use of protein supplements reduces muscle damage and helps muscle recovery by remodeling skeletal muscle and is strongly recommended for muscle recovery after submaximal exercise [32]. Two recent randomized controlled trials examined the effects of amino acid or protein supplementation on joint pain [12,33]. Third, the protein source for muscle building was regarded as a promising factor. There was a sex difference in the association between each protein source and lean mass. The intake of total protein foods was positively associated with the appendicular lean mass index in both men and women, but consumption of seafood and plant protein foods were positively associated with appendicular lean mass index in women only [34]. Further studies are needed to investigate the impact of each protein source on LBP.

Although chronic pain is an important health issue in the older population, few studies have evaluated the effect of exercise or nutrition on LBP in aging populations. To the best of our knowledge, this is the first representative nationwide study to evaluate the combined associations between exercise, dietary protein intake, and LBP. We demonstrated that engagement in exercise and sufficient protein intake are associated with a low probability of LBP in middle-aged and older adults in the general Korean population.

This study had several limitations. First, the causal relationship between exercise and progression of symptoms was unclear because the KNHANES only records cross-sectional data. The American Physical Therapy Association recommends strengthening exercises and progressive walking in older patients with LBP [35] because regular exercise may help to relieve LBP and prevent further damage. Second, we did not have data on the history of pharmacological or surgical treatment of LBP in the study participants. To minimize the possible confounding effect of medical treatment on LBP, we excluded subjects with vertebral fracture and those with advanced arthritic changes in the lumbar spine as identified on plain radiography. Degeneration of the lumbar spine affects LBP, and an association between vertebral OA and LBP has already been reported [36,37]. These degenerative changes in the spine are highly likely to cause chronic intractable LBP that cannot be managed by lifestyle modifications, such as regular exercise and daily nutrient control; in such cases, timely medical intervention helps reduce the pain induced by severely progressive arthritis of the lumbar spine. Third, the KNHANES collected dietary data by 24 h recall. One day of data may not have accurately reflected the average amount of nutrients ingested by the study participants. However, to increase the accuracy of this large population-based survey, the frequency of food intake and portion size for each item were estimated using the semi-quantitative food intake frequency survey table, which verified the validity of 112 food items, and the food intake frequency survey, which consists of 63 food items. Furthermore, trained dietitians helped the study participants recall their dietary information. A further prospective study over a longer period will be needed to evaluate the association between regular exercise, dietary protein intake, and LBP in the older population.

5. Conclusions

In this study, we found that a combination of sufficient dietary protein intake (≥ 0.8 g/kg/day) and regular exercise was associated with a low probability of LBP in middle-aged and older Korean adults. Regular exercise and a daily dietary protein intake equivalent to the RDA should be maintained in everyday life to prevent LBP. Women who are middle-aged or older who cannot exercise regularly, including walking as a physical activity, should be encouraged to consume adequate dietary protein to reduce their risk of LBP.

Author Contributions: Conceptualization, Y.H.C. and H.-M.N.; methodology, H.-M.N. and Y.S.P.; formal analysis, H.-M.N.; data curation, Y.H.C. and H.-M.N.; writing—original draft preparation, Y.H.C. and H.-M.N.; evidence collection and manuscript preparation, N.K. and J.C.; writing—review and editing, Y.H.C., H.J.S., S.K.L. and H.-M.N.; supervision, H.J.S. and S.K.L. All authors have read and agreed to the published version of the manuscript.

Funding: This research received no external funding.

Institutional Review Board Statement: This study was approved by the Institutional Review Board of the Korea Centers for Disease Control and Prevention (2010-02CON-21-C and 2011-02CON-06-C).

Informed Consent Statement: Informed consent was obtained from all subjects involved in the study.

Data Availability Statement: The KNHANES data can be downloaded from the website (https://knhanes.kdca.go.kr/knhanes/main.do (accessed on 21 December 2021).

Conflicts of Interest: The authors declare no conflict of interest.

References

1. Hoy, D.; Brooks, P.; Blyth, F.; Buchbinder, R. The epidemiology of low back pain. *Best Pract. Res. Clin. Rheumatol.* **2010**, *24*, 769–781. [CrossRef] [PubMed]
2. Dagenais, S.; Caro, J.; Haldeman, S. A systematic review of low back pain cost of illness studies in the United States and internationally. *Spine J.* **2008**, *8*, 8–20. [CrossRef]
3. Reid, M.C.; Eccleston, C.; Pillemer, K. Management of chronic pain in older adults. *BMJ* **2015**, *350*, h532. [CrossRef]

4. Shiri, R.; Coggon, D.; Falah-Hassani, K. Exercise for the prevention of low back pain: Systematic review and meta-analysis of controlled trials. *Am. J. Epidemiol.* **2018**, *187*, 1093–1101. [CrossRef] [PubMed]
5. Hayden, J.A.; van Tulder, M.W.; Malmivaara, A.; Koes, B.W. Exercise therapy for treatment of non-specific low back pain. *Cochrane Database Syst. Rev.* **2005**, *3*, CD000335. [CrossRef] [PubMed]
6. van Middelkoop, M.; Rubinstein, S.M.; Verhagen, A.P.; Ostelo, R.W.; Koes, B.W.; van Tulder, M.W. Exercise therapy for chronic nonspecific low-back pain. *Best Pract. Res. Clin. Rheumatol.* **2010**, *24*, 193–204. [CrossRef]
7. Mustafa, J.; Ellison, R.C.; Singer, M.R.; Bradlee, M.L.; Kalesan, B.; Holick, M.F.; Moore, L.L. Dietary protein and preservation of physical functioning among middle-aged and older adults in the Framingham Offspring Study. *Am. J. Epidemiol.* **2018**, *187*, 1411–1419. [CrossRef]
8. Morley, J.E.; Argiles, J.M.; Evans, W.J.; Bhasin, S.; Cella, D.; Deutz, N.E.; Doehner, W.; Fearon, K.C.; Ferruci, L.; Hellerstein, M.K.; et al. Nutritional recommendations for the management of sarcopenia. *J. Am. Med. Dir. Assoc.* **2010**, *11*, 391–396. [CrossRef]
9. Bauer, J.; Biolo, G.; Cederholm, T.; Cesari, M.; Cruz-Jentoft, A.J.; Morley, J.E.; Phillips, S.; Sieber, C.; Stehle, P.; Teta, D.; et al. Evidence-based recommendations for optimal dietary protein intake in older people: A position paper from the PROT-AGE Study Group. *J. Am. Med. Dir. Assoc.* **2013**, *14*, 542–559. [CrossRef]
10. Deutz, N.E.; Bauer, J.M.; Barazzoni, R.; Biolo, G.; Boirie, Y.; Bosy-Westphal, A.; Cederholm, T.; Cruz-Jentoft, A.; Krznariç, Z.; Nair, K.S.; et al. Protein intake and exercise for optimal muscle function with aging: Recommendations from the ESPEN Expert Group. *Clin. Nutr.* **2014**, *33*, 929–936. [CrossRef] [PubMed]
11. Karunanayake, A.L.; Pathmeswaran, A.; Kasturiratne, A.; Wijeyaratne, L.S. Risk factors for chronic low back pain in a sample of suburban Sri Lankan adult males. *Int. J. Rheum. Dis.* **2013**, *16*, 203–210. [CrossRef] [PubMed]
12. Shell, W.E.; Pavlik, S.; Roth, B.; Silver, M.; Breitstein, M.L.; May, L.; Silver, D. Reduction in pain and inflammation associated with chronic low back pain with the use of the medical food theramine. *Am. J. Ther.* **2016**, *23*, e1353–e1362. [CrossRef] [PubMed]
13. Craig, C.L.; Marshall, A.L.; Sjöström, M.; Bauman, A.E.; Booth, M.L.; Ainsworth, B.E.; Pratt, M.; Ekelund, U.; Yngve, A.; Sallis, J.F.; et al. International Physical Activity Questionnaire: 12-country reliability and validity. *Med. Sci. Sports Exerc.* **2003**, *35*, 1381–1395. [CrossRef] [PubMed]
14. Yoshimura, N.; Muraki, S.; Oka, H.; Mabuchi, A.; En-Yo, Y.; Yoshida, M.; Saika, A.; Yoshida, H.; Suzuki, T.; Yamamoto, S.; et al. Prevalence of knee osteoarthritis, lumbar spondylosis, and osteoporosis in Japanese men and women: The Research on Osteoarthritis/Osteoporosis Against Disability Study. *J. Bone Miner. Metab.* **2009**, *27*, 620–628. [CrossRef]
15. Jeon, H.; Lee, S.U.; Lim, J.Y.; Chung, S.G.; Lee, S.J.; Lee, S.Y. Low skeletal muscle mass and radiographic osteoarthritis in knee, hip, and lumbar spine: A cross-sectional study. *Aging Clin. Exp. Res.* **2019**, *31*, 1557–1562. [CrossRef]
16. Chen, L.K.; Woo, J.; Assantachai, P.; Auyeung, T.W.; Chou, M.Y.; Iijima, K.; Jang, H.C.; Kang, L.; Kim, M.; Kim, S.; et al. Consensus update on sarcopenia diagnosis and treatment. *J. Am. Med. Dir. Assoc.* **2019**, *21*, 300–307.e2. [CrossRef]
17. Assessment of fracture risk and its application to screening for postmenopausal osteoporosis: Report of a WHO Study Group. *World Health Organ. Tech. Rep. Ser.* **1994**, *843*, 1–129.
18. National Rural Resources Development Institute; Rural Development Administration. *Food Composition Table*, 7th ed.; Medpharm: Guildford, UK, 2006.
19. Trumbo, P.; Schlicker, S.; Yates, A.A.; Poos, M.; Food and Nutrition Board of the Institute of Medicine, The National Academies. Dietary reference intakes for energy, carbohydrate, fiber, fat, fatty acids, cholesterol, protein and amino acids. *J. Am. Diet. Assoc.* **2002**, *102*, 1621–1630. [CrossRef]
20. Gordon, R.; Bloxham, S. A systematic review of the effects of exercise and physical activity on non-specific chronic low back pain. *Healthcare* **2016**, *4*, 22. [CrossRef]
21. Smeets, R.J.; Severens, J.L.; Beelen, S.; Vlaeyen, J.W.; Knottnerus, J.A. More is not always better: Cost-effectiveness analysis of combined, single behavioral and single physical rehabilitation programs for chronic low back pain. *Eur. J. Pain* **2009**, *13*, 71–81. [CrossRef]
22. Liu, J.; Yeung, A.; Xiao, T.; Tian, X.; Kong, Z.; Zou, L.; Wang, X. Chen-style Tai Chi for individuals (aged 50 years old or above) with chronic non-specific low back pain: A randomized controlled trial. *Int. J. Environ. Res. Public Health* **2019**, *16*, 517. [CrossRef] [PubMed]
23. Zou, L.; Zhang, Y.; Liu, Y.; Tian, X.; Xiao, T.; Liu, X.; Yeung, A.S.; Liu, J.; Wang, X.; Yang, Q. The effects of Tai Chi Chuan versus core stability training on lower-limb neuromuscular function in aging individuals with non-specific chronic lower back pain. *Medicina* **2019**, *55*, 60. [CrossRef] [PubMed]
24. Walrand, S.; Guillet, C.; Salles, J.; Cano, N.; Boirie, Y. Physiopathological mechanism of sarcopenia. *Clin. Geriatr. Med.* **2011**, *13*, 27365–27385. [CrossRef]
25. Kim, I.Y.; Park, S.; Jang, J.; Wolfe, R.R. Understanding muscle protein dynamics: Technical considerations for advancing sarcopenia research. *Ann. Geriatr. Med. Res.* **2020**, *24*, 157–165. [CrossRef] [PubMed]
26. Coelho-Júnior, H.J.; Rodrigues, B.; Uchida, M.; Marzetti, E. Low protein intake is associated with frailty in older adults: A systematic review and meta-analysis of observational studies. *Nutrients* **2018**, *10*, 1334. [CrossRef] [PubMed]
27. Fulgoni, V.L., 3rd. Current protein intake in America: Analysis of the National Health and Nutrition Examination Survey, 2003–2004. *Am. J. Clin. Nutr.* **2008**, *87*, 1554S–1557S. [CrossRef] [PubMed]
28. Park, H.A. Adequacy of protein intake among Korean elderly: An analysis of the 2013–2014 Korea National Health and Nutrition Examination Survey Data. *Korean J. Fam. Med.* **2018**, *39*, 130–134. [CrossRef]

29. Beasley, J.M.; LaCroix, A.Z.; Neuhouser, M.L.; Huang, Y.; Tinker, L.; Woods, N.; Michael, Y.; Curb, J.D.; Prentice, R.L. Protein intake and incident frailty in the Women's Health Initiative observational study. *J. Am. Geriatr. Soc.* **2010**, *58*, 1063–1071. [CrossRef]
30. Cho, K.H.; Beom, J.W.; Lee, T.S.; Lim, J.H.; Lee, T.H.; Yuk, J.H. Trunk muscle strength as a risk factor for non-specific low back pain: A pilot study. *Ann. Rehabil. Med.* **2014**, *38*, 234–240. [CrossRef]
31. Park, S.M.; Kim, G.U.; Kim, H.J.; Kim, H.; Chang, B.S.; Lee, C.K.; Yeom, J.S. Low handgrip strength is closely associated with chronic low back pain among women aged 50 years or older: A cross-sectional study using a national health survey. *PLoS ONE* **2018**, *13*, e0207769. [CrossRef]
32. Pasiakos, S.M.; Lieberman, H.R.; McLellan, T.M. Effects of protein supplements on muscle damage, soreness and recovery of muscle function and physical performance: A systematic review. *Sports Med.* **2014**, *44*, 655–670. [CrossRef] [PubMed]
33. Delitto, A.; George, S.Z.; Van Dillen, L.; Whitman, J.M.; Sowa, G.; Shekelle, P.; Denninger, T.R.; Godges, J.J. Orthopaedic Section of the American Physical Therapy Association: Low back pain. *J. Orthop. Sports Phys. Ther.* **2012**, *42*, A1-57. [CrossRef] [PubMed]
34. Xu, F.; Earp, J.E.; Vadiveloo, M.; Adami, A.; Delmonico, M.J.; Lofgren, I.E.; Greaney, M.L. The relationships between total protein intake, protein sources, physical activity, and lean mass in a representative sample of the US Adults. *Nutrients* **2020**, *12*, 3151. [CrossRef] [PubMed]
35. Ziegenfuss, T.N.; Kerksick, C.M.; Kedia, A.W.; Sandrock, J.; Raub, B.; Lopez, H.L. Proprietary milk protein concentrate reduces joint discomfort while improving exercise performance in non-osteoarthritic individuals. *Nutrients* **2019**, *11*, 283. [CrossRef] [PubMed]
36. Muraki, S.; Oka, H.; Akune, T.; Mabuchi, A.; En-Yo, Y.; Yoshida, M.; Saika, A.; Suzuki, T.; Yoshida, H.; Ishibashi, H.; et al. Prevalence of radiographic lumbar spondylosis and its association with low back pain in elderly subjects of population-based cohorts: The ROAD study. *Ann. Rheum. Dis.* **2009**, *68*, 1401–1406. [CrossRef]
37. Borenstein, D. Does osteoarthritis of the lumbar spine cause chronic low back pain? *Curr. Pain Headache Rep.* **2004**, *8*, 512–517. [CrossRef]

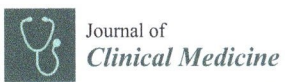

Article

Opioid Consumption in Chronic Pain Patients: Role of Perceived Injustice and Other Psychological and Socioeconomic Factors

Barbara Kleinmann and Tilman Wolter *

Interdisciplinary Pain Center, Faculty of Medicine, University of Freiburg, 79106 Freiburg, Germany; barbara.kleinmann@uniklinik-freiburg.de
* Correspondence: tilman.wolter@uniklinik-freiburg.de; Tel.: +49-761-27054801; Fax: +49-761-27050130

Abstract: Background: Chronic pain is a complex biopsychosocial phenomenon. Lifestyle, behavioral, socioeconomic, and psychosocial factors such as depression and perceived injustice are often associated with the development of chronic pain and vice versa. We sought to examine the interaction of these factors with opioid intake. Methods: At our institution, 164 patients with chronic pain undergoing an interdisciplinary assessment within a three-month period participated in the study and completed the Injustice Experience Questionnaire (IEQ). Data regarding opioid intake, pain levels, pain diagnosis, depression, anxiety, stress, quality of life, pain-related disability, habitual well-being, occupational status, and ongoing workers compensation litigation were extracted from the patients' charts. Results: Approximately one-fourth of the patients used opioids. The IEQ total was significantly higher in patients using Schedule III opioids. Depression, but not the anxiety and stress scores, were significantly higher in patients using opioids. There were no significant differences regarding pain-related disability, habitual well-being, and the coded psychosocial diagnoses. In the patient group without opioids, the percentage of employed persons was significantly higher but there were no significant differences regarding work leave, pension application, or professional education. Conclusions: Opioid use appears to be more closely related to psychological factors and single social determinants of pain than to somatic factors.

Keywords: chronic pain; perceived injustice; opioid use; socioeconomic factors; psychological factors; lifestyle

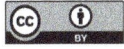

1. Introduction

Chronic pain affects many aspects of daily activities, physical and mental health, family, social relationships, and workplace interactions [1]. In turn, all of these factors can also influence the perception of chronic pain [2]. Opioids can be an important tool in the management of chronic pain. However, the experience of recent years has shown that benefit and harm in treatment of non-cancer pain can be closely related, and that opioid consumption is influenced by different factors [3–5].

Studies on opioid prescriptions show that besides compromised lifestyle factors such as physical activity and functioning, psychological and socioeconomic factors such as work force participation and social capital contribute to the amount of opioid consumption and the number of opioid-related deaths [1,6–8]. Opioid use is associated with statistically significant but small improvements in pain and physical functioning [9]. Numerous studies exist demonstrating that psychological comorbidities such as depression and anxiety are prevalent among patients with chronic non-cancer pain [3,6], and that these patients are more likely to receive long-term opioid therapy for pain [4]. A proposed reason for this phenomenon is that mental health conditions and chronic non-cancer pain are closely correlated concerning severity [5]. Moreover, patients with psychological comorbidities have a tendency to use opioids earlier and to use higher dosages of opioids [6], and opioid use may be a contributing factor for the development of depression [2].

Perceived injustice is a novel psychological variable interacting with chronic pain and opioid use. Scott et al. and Sullivan et al. showed that high levels of perceived injustice as measured with the Injustice Experience Questionnaire (IEQ) may also increase pain severity and depressive symptoms [10,11]. Sullivan et al. showed that high scores on perceived injustice are correlated negatively with recovery from mental health problems, poor rehabilitation outcomes, and prolonged work disability, and that the IEQ could possibly be used as a prognostic factor in the treatment of patients with chronic pain [12]. High scores on perceived injustice also predicted work disability, even if the initial pain intensity, functional limitations after the injury, catastrophizing, depression, and pain-related fears are controlled. Perceived injustice was more related to disability than to pain severity and it was the best predictor for occupational disability. Interestingly, catastrophizing was the best predictor for pain severity. Sullivan et al. suggested that perceived injustice should be further investigated in terms of its prognostic value for recovery [13].

Carriere et al. reported a correlation between perceived injustice and opioid prescription in patients with chronic pain [14]. They found that pain behavior, rather than pain intensity and depressive symptoms, mediated the association between perceived injustice and opioid prescription in patients with chronic pain. They discussed perceived injustice as a risk factor for adverse pain-related outcomes [14] and recommended future research in this area in order to identify more details and factors influencing the relationship of perceived injustice and opioid prescription. Moreover, Nijs et al. recently proposed that the assessment of perceived injustice, by means of the IEQ, should be included in the screening of cancer survivors with chronic pain because of its potential relevance for different treatment strategies including opioid medication [15]. While the correlation between depression, perceived injustice, and opioid use in chronic pain is well established, there is little knowledge about the possibly contributing socioeconomic factors. High perceived stress, e.g., due to high job demands and low control of decisions at work, was associated with more neck pain and decreased work productivity [16–19]. Occupational factors can also have a significant influence on the development of low back pain disorders [20]. Recently, Serra-Pujadas et al. [21] showed that socioeconomic status has a major influence on opioid use but their study was based only on regional insurance data.

The aim of this prospective study was to evaluate a possible correlation of opioid therapy in particular with socioeconomic factors and psychological factors such as the feeling of perceived injustice. For this purpose, we examined a representative group of patients with chronic non-cancer pain in a tertiary pain center.

2. Material and Methods

2.1. Patients

Inclusion criteria were: appointment in our institution for an interdisciplinary assessment between 1 October 2020 and 31 December 2020, age above 18 years, ability to understand and fill in the study questionnaires. Patients are treated in this department on an outpatient, inpatient and inpatient day-care basis. Prior to first presentation, patients routinely fill out the German Pain Questionnaire before then being admitted to our institution [22]. Assessment examinations are only given to patients who, based on the evaluation of the German Pain Questionnaire and the available medical findings, suffer from chronic pain with psychosocial stress factors and who have already undergone multiple frustrating pain therapies. This assessment is carried out in one day, i.e., the patient is inpatient for one day and is being looked after by an interprofessional team of doctors, physiotherapists, and psychologists during this time. [23]. Specialists from each discipline examine the patients for the causes of their chronic pain and the contributing chronification factors with the aim of appropriate, generally multimodal treatment [24].

Exclusion criteria were: insufficiently completed questionnaires, acute pain syndromes.

Of the 191 patients initially fulfilling the inclusion criteria, 164 gave written content to participate in this cross-sectional study. The IEQ (Injustice Experience Questionnaire, German version) was distributed to the patients, during their stay for the assessment [25].

2.2. Questionnaires and Data Extraction

The IEQ examines perceived injustice (sense of unfairness, severity of loss) as a contributing factor for the development of chronic pain [12,26]. The IEQ consists of 12 items with a 5-point scale (0–4), so that a maximal 48 points can be reached in total. Six items each form the subscale blame and the subscale severity. The cut-off value for the IEQ total score is 30; 14 for the subscale blame and 16 for the subscale severity [13,27]. The IEQ total score and the scores for the subscales blame and severity were calculated from the IEQ [13].

The German Pain Questionnaire was developed and validated by the German Chapter of the International Association for the Study of Pain (DGSS) [22,28]. The concept of this questionnaire is based on a bio-(medical)-psycho-social pain model. This questionnaire generates pain ratings on the 11-point numerical rating scale (NRS) and anxiety/depression/stress scores as measured by the German version of the Depression Anxiety Stress Scale (DASS) [29]. Patients rate their current, mean, maximum pain in the last four weeks and their bearable pain in case of successful pain treatment. The DASS consists of seven items each for depression, anxiety, and stress. In each of these items, 0–3 points can be reached. Values above 10 indicate an increased probability of the presence of chronic stress or a depressive disorder, while values above 6 are suspicious for anxiety. Moreover, for the experience of impairment, the German Pain Questionnaire contains a disability score, a shortened version of the Pain Disability Index (PDI) in which scale items are rated on an 11-point scale ranging from 0–10 [30]. The mean value of these 3 items multiplied by 10 gives the value for the disability score. The German Pain Questionnaire further includes the Marburg Questionnaire on Habitual Health Findings (FW 7), a 7-item questionnaire with a 6-point scale for each item [31].

Data on employment status, current sick leave, pension application, education, and marital status were also collected from the German Pain Questionnaire. Furthermore, personal data, medication, as well as coded diagnoses were extracted from the charts. Moreover, diagnoses based on the ICD-10 (International Classification of Diseases) [32,33] were derived from the patients' charts.

The study was approved by the local Ethics Committee (IRB number: 20-1061). The datasets generated and/or analyzed during the current study are available from the corresponding author on reasonable request. The analysis of the contributing factors to the IEQ will be published separately.

2.3. Coded Diagnoses

For the analysis, pain diagnoses were further grouped by body region in the following categories: headache, facial pain, neck pain, low back pain, neuropathic pain, and widespread pain. Psychological diagnoses were grouped in the following categories: Chronic Pain Disorder with Somatic and Psychological Factors (ICD-10: F45.41) [34], depression, anxiety, sleep disorder. Psychosocial factors are coded under Z-diagnoses (factors influencing health status and contact with health services). These diagnoses were grouped in four categories: family (Z63), work (Z56), biography (Z61), and finance (Z59). For instance, Z-diagnoses pertaining to the family are coded in case of severe conflicts within the family. Work factors are coded in case of imminent loss of employment or severe conflicts in the working environment. Biographical Z-diagnoses are coded in case of childhood trauma, parental neglect, or in some cases loss of parents during childhood, while financial Z-diagnoses are coded in case of severe financial problems, i.e., massive debts or imminent loss of housing.

2.4. Statistical Analysis

A computer software package (GraphPad Prism, Version 5.01, GraphPad Software, Inc., La Jolla, CA, USA) was used to conduct statistical analyses other than the regression analysis, which was performed with SPSS (IBM SPSS Statistics for Windows, Version 27.0, Armonk, NY, USA). Initially, descriptive statistics were applied to all measures. An unpaired t-test (in case of normally distributed variables) and, in the more frequent case of missing Gaussian distribution, the Mann–Whitney Test were used to determine the statistical significance of the differences in mean scores. Comparisons with categorical variables were made by means of the chi-squared test and, if indicated, Fisher's exact test. Statistical significance was considered when $p < 0.05$. The sample size estimation was performed with G*Power [35]. The sample size was 164 for the Mann–Whitney Test with $\alpha = 0.05$ and a power of 0.8 and an effect size of 0.4. Logistic regression analysis was used to investigate the relation between the variables found significant in the individual comparisons between patients with and without opioid use (plus age and sex).

3. Results

3.1. Patients

Of the 191 patients initially fulfilling the inclusion criteria, 164 were included in the analysis (Figure 1).

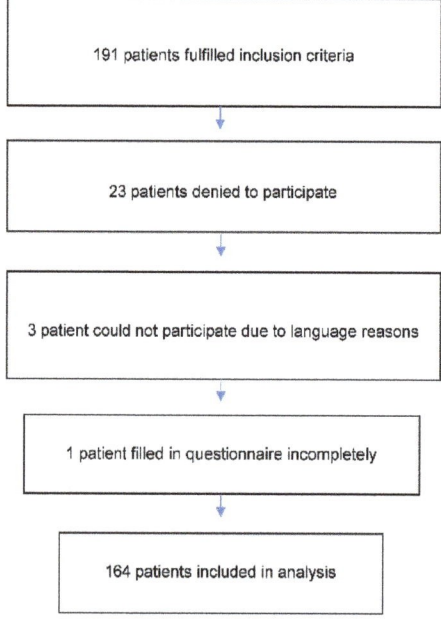

Figure 1. Flowsheet of patients eligible and patients analyzed.

Mean age was 50.3 years and nearly two-thirds of the patients included were female. Among the pain localizations, lumbar pain (low back pain) was most frequent followed by head and face pain, cervical pain, and widespread pain.

The median total pain score was 7.33 (IQR: 6.33–8.0). Almost 25% of the patients used opioids (39/164) equally divided between Schedule II and Schedule III opioids. Most of the patients (59.1%) used non-opioids or a single compound (55.5%). The proportion of patients who took anticonvulsants (18.3%) and antidepressants (21.9%) was roughly evenly distributed (Table 1).

Table 1. Patient characteristics: Personal data, pain localizations, socioeconomic data, coded diagnoses and scales, and analgesic medications, WSP = widespread pain, IEQ = Injustice Experience Questionnaire, DASS = Depression, Anxiety and Stress Scale, FW7 = Marburg questionnaire on habitual health findings, * during the last 4 weeks, ** total = (current + mean + highest)/3.

		Patients/n (%)
Age *		50.3 (SD 14.2)
Sex (m/f)		67/97
Pain localization	Head and Face	30 (18.3%)
	Cervical	23 (14.0%)
	Lumbar	66 (40.3%)
	Extremities	15 (9.1%)
	Abdominal	5 (3.0%)
	WSP	25 (15.2%)
Occupational Status	Retired	19 (11.5%)
	Disability pension	31 (18.9%)
	Unemployed	29 (17.6%)
	Employed	85 (51.9%)
Work leave	Yes	58 (35.7%)
	No	66 (40.2%)
	n.a.	40 (24.4%)
Pension application	Yes	12 (7.3%)
	No	123 (75.0%)
	n.a.	29 (17.6%)
Professional education	Academic	27 (16.4%)
	Non-academic	128 (78.0%)
	None	10 (6%)
Marital status	married	100 (60.9%)
	divorced	13 (7.9%)
	widowed	3 (1.8%)
	unwedded	48 (29.3%)
Analgesic medication	Opioids schedule II	16 (9.85)
	Opioids schedule III	26 (15.8%)
	Non-opioids	97 (59.1%)
	Antidepressants	36 (21.9%)
	Anticonvulsants	30 (18.3%)
	Muscle relaxants	5 (3.0%)
	Others	26 (15.8%)
Number of compounds	One compound	91 (55.5%)
	Two compounds	30 (18.3%)
	Three compounds	23 (14.0%)
	>Three compounds	18 (11.0%)
Coded psychological Diagnoses	Patients (n)	Patients (n)
Pain Disorder with Somatic and Psychological Factors	Yes: 149	No: 15
Depression	Yes: 79	No: 85
Anxiety	Yes: 12	No: 152
Somatization disorder	Yes: 7	No: 157
Sleep disorder	Yes: 83	No: 81
Coded Z-diagnoses		
family	Yes: 52	No: 112
work	Yes: 88	No: 76
biography	Yes: 37	No: 127

Table 1. Cont.

		Patients/n (%)
finance	Yes: 26	No: 138
any Z-diagnose	Yes: 129	No: 35
Pain scores		Median (IQR)
	Current	7.0 (5.0–8.0)
	Mean *	7.0 (6.0–8.0)
	Highest	9.0 (8.0–10.0)
	Bearable	3.0 (2.0–4.0)
	Total **	7.33 (6.33–8.0)
IEQ	Blame	8.0 (4.0–13.75)
	Severity	15.0 (12.0–18.0)
	Total	24.0 (17.0–31.0)
DASS	Depression	9.0 (4.0–14.0)
	Anxiety	5.0 (2.0–9.0)
	Stress	10.0 (7.0–14.0)
	Total	25.0 (15.0–34.0)
FW 7		10.0 (4.0–14.75)
Disability score		77.33 (56.67–83.33)

The median scores for depression, anxiety, and stress within the study population were below the cutoffs for conspicuous or probable disorder. With regard to education, marital, and professional status, the following results were obtained: More than half of the patients were employed, one-third of the patients were unemployed or retired, and the rest of the patients received a disability pension. Most of the patients had no pension application, while 12 patients had. A non-academic professional education was reported by 78.05% of the patients (128/164). Two-thirds of the patients were married (Table 1).

3.2. Opioid Use, Gender, Age, Pain Localization, and Pain Diagnosis

No statistically significant differences were found among the proportion of opioid users between male and female patients. Moreover, there were no differences in age between patients with and without opioid use (Table 2).

Table 2. Opioids and Age (years), sex, and different pain localizations, percentages represent within group values, * Mann–Whitney Test, ** Fisher's exact test, *** chi-squared test, $p < 0.05$ = significant, [a] WSP = widespread pain.

		Opioids	No Opioids	p
Age *	50.3 (SD 14.2)	56.30 (35.30–67.70)	51.40 (40.30–58.25)	0.1727
Sex (m/f) **	67/97	18/21	49/76	0.4606
Pain *** localization				0.1551
Head and Face		4 (10.3%)	26 (20.8%)	
Cervical		6 (15.4%)	17 (13.6%)	
Lumbar		19 (48.7%)	48 (29.3%)	
Extremities		4 (10.3%)	11 (6.7%)	
Abdominal		3 (7.7%)	2 (1.2%)	
WSP [a]		3 (7.7%)	21 (12.8%)	

There were no statistically significant differences found in pain localizations among patients with and without opioid use (Table 2).

Mean pain scores were higher in the group of patients taking opioids compared to those without opioid therapy. No statistically significant correlations between the other pain scores were found (Table 3).

Table 3. Opioids and pain scores, * during the last 4 weeks, $p < 0.05$ = significant, Mann–Whitney Test.

Pain Scores	Opioids	No Opioids	
Current	7.0 (5.0–8.0)	6.5 (5.0–8.0)	0.5181
Mean *	8.0 (7.0–9.0)	7.0 (6.0–8.0)	0.0047
Highest	9.0 (8.0–10.0)	9.0 (8.0–10.0)	0.3952
Bearable	3.0 (2.0–4.0)	3.0 (2.0–4.0)	0.4854
Total NRS	7.67 (6.67–8.33)	7.33 (6.33–8.0)	0.2215

3.3. Opioid Use and Psychological Factors

The IEQ total, but not the subscales blame and severity, was significantly higher in patients using Schedule III opioids than in those using no opioids. Considering all opioids (Schedule II and Schedule III opioids), this difference was no longer statistically significant. This was the only item which yielded different significance in patients taking Schedule III opioids than in patients taking Schedule II or III opioids, or both. The DASS depression and the DASS total score, but not the DASS anxiety and stress scores, were significantly higher in patients with opioid therapy compared to patients with no opioid therapy. There were no differences regarding pain-related disability and habitual well-being (Table 4), and no statistically significant differences in the frequency of coding of diagnoses such as "Pain Disorder with Somatic and Psychological Factors" (ICD-10: F45.41) [34], depression, anxiety, or sleep disorder (Table 5).

Table 4. Opioids and psychological factors, Fisher's exact test, *p*-values = opioids (strong and weak) vs. no opioids.

	Opioids	No Opioids	*p*
IEQ			
IEQ total (all opioids)	26.0 (19.0–33.0)	23.0 (17.0–29.5)	0.1342
IEQ total (only Schedule III opioids)	28.0 (22.5–33.5)	23.0 (17.0–29.5)	$p = 0.0417$
IEQ blame	10.0 (6.0–15.0)	8.00 (4.0–13.0)	0.1270
IEQ severity	16.0 (12.0–19.0)	15.9 (12.0–18.0)	0.2407
DASS			
Depression	13.0 (6.0–18.0)	8.0 (4.0–13.0)	0.0094
Anxiety	6.0 (2.0–11.0)	4.0 (1.0–8.0)	0.0522
Stress	12.0 (8.0–16.0)	10.0 (7.0–14.0)	0.0618
Total	32.0 (17.0–42.0)	22.0 (14.5–33.0)	0.0182
PDI	76.67 (53.33–86.67)	73.33 (56.67–83.33)	0.5097
FW 7	9.0 (3.0–14.0)	10.0 (5.0–15.0)	0.4544
Coded diagnoses			
Pain Disorder with Somatic and Psychological Factors	Yes: 35 No: 4	Yes: 114 No: 11	0.7556
Depression	Yes: 17 No: 22	Yes: 49 No: 76	0.7091
Anxiety	Yes: 3 No: 36	Yes: 9 No: 116	1.0
Sleep disorder	Yes: 22 No: 17	Yes: 61 No: 64	0.4651

Table 5. Opioids and social factors ** values missing to 164: n.a., chi-squared test, *p*-values = opioids vs. no opioids.

	All Opioids	No Opioids	*p*
Occupational status			
employed	6	71	
unemployed	15	21	<0.0001
retired	10	9	
disability pension	8	21	
Work leave **	Yes: 12	Yes: 44	0.6430
	No: 11	No: 55	
Pension application	Yes: 0	Yes: 12	0.0714
	No: 28	No: 95	
Professional education			
academic	3	24	
nonacademic	32	96	0.0994
none	4	5	
Marital status			
divorced	3	10	
married	24	76	0.9862
unwedded	12	36	
Coded psychosocial diagnoses			
Finance	Yes: 5	Yes: 21	0.6256
	No: 34	No: 104	
Family	Yes: 9	Yes: 43	0.2378
	No: 30	No: 82	
Workplace	Yes: 20	Yes: 69	0.7149
	No: 19	No: 56	
Biography	Yes: 11	Yes: 25	0.2773
	No: 28	No: 100	

3.4. Opioid Use and Social Factors

There were significant differences in the occupational status between the patient groups with and without opioids. Logistic regression analysis showed that occupational status had a high correlation to opioid use. The overall model was significant, $p < 0.001$ (Table 6). No differences were found in the incidence of work leave or pension application or with different educational levels. Among the coded psychosocial diagnoses, there were no statistically significant differences between the patient groups with and without opioids (Table 5).

Table 6. Logistic regression analysis examining the relation between opioid use (dependent variable) and IEQ total, DASS Depression, mean pain, B: regression coefficient, SE: Standard error.

	B	SE	Wald	df	*p*	Odds Ratio
Regression						
Constant	−0.3441	1.060	10.541	1	0.001	0.032
Age	0.015	0.014	1.020	1	0.313	1.015
Sex	−0.394	0.394	1.002	1	0.317	0.674
IEQ total	−0.016	0.026	0.365	1	0.545	0.984
DASS D	0.094	0.042	4.875	1	0.027	1.098
NRS mean	0.168	0.106	2.508	1	0.113	1.184
Occupation status	−0.146	0.539	0.073	1	0.787	0.864

4. Discussion

In this prospective study, 24% of all investigated patients with chronic pain consumed opioids. There was no significant correlation between age, gender, and opioid consumption

(Table 2). In contrast, other studies on the subject of gender-specific differences in patients with chronic pain found that women suffer from pain more often and also report higher pain intensity and more pain problems. This led to the conclusion that women were prescribed more opioids than men [36,37]. In our study, there were also no statistically significant age-related differences in opioid consumption behavior. However, a national population-based survey by Hudson et al. found that individuals older than 60 years were less likely to receive opioids than younger individuals [38].

Also pain localization showed no differences in the frequency of opioid consumption. In our study the majority complained of lumbar back pain (Table 3). In agreement with our study result, lumbar back pain is one of the most complained of pain syndromes in the western countries, with a global point prevalence estimated to be 9.4% [39]. We found no other references examining the relationship between different pain localizations and opioid consumption.

Opioid consumption was not related to most of the pain scores (Table 4), but interestingly, only mean pain was significantly higher in the group of patients taking opioids than in those without opioids. This result could confirm previous study results which report that opioid users were more likely than non-users to report high levels of pain interference with their daily lives [38]. On the other hand, Chen et al. reported on the lack of connection between the opioid dose change (increase or decrease) and the clinical pain score in a group of patients with chronic pain, regardless of age or gender [40]. These results were confirmed in further studies. Escalation of opioid dose was either not associated with improvements in NRS pain scores or with mild but clinically insignificant improvements [41].

In contrast to other study data, our study results show no difference in the mean values of the habitual well-being or the disability score of patients taking opioids and those not taking opioids [42]. This could possibly be a dose-dependent or habituation effect. Possible underlying mechanisms of a loss of efficacy of opioids in the sense of developing tolerance remain elusive, despite intensive research to understand the phenomenon [43]. Opioids may impair the assessment of one's own quality of life through central nervous system side effects depending on the dose, speed of dose escalation and on comorbidities and co-medication [44]. Patients' self-reported physical and psychological effects of opioid use in chronic non-cancer pain showed that improvement in general well-being irrespective of pain relief was experienced by 40% of the patients with chronic pain and opioid intake [45].

Wakaizumi et al. compared psychosocial, functional, and psychological measures between patients with chronic back pain who were managing their pain with or without opioids. Patients on opioids displayed poorer physical function [46]. In this context, it is important to know that our own non-pharmacological measures to improve the pain consist of self-reliant health attitudes and physical activities. Self-reliant health attitude, exercise, and physical activity have been shown to be a successful tool in avoiding opioids or discontinuing opioid use [47]. Further, a systematic review on opioids in patients with chronic non-cancer pain found small improvements in social functioning which were, however, far below the minimally important difference, and no improvements in emotional or role functioning [9].

The coded ICD-10 diagnoses of our study population, such as chronic pain disorder, depression, anxiety, and sleep disorder, had no significant correlation with opioid consumption. It is theorized that this could be the consequence of a relatively unspecific coding or diagnosis. An electronic health record such as the International Statistical Classification of Diseases and Related Health Problems, 10th Revision, German Modification (ICD-10-GM) is the official classification for coding diagnoses in outpatient and inpatient care in Germany. ICD-10 may receive insufficient underdiagnosis or outdated data if it is not updated regularly.

Depression showed a significant dependency on opioid intake in contrast to anxiety and stress. This result is partially consistent with Jamison et al., who reported that 40% of chronic pain patients treated with opioids suffer from additional affective disorders (depression and anxiety), which in turn are associated with a significantly increased misuse of opioids [36]. There are a number of studies demonstrating that people with psychological comorbidities such as depression and anxiety are prevalent among patients with chronic non-cancer pain [6,48–50], and that they are more likely to receive long-term opioid therapy for non-cancer pain than those without such comorbidities [4]. One reason for that could be that mental health conditions and chronic non-cancer pain are closely correlated concerning severity [5]. Moreover, patients with psychological comorbidities have a tendency to use opioids earlier and to use higher dosages of opioids [6]. Opioid use may be a factor for the new onset of depression, although the risk of depression is associated with longer duration of use but not with dose [2].

Consistent with previous research by Carriere et al. [14] we found a significant correlation between opioid consumption and perceived injustice (IEQ total) in our study population. Interestingly, this relationship was only confirmed for Schedule III opioids. If one assumes that patients with severe pain also prefer Schedule III opioids, this fits well with the results published by Carriere et al. This study group discussed that perceived injustice might contribute to higher levels of pain and as a consequence might increase the likelihood of opioid prescription [14]. For Carriere et al., pain behavior plays an important role in mediating between perceived injustice and opioid prescription. In a longitudinal study, Dickman et al. found that perceived injustice predicted increases in reported opioid use over three months, at least in patients without a high score in the PMQ (pain medicine questionnaire), thus in patients who did not take many other analgesics [51].

In our opinion, a therapeutic consequence for the reduction of opioids could be that patients should be screened for perceived injustice and receive psychoeducation or be counselled on that subject as appropriate. Other studies show that perceived injustice is a pain-influencing factor even in cancer survivors. Therefore, such patients should also be screened for perceived injustice as a trigger for behavioral patterns associated with opioid use [15]. Scott et al. even showed that perceived injustice augments the relationship between pain severity and depressive symptoms [10]. Based on the well-known relationships between depression and opioid consumption, one could argue that this observation could also be a cause of changed opioid consumption behavior.

As we already mentioned, there is a strong relationship between emotional stress and chronic pain. Furthermore, physical pain and negative emotions reinforce each other. This correlation is also shown in the fact that physical pain and negative emotions activate the same areas of the brain [52]. Opioids could be one way to treat not only physical pain but also social stress, and this could be a reason for the development of opioid abuse. Mark D. Sullivan emphasizes that "long-term opioid therapy impairs human social and emotional functions" [8]. Pain-related distress has been shown to increase pain intensity and interference [53–55] and to be associated with worse outcomes in treatment studies [56].

Concerning socioeconomic factors, only occupational status showed a significant correlation to opioid consumption. In addition, the logistic regression analysis showed that among the variables examined, occupational status had the strongest correlation with opioid use.

Employment status, education level, income, and occupational factors have already been discussed as risk factors for chronic pain [52,57]. To our knowledge, there are no proven correlations between opioid consumption and occupational status up to now. However, if one assumes that psychosocial stress, e.g., professional problems or problems in the workplace, is a risk for chronicity, and one knows that psychological stress can be associated with higher pain perception, a correlation between occupation and opioid consumption would be possible [57].

Limitations

One limitation of this study could be that we do not know for sure whether there has been a change of medication or dosage between data collection from the German Pain Questionnaire and the IEQ. Since the time between data collection was only few weeks, clinical experience indicates that a substantial change is unlikely. Further, it should be taken into account that the socioeconomic data were submitted subjectively by the patients, e.g., patients may have classified themselves as incapacitated without stating whether this is an official assessment or an estimation. A type 2 error cannot be ruled out completely, as multiple items have been tested, but it seems rather unlikely. Some of the ICD-10 coded diagnoses, such as depression or sleep disorder, were rarely recorded and, therefore, may not have enough power to determine statistical differences.

A strength of this study is the prospective study design with the inclusion at a university tertiary pain center of patients with chronic pain and high impairment of their quality of life. Contributing to the strength are the variety of several potentially important psychosocial, socioeconomic, and somatic factors and a broad analysis of the subject.

5. Conclusions

In summary, our study again highlights that opioid use is strongly interwoven with a variety of psychological and socioeconomic factors. In addition to the psychological factors of opioid consumption in patients with chronic pain, we found a correlation of opioid use with the occupational status and the IEQ total. Taking occupational status and IEQ into account could be useful for weighting the treatment of pain, e.g., for special psychological, social, and medical support. Therefore, further screening models, e.g., with the help of assessments, could be a requirement for successful multimodal treatment schemes.

Author Contributions: Conceptualization, B.K. and T.W.; Data curation, B.K. and T.W.; Formal analysis, T.W.; Project administration, B.K.; Writing—original draft, B.K. and T.W.; Writing—review & editing, B.K. and T.W. All authors have read and agreed to the published version of the manuscript.

Funding: This research received no external funding.

Institutional Review Board Statement: The study was conducted according to the guidelines of the Declaration of Helsinki, and approved by the Ethics Committee of the Albert-Ludwigs-Univerität (protocol code 20-1061, date of approval: 27 August 2020).

Informed Consent Statement: Informed consent was obtained from all subjects involved in the study.

Data Availability Statement: The data presented in this study are available on request from the corresponding author. The data are not publicly available for reasons of data protection.

Conflicts of Interest: The authors declare that they have no conflict of interest.

References

1. Heyman, G.M.; McVicar, N.; Brownell, H. Evidence that social-economic factors play an important role in drug overdose deaths. *Int. J. Drug Policy* **2019**, *74*, 274–284. [CrossRef]
2. Scherrer, J.F.; Salas, J.; Copeland, L.A.; Stock, E.M.; Ahmedani, B.K.; Sullivan, M.D.; Burroughs, T.; Schneider, F.D.; Bucholz, K.K.; Lustman, P.J. Prescription Opioid Duration, Dose, and Increased Risk of Depression in 3 Large Patient Populations. *Ann. Fam. Med.* **2016**, *14*, 54–62. [CrossRef]
3. Petzke, F.; Bock, F.; Huppe, M.; Nothacker, M.; Norda, H.; Radbruch, L.; Schiltenwolf, M.; Schuler, M.; Tolle, T.; Viniol, A.; et al. Long-term opioid therapy for chronic noncancer pain: Second update of the German guidelines. *Pain Rep.* **2020**, *5*, e840. [CrossRef]
4. Braden, J.B.; Sullivan, M.D.; Ray, G.T.; Saunders, K.; Merrill, J.; Silverberg, M.J.; Rutter, C.M.; Weisner, C.; Banta-Green, C.; Campbell, C.; et al. Trends in long-term opioid therapy for noncancer pain among persons with a history of depression. *Gen. Hosp. Psychiatry* **2009**, *31*, 564–570. [CrossRef]
5. Sellinger, J.J.; Sofuoglu, M.; Kerns, R.D.; Rosenheck, R.A. Combined Use of Opioids and Antidepressants in the Treatment of Pain: A Review of Veterans Health Administration Data for Patients with Pain Both With and Without Co-morbid Depression. *Psychiatr. Q.* **2016**, *87*, 585–593. [CrossRef]
6. Elrashidi, M.Y.; Philpot, L.M.; Ramar, P.; Leasure, W.B.; Ebbert, J.O. Depression and Anxiety Among Patients on Chronic Opioid Therapy. *Health Serv. Res. Manag. Epidemiol.* **2018**, *5*, 2333392818771243. [CrossRef]
7. Hung, H.Y.; Chien, W.C.; Chung, C.H.; Kao, L.T.; Chow, L.H.; Chen, Y.H.; Kotlinska, J.H.; Silberring, J.; Huang, E.Y. Patients with alcohol use disorder increase pain and analgesics use: A nationwide population-based cohort study. *Drug Alcohol Depend.* **2021**, *229*, 109102. [CrossRef]
8. Sullivan, M.D.; Ballantyne, J.C. When Physical and Social Pain Coexist: Insights Into Opioid Therapy. *Ann. Fam. Med.* **2021**, *19*, 79–82. [CrossRef]
9. Busse, J.W.; Wang, L.; Kamaleldin, M.; Craigie, S.; Riva, J.J.; Montoya, L.; Mulla, S.M.; Lopes, L.C.; Vogel, N.; Chen, E.; et al. Opioids for Chronic Noncancer Pain: A Systematic Review and Meta-analysis. *JAMA* **2018**, *320*, 2448–2460. [CrossRef]

10. Scott, W.; Sullivan, M. Perceived injustice moderates the relationship between pain and depressive symptoms among individuals with persistent musculoskeletal pain. *Pain Res. Manag.* **2012**, *17*, 335–340. [CrossRef]
11. Sullivan, M.J.L.; Thibault, P.; Simmonds, M.J.; Milioto, M.; Cantin, A.P.; Velly, A.M. Pain, perceived injustice and the persistence of post-traumatic stress symptoms during the course of rehabilitation for whiplash injuries. *Pain* **2009**, *145*, 325–331. [CrossRef]
12. Sullivan, M.J.; Scott, W.; Trost, Z. Perceived injustice: A risk factor for problematic pain outcomes. *Clin. J. Pain* **2012**, *28*, 484–488. [CrossRef]
13. Sullivan, M.J.; Adams, H.; Horan, S.; Maher, D.; Boland, D.; Gross, R. The role of perceived injustice in the experience of chronic pain and disability: Scale development and validation. *J. Occup. Rehabil.* **2008**, *18*, 249–261. [CrossRef]
14. Carriere, J.S.; Martel, M.O.; Kao, M.C.; Sullivan, M.J.; Darnall, B.D. Pain behavior mediates the relationship between perceived injustice and opioid prescription for chronic pain: A Collaborative Health Outcomes Information Registry study. *J. Pain Res.* **2017**, *10*, 557–566. [CrossRef]
15. Nijs, J.; Roose, E.; Lahousse, A.; Mostaqim, K.; Reynebeau, I.; De Couck, M.; Beckwee, D.; Huysmans, E.; Bults, R.; van Wilgen, P.; et al. Pain and Opioid Use in Cancer Survivors: A Practical Guide to Account for Perceived Injustice. *Pain Physician* **2021**, *24*, 309–317.
16. Jun, D.; Johnston, V.; McPhail, S.M.; O'Leary, S. A Longitudinal Evaluation of Risk Factors and Interactions for the Development of Nonspecific Neck Pain in Office Workers in Two Cultures. *Hum. Factors* **2021**, *63*, 663–683. [CrossRef]
17. Svedmark, A.; Bjorklund, M.; Hager, C.K.; Sommar, J.N.; Wahlstrom, J. Impact of Workplace Exposure and Stress on Neck Pain and Disabilities in Women-A Longitudinal Follow-up After a Rehabilitation Intervention. *Ann. Work Expo. Health* **2018**, *62*, 591–603. [CrossRef]
18. Elfering, A.; Grebner, S.; Gerber, H.; Semmer, N.K. Workplace observation of work stressors, catecholamines and musculoskeletal pain among male employees. *Scand. J. Work Environ. Health* **2008**, *34*, 337–344. [CrossRef]
19. Arvidsson, I.; Gremark Simonsen, J.; Lindegard-Andersson, A.; Bjork, J.; Nordander, C. The impact of occupational and personal factors on musculoskeletal pain-a cohort study of female nurses, sonographers and teachers. *BMC Musculoskelet. Disord.* **2020**, *21*, 621. [CrossRef]
20. Pranjic, N.; Males-Bilic, L. Low Back Pain at New Working Ambient in Era of New Economy: A Systematic Review About Occupational Risk Factors. *Acta Med. Croat.* **2015**, *69*, 49–58.
21. Serra-Pujadas, S.; Alonso-Buxade, C.; Serra-Colomer, J.; Folguera, J.; Carrilero, N.; Garcia-Altes, A. Geographical, Socioeconomic, and Gender Inequalities in Opioid Use in Catalonia. *Front. Pharm.* **2021**, *12*, 750193. [CrossRef]
22. Nagel, B.; Gerbershagen, H.U.; Lindena, G.; Pfingsten, M. Development and evaluation of the multidimensional German pain questionnaire. *Schmerz* **2002**, *16*, 263–270. [CrossRef]
23. Casser, H.R.; Arnold, B.; Brinkschmidt, T.; Gralow, I.; Irnich, D.; Klimczyk, K.; Nagel, B.; Pfingsten, M.; Sabatowski, R.; Schiltenwolf, M.; et al. Multidisciplinary assessment for multimodal pain therapy. Indications and range of performance. *Schmerz* **2013**, *27*, 363–370. [CrossRef]
24. Dale, R.; Stacey, B. Multimodal Treatment of Chronic Pain. *Med. Clin. N. Am.* **2016**, *100*, 55–64. [CrossRef]
25. Niederstrasser, N.; Steiger, B.; Welsch, K.; Hartmann, S.; Nilges, P.; Ljutow, A.; Ettlin, D. German transcultural translation of the Injustice Experience Questionnaire. *Schmerz* **2018**, *32*, 442–448. [CrossRef]
26. Steiger, B.; Welsch, K.; Niederstrasser, N.; Hartmann, S.; Nilges, P.; Ljutow, A.; Ettlin, D. Validation of the German-language version of the Injustice Experience Questionnaire (IEQ) in five outpatient clinics. *Schmerz* **2019**, *33*, 106–115. [CrossRef]
27. Sullivan, M.J. User Manual for the Injustice Experience Questionnaire IEQ. Available online: https://sullivan-painresearch.mcgill.ca/ieq.php2017 (accessed on 30 August 2021).
28. Petzke, F.; Hüppe, M.; Kohlmann, T.; Kükenshöner, S.; Lindena, G.; Pfingsten, M.; Nagel, N. Handbuch Deutscher Schmerz-Fragebogen. Available online: https://www.schmerzgesellschaft.de/fileadmin/pdf/DSF_Handbuch_2020_final.pdf (accessed on 30 August 2021).
29. Nilges, P.; Essau, C. Depression, anxiety and stress scales: DASS—A screening procedure not only for pain patients. *Schmerz* **2015**, *29*, 649–657. [CrossRef]
30. Pollard, C.A. Preliminary validity study of the pain disability index. *Percept. Mot. Ski.* **1984**, *59*, 974. [CrossRef]
31. Basler, H.D. The Marburg questionnaire on habitual health findings—A study on patients with chronic pain. *Schmerz* **1999**, *13*, 385–391. [CrossRef]
32. Boleloucky, Z. Aspects of the 10th decennial revision of the international statistical classification of diseases (ICD-10). *Cesk Psychiatr.* **1989**, *85*, 183–193.
33. Ewert, T.; Stucki, G. The international classification of functioning, disability and health. Potential applications in Germany. *Bundesgesundheitsblatt Gesundh. Gesundh.* **2007**, *50*, 953–961. [CrossRef] [PubMed]
34. Nilges, P.; Rief, W. F45.41: Chronic pain disorder with somatic and psychological factors: A coding aid. *Schmerz* **2010**, *24*, 209–212. [CrossRef] [PubMed]
35. Erdfelder, E.; Faul, F.; Buchner, A. GPOWER: A general power analysis program. *Behav. Res. Methods Instrum. Comput.* **1996**, *28*, 1–11. [CrossRef]
36. Jamison, R.N.; Butler, S.F.; Budman, S.H.; Edwards, R.R.; Wasan, A.D. Gender differences in risk factors for aberrant prescription opioid use. *J. Pain* **2010**, *11*, 312–320. [CrossRef]

37. Campbell, C.I.; Weisner, C.; Leresche, L.; Ray, G.T.; Saunders, K.; Sullivan, M.D.; Banta-Green, C.J.; Merrill, J.O.; Silverberg, M.J.; Boudreau, D.; et al. Age and gender trends in long-term opioid analgesic use for noncancer pain. *Am. J. Public Health* **2010**, *100*, 2541–2547. [CrossRef]
38. Hudson, T.J.; Edlund, M.J.; Steffick, D.E.; Tripathi, S.P.; Sullivan, M.D. Epidemiology of regular prescribed opioid use: Results from a national, population-based survey. *J. Pain Symptom Manag.* **2008**, *36*, 280–288. [CrossRef]
39. Petzke, F.; Klose, P.; Welsch, P.; Sommer, C.; Hauser, W. Opioids for chronic low back pain: An updated systematic review and meta-analysis of efficacy, tolerability and safety in randomized placebo-controlled studies of at least 4 weeks of double-blind duration. *Eur. J. Pain* **2020**, *24*, 497–517. [CrossRef]
40. Chen, L.; Vo, T.; Seefeld, L.; Malarick, C.; Houghton, M.; Ahmed, S.; Zhang, Y.; Cohen, A.; Retamozo, C.; St Hilaire, K.; et al. Lack of correlation between opioid dose adjustment and pain score change in a group of chronic pain patients. *J. Pain* **2013**, *14*, 384–392. [CrossRef]
41. Hayes, C.J.; Krebs, E.E.; Hudson, T.; Brown, J.; Li, C.; Martin, B.C. Impact of opioid dose escalation on pain intensity: A retrospective cohort study. *Pain* **2020**, *161*, 979–988. [CrossRef]
42. Fishman, M.A.; Antony, A.B.; Hunter, C.W.; Pope, J.E.; Staats, P.S.; Agarwal, R.; Connolly, A.T.; Dalal, N.; Deer, T.R. The Cost of Lost Productivity in an Opioid Utilizing Pain Sample. *J. Pain Res.* **2021**, *14*, 2347–2357. [CrossRef]
43. Ballantyne, J.C.; Shin, N.S. Efficacy of opioids for chronic pain: A review of the evidence. *Clin. J. Pain* **2008**, *24*, 469–478. [CrossRef] [PubMed]
44. Benyamin, R.; Trescot, A.M.; Datta, S.; Buenaventura, R.; Adlaka, R.; Sehgal, N.; Glaser, S.E.; Vallejo, R. Opioid complications and side effects. *Pain Physician* **2008**, *11*, S105–S120. [CrossRef] [PubMed]
45. Schulte, E.; Spies, C.; Denke, C.; Meerpohl, J.J.; Donner-Banzhoff, N.; Petzke, F.; Hertwig, R.; Schafer, M.; Wegwarth, O. Patients' self-reported physical and psychological effects of opioid use in chronic noncancer pain-A retrospective cross-sectional analysis. *Eur. J. Pain* **2022**, *26*, 417–427. [CrossRef] [PubMed]
46. Wakaizumi, K.; Vigotsky, A.D.; Jabakhanji, R.; Abdallah, M.; Barroso, J.; Schnitzer, T.J.; Apkarian, A.V.; Baliki, M.N. Psychosocial, Functional, and Emotional Correlates of Long-Term Opioid Use in Patients with Chronic Back Pain: A Cross-Sectional Case-Control Study. *Pain* **2021**, *10*, 691–709. [CrossRef]
47. Geneen, L.J.; Moore, R.A.; Clarke, C.; Martin, D.; Colvin, L.A.; Smith, B.H. Physical activity and exercise for chronic pain in adults: An overview of Cochrane Reviews. *Cochrane Database Syst. Rev.* **2017**, *4*, CD011279. [CrossRef]
48. Tumenta, T.; Ugwendum, D.F.; Chobufo, M.D.; Mungu, E.B.; Kogan, I.; Olupona, T. Prevalence and Trends of Opioid Use in Patients With Depression in the United States. *Cureus* **2021**, *13*, e15639. [CrossRef]
49. Dufort, A.; Samaan, Z. Problematic Opioid Use Among Older Adults: Epidemiology, Adverse Outcomes and Treatment Considerations. *Drugs Aging* **2021**, *38*, 1043–1053. [CrossRef]
50. Rus Makovec, M.; Vintar, N.; Makovec, S. Level of Depression, Anxiety and Impairment of Social Relations with Regard to Pain Intensity in a Naturalistic Sample of Patients at the Outpatient Chronic Pain Clinic. *Psychiatr. Danub.* **2021**, *33*, 558–564.
51. Dickman, J.; Slepian, P.; Ankawi, B.; France, C. Perceived injustice moderates the relationship between pain medication questionnaire scores and opioid use over three months. *J. Pain* **2018**, *19*, S54. [CrossRef]
52. Gureje, O.; Simon, G.E.; Von Korff, M. A cross-national study of the course of persistent pain in primary care. *Pain* **2001**, *92*, 195–200. [CrossRef]
53. Barke, A.; Koechlin, H.; Korwisi, B.; Locher, C. Emotional distress: Specifying a neglected part of chronic pain. *Eur. J. Pain* **2020**, *24*, 477–480. [CrossRef] [PubMed]
54. Nordstoga, A.L.; Vasseljen, O.; Meisingset, I.; Nilsen, T.I.L.; Unsgaard-Tondel, M. Improvement in Work Ability, Psychological Distress and Pain Sites in Relation to Low Back Pain Prognosis: A Longitudinal Observational Study in Primary Care. *Spine (Phila Pa 1976)* **2019**, *44*, E423–E429. [CrossRef] [PubMed]
55. Smedbraten, K.; Oiestad, B.E.; Roe, Y. Emotional distress was associated with persistent shoulder pain after physiotherapy: A prospective cohort study. *BMC Musculoskelet. Disord.* **2018**, *19*, 304. [CrossRef] [PubMed]
56. Helminen, E.E.; Sinikallio, S.H.; Valjakka, A.L.; Vaisanen-Rouvali, R.H.; Arokoski, J.P. Determinants of pain and functioning in knee osteoarthritis: A one-year prospective study. *Clin. Rehabil.* **2016**, *30*, 890–900. [CrossRef]
57. Mills, S.E.E.; Nicolson, K.P.; Smith, B.H. Chronic pain: A review of its epidemiology and associated factors in population-based studies. *Br. J. Anaesth.* **2019**, *123*, e273–e283. [CrossRef]

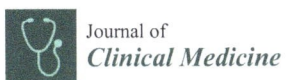

Article

Is Central Sensitisation the Missing Link of Persisting Symptoms after COVID-19 Infection?

Lisa Goudman [1,2,3,4,5,*], Ann De Smedt [2,3,6], Marc Noppen [7] and Maarten Moens [1,2,3,4,8]

1. Department of Neurosurgery, Universitair Ziekenhuis Brussel, Laarbeeklaan 101, 1090 Brussels, Belgium; maarten.moens@uzbrussel.be
2. STIMULUS Research Group (reSearch and TeachIng neuroModULation Uz bruSsel), Vrije Universiteit Brussel, Laarbeeklaan 103, 1090 Brussels, Belgium; Ann.DeSmedt@uzbrussel.be
3. Center for Neurosciences (C4N), Vrije Universiteit Brussel, Laarbeeklaan 103, 1090 Brussels, Belgium
4. Pain in Motion (PAIN) Research Group, Department of Physiotherapy, Human Physiology and Anatomy, Faculty of Physical Education and Physiotherapy, Vrije Universiteit Brussel, Laarbeeklaan 103, 1090 Brussels, Belgium
5. Research Foundation—Flanders (FWO), 1090 Brussels, Belgium
6. Department of Physical Medicine and Rehabilitation, Universitair Ziekenhuis Brussel, Laarbeeklaan 101, 1090 Brussels, Belgium
7. Chief Executive Officer, Universitair Ziekenhuis Brussel, Laarbeeklaan 101, 1090 Brussels, Belgium; marc.noppen@uzbrussel.be
8. Department of Radiology, Universitair Ziekenhuis Brussel, Laarbeeklaan 101, 1090 Brussels, Belgium
* Correspondence: lisa.goudman@vub.be; Tel.: +32-2477-5514

Abstract: Patients recovered from a COVID-19 infection often report vague symptoms of fatigue or dyspnoea, comparable to the manifestations in patients with central sensitisation. The hypothesis was that central sensitisation could be the underlying common aetiology in both patient populations. This study explored the presence of symptoms of central sensitisation, and the association with functional status and health-related quality of life, in patients post COVID-19 infection. Patients who were previously infected with COVID-19 filled out the Central Sensitisation Inventory (CSI), the Post-COVID-19 Functional Status (PCFS) Scale and the EuroQol with five dimensions, through an online survey. Eventually, 567 persons completed the survey. In total, 29.73% of the persons had a score of <40/100 on the CSI and 70.26% had a score of ≥40/100. Regarding functional status, 7.34% had no functional limitations, 9.13% had negligible functional limitations, 37.30% reported slight functional limitations, 42.86% indicated moderate functional limitations and 3.37% reported severe functional limitations. Based on a one-way ANOVA test, there was a significant effect of PCFS Scale group level on the total CSI score ($F(4,486) = 46.17$, $p < 0.001$). This survey indicated the presence of symptoms of central sensitisation in more than 70% of patients post COVID-19 infection, suggesting towards the need for patient education and multimodal rehabilitation, to target nociplastic pain.

Keywords: COVID-19; persisting symptoms; fatigue; nociplastic pain; functional status; central sensitisation

Citation: Goudman, L.; De Smedt, A.; Noppen, M.; Moens, M. Is Central Sensitisation the Missing Link of Persisting Symptoms after COVID-19 Infection? *J. Clin. Med.* **2021**, *10*, 5594. https://doi.org/10.3390/jcm10235594

Academic Editor: Tomoyuki Kawamata

Received: 26 October 2021
Accepted: 26 November 2021
Published: 28 November 2021

Publisher's Note: MDPI stays neutral with regard to jurisdictional claims in published maps and institutional affiliations.

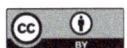

Copyright: © 2021 by the authors. Licensee MDPI, Basel, Switzerland. This article is an open access article distributed under the terms and conditions of the Creative Commons Attribution (CC BY) license (https://creativecommons.org/licenses/by/4.0/).

1. Introduction

Currently, the outbreak of the coronavirus disease 2019 (COVID-19) pandemic is still a serious global public health concern. This novel coronavirus, was first discovered in Wuhan, China, in 2019 and afterwards rapidly spread throughout the world, causes a disease that manifested itself with fever, cough, encephalitis, myalgia, fatigue, muscle weakness, arthralgia, anosmia, and impairment in other bodily functions in the acute phase [1–5]. While mild symptoms are reported in approximately 85% of the cases, a substantial proportion of patients with COVID-19 develop acute respiratory distress syndrome (ARDS) and critical illness [6]. Up to 17% of cases needed high-dependency/intensive care unit treatment due to hypoxemic pulmonary failure [7]. Besides the impact on the respiratory system, coronaviruses had an effect on other systems as well including the central nervous system, cardiovascular system, musculoskeletal system, and gastrointestinal system [2,3,8–11]. As the COVID-19 pandemic continues, signs and symptoms, such as persistent fatigue or depression, which continue or develop after acute COVID-19 are reported, and are denoted as "long COVID" [12].

In patients who are suffering from chronic non-specific pain, central sensitisation (i.e., an amplification of neural signalling within the central nervous system that elicits pain hypersensitivity [13]) often serves as an underlying neurophysiological mechanism to explain the manifestations [14]. Especially, in patients in whom there is an absence of a clear origin of nociceptive input or absence of enough tissue damage to explain the experienced pain, disability, and other symptoms, central nervous system sensitisation is often proposed. Central sensitisation has been denoted as an important contributor or a common aetiology in a variety of chronic musculoskeletal conditions, including fibromyalgia, chronic fatigue syndrome, and irritable bowel syndrome [15]. Despite the lack of a solid outcome measurement, the Central Sensitization Inventory (CSI) was previously introduced as a screening instrument for clinicians to help identify patients with central sensitisation [15]. In post COVID-19 patients, potential long-term secondary effects on the musculoskeletal system such as muscle weakness, decreased muscle mass, and myopathies have been brought to attention [16]. Persisting symptoms are a frequently reported complaint in patients recovered from COVID-19 infection with at least one symptom, particularly fatigue and dyspnoea [17]. Fatigue is also one of the core symptoms in central sensitisation disorders [18], leading to the hypothesis that central sensitisation might be the underlying common aetiology in patients with chronic pain and patients post COVID-19 infection.

The goal of this study was to gain further insight in the presence of central sensitisation as underlying factor for long-term secondary effects in post COVID-19 patients. Additionally, we evaluated whether there was an association between total scores on the CSI and the functional status after COVID-19 infection. Therefore, the aim of this study was to explore the presence of symptoms of central sensitisation, and the association with functional status and health-related quality of life, in patients post COVID-19 infection.

2. Materials and Methods

2.1. Study Participants

This study used a cross-sectional online survey design with a convenience sample of individuals self-reporting the presence of a post COVID-19 infection state. The survey population comprised all Dutch speaking adults, living in Belgium. The sampling frame consisted of all post COVID-19 patients who were active on social media since the survey was spread on LinkedIn, Facebook and Instagram several times between 4 June 2021 and 22 August 2021. Additionally, personal contacts of the research group members who were infected with COVID-19 were asked to complete the online survey. No specific criteria were imposed regarding the time frame after infection.

On the first page of the survey, all respondents were informed that the survey was completely anonymous and that the information would only be used for this study. Additionally, they were informed about the main goal of this survey. No financial or other incentives were provided. The survey took around 10 min to complete.

The study protocol was approved by the central ethics committee of Universitair Ziekenhuis Brussels (B.U.N. 1432021000484) on 26 May 2021. The study was registered on clinicaltrials.gov (NCT04912778). The study was conducted according to the revised Declaration of Helsinki (1998).

2.2. Data Collection

The online survey consisted of three validated questionnaires (in a random order) to evaluate the functional status, health-related quality of life and symptoms of central sensitisation. Additionally, demographics were questioned (age, sex, time of COVID-19 infection (based on symptoms), availability of a test, length, and weight). In the case that respondents underwent a test to confirm a COVID-19 infection, this was denoted as a confirmatory diagnosis. Respondents without the availability of a COVID-19 test result were denoted as a presumptive diagnosis.

Symptoms of central sensitisation were assessed with the Central Sensitization Inventory (CSI). The CSI consists of 25 symptom-related opinions that the patient had to score on a 5-point Likert scale [15]. A total score of $\geq 40/100$ indicated the presence of central sensitisation (sensitivity: 81%, specificity: 75%) [15]. The CSI has good clinimetric properties for assessing symptoms of central sensitisation and is validated in Dutch [19,20]. Additionally, respondents were categorised based on central sensitisation-related severity into three subgroups: (i) low level, (ii) medium level, or (iii) high level of central sensitisation-related symptom severity using the freely accessible online calculator (https://www.pridedallas.com/questionnaires, accessed on 19 November 2021) [21].

The post COVID-19 functional status was evaluated by the Post-COVID-19 Functional Status (PCFS) Scale, using the self-reporting version of this questionnaire [22,23]. This intuitive scale is ordinal, with 6 steps ranging from grade 0 (no functional limitations) to grade 4 (severe functional limitations) and grade 5 (death), and covers the entire range of functional outcomes by focusing on limitations in usual duties/activities either at home or at work/study, as well as changes in lifestyle.

The EuroQol with five dimensions and three levels (EQ5D-3L) [24] is a standardised health-related quality of life questionnaire to provide a generic measure of health for clinical and economic appraisal [25]. The EQ5D-3L consists of a descriptive system and a visual analogue scale (VAS). The descriptive system contains five dimensions (mobility, self-care, usual activities, pain/discomfort, anxiety/depression). Each dimension has three response levels. In the second part of the questionnaire, a standard vertical 20 cm VAS was implemented to record an individual's rating for their current health-related quality of life state. The responses to the EQ-5D dimensions were converted into a single index value for all health states [26]. Health state index scores generally range from less than zero (where zero is a health state equivalent to death; negative values are valued as worse than death) to one (perfect health), with higher scores indicating a higher health utility.

2.3. Statistical Analysis

Survey data were collected through LimeSurvey. All analyses were performed in R Studio version 1.4.1106 (R version 4.0.5). *P*-values of 0.05 or less were considered statistically significant. Descriptive statistics were provided as means with corresponding standard deviation (SD). Two-sample *t*-tests were performed to evaluate the effect of sex and the presence of a test on CSI, EQ5D and EQ5D VAS scores. Pearson correlation coefficients were calculated between total CSI scores, EQ5D scores and EQ5D VAS scores on the one hand and time since infection and body mass index (BMI) on the other hand. A point-biserial correlation was calculated between PCFS Scale scores and CSI total scores and between PCFS Scale scores and EQ5D scores. One-way ANOVA testing was used to explore the effect of PCFS Scale scores on CSI total scores and EQ5D scores, with corresponding Tukey HSD test for post hoc comparisons. All analyses were performed on data as observed, meaning that for respondents with incomplete data, all data that were available was used.

3. Results

3.1. Demographic Statistics

In total, 741 respondents who were previously infected with COVID-19 opened the survey between 4 June 2021 and 30 August 2021. Of those 741 respondents, 567 started to complete the survey. Demographics were available for 567 respondents; the CSI was filled in by 491 persons, the EQ5D-3L by 547 respondents, the EQ5D VAS by 537 persons and the PCFS Scale by 504 persons. Seventy-seven (13.58%) males and 490 (86.42%) females completed the survey. Respondents had a mean age of 46.5 (SD: 11.4) years and a BMI of 26.5 (SD: 5.42) kg/m^2. Respondents were infected with COVID-19 between 22 January

2020 and 25 July 2021. The mean time between the infection and the time of completing this survey was 287 days (SD: 150).

3.2. Symptoms of Central Sensitisation, Functional Status and Health-Related Quality of Life

The mean score on the CSI was 45.9 (SD: 13.1), where 146 (29.73%) of the persons had a score of <40/100 on the CSI and 345 (70.26%) of a score $\geq$40/100. In total, 21 respondents (4.28%) could be classified with a low level of central sensitisation-related symptom severity, 152 (30.96%) with a medium level and 318 (64.76%) with a high level of central sensitisation-related symptom severity. Table 1 presents CSI scores for the full sample, separated by sex, the presence of a Covid test and PCFS Scale score. There was a significant difference in CSI score between males (41.2 (SD 13.8)) and females (46.6 (SD 12.8), $t(86.54) = -3.01, p = 0.003$), but not between respondents with a confirmatory or presumptive COVID-19 diagnosis ($t(163.1) = 1.35, p = 0.18$). There was a positive correlation (r = 0.09, 95% CI from 0.003 to 0.18) between BMI and the total CSI score ($p = 0.04$). Additionally, a positive significant correlation was revealed between total CSI score and time since infection (r = 0.14, 95% CI from 0.05 to 0.23, $p = 0.002$).

Table 1. Total scores on the CSI, separated for categorical variables. Abbreviations. N: number of respondents; PCFS: Post-COVID-19 Functional Status Scale, SD: standard deviation.

Variable	Level	Mean CSI Score	Mean EQ5D	Mean EQ5D Vas
Sample		45.9 (SD 13.1) (N = 491)	0.57 (SD 0.23) (N = 547)	56.6 (SD 18.2) (N = 537)
Sex	Male	41.2 (SD 13.8) (N = 68)	0.60 (SD 0.23) (N = 75)	61.8 (SD 18.6) (N = 74)
	Female	46.6 (SD 12.8) (N = 423)	0.56 (SD 0.23) (N = 472)	55.8 (SD 18.1) (N = 463)
COVID-19 DIAGNOSIS	Confirmatory	45.5 (SD 13.2) (N = 390)	0.57 (SD 0.24) (N = 433)	56.6 (SD 17.9) (N = 112)
	Presumptive	47.4 (SD 12.5) (N = 101)	0.57 (SD 0.22) (N = 114)	57.0 (SD 19.5) (N = 425)
PCFS	Score 0	28.5 (SD 11.8) (N = 35)	0.87 (SD 0.15) (N = 37)	78.4 (SD 15.8) (N = 37)
	Score 1	37.3 (SD 13.1) (N = 44)	0.73 (SD 0.12) (N = 46)	72.3 (SD 12.7) (N = 46)
	Score 2	44.4 (SD 10.8) (N = 187)	0.63 (SD 0.15) (N = 188)	60.7 (SD 13.1) (N = 188)
	Score 3	50.7 (SD 11.1) (N = 208)	0.45 (SD 0.22) (N = 216)	47.3 (SD 15.2) (N = 216)
	Score 4	61.3 (SD 10.9) (N = 17)	0.15 (SD 0.11) (N = 17)	34.1 (SD 14.5) (N = 17)

Concerning the PCFS, 37 persons (7.34%) had no functional limitations (grade 0), 46 (9.13%) had negligible functional limitations (grade 1), 188 (37.30%) reported slight functional limitations (grade 2), 216 (42.86%) indicated moderate functional limitations (grade 3) and 17 (3.37%) reported severe functional limitations (grade 4). Figure 1 presents the CSI scores for each level of the PCFS Scale.

The mean EQ5D-3L index score was 0.57 (SD: 0.23) and the EQ5D VAS mean score was 56.6 (SD: 18.2) (Table 1). For the mobility component of the EQ5D-3L, 56.96% of the respondents had no problems, 40.36% had some problems with mobility and 2.68% was confined to bed. For the self-care component, 86.98% reported no problems, 12.30% some problems and 0.72% was unable to wash or dress himself/herself. For usual activities, 17.67% had no problems, 62.66% some problems and 19.67% was unable to perform usual activities. No pain or discomfort was reported by 10.42%, moderate pain or discomfort by 74.59% and extreme pain or discomfort by 14.99%. For anxiety/depression, 57.40% indicated not being anxious or depressed, 38.39% was moderately anxious or depressed and 4.20% was extremely anxious or depressed. There were no statistically significant correlations between EQ5D or EQ5D VAS scores and BMI or time since infection. There was a significant difference in EQ5D VAS scores between males (61.8 (SD 18.6)) and females (55.8 (SD 18.1), $t(96.51) = 2.56, p = 0.01$), but not between respondents with a confirmatory or presumptive COVID-19 diagnosis ($t(163.5) = 0.20, p = 0.84$). No significant differences in EQ5D scores were found for sex ($t(100.1) = 1.14, p = 0.26$) or COVID-19 diagnosis ($t(185.2) = -0.03, p = 0.98$).

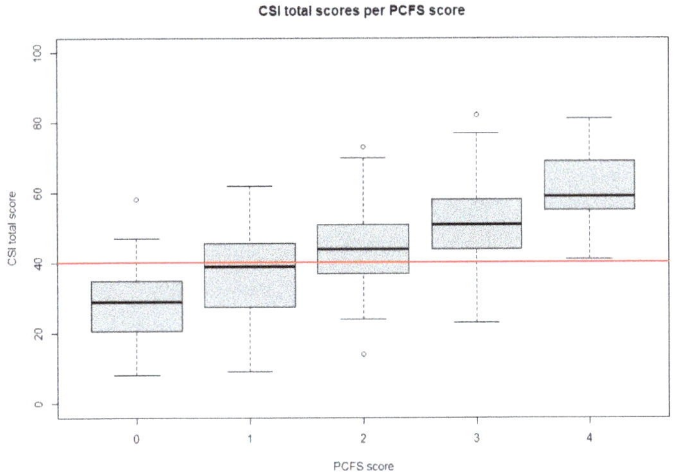

Figure 1. Boxplot of total score on the CSI by PCFS Scale score for all respondents. The red line is presents the cut-off value of the CSI at 40/100 to denote a person as having symptoms of central sensitisation. Abbreviations. CSI: Central Sensitization Inventory, PCFS: Post-COVID-19 Functional Status Scale.

3.3. Association between Symptoms of Central Sensitisation, Functional Status and Health-Related Quality of Life

A significant positive correlation was revealed between PCFS Scale scores and CSI scores (r = 0.52, 95% CI from 0.45 to 0.58, $p < 0.001$). Statistically significant negative correlations were revealed between CSI scores and EQ5D scores (r = −0.58, 95% CI from −0.51 to −0.63, $p < 0.001$), CSI scores and EQ5D VAS scores (r = −0.50, 95% CI from −0.43 to −0.56, $p < 0.001$) and PCFS Scale scores and EQ5D scores (r = −0.61, 95% CI from −0.56 to −0.67, $p < 0.001$) (Figure 2).

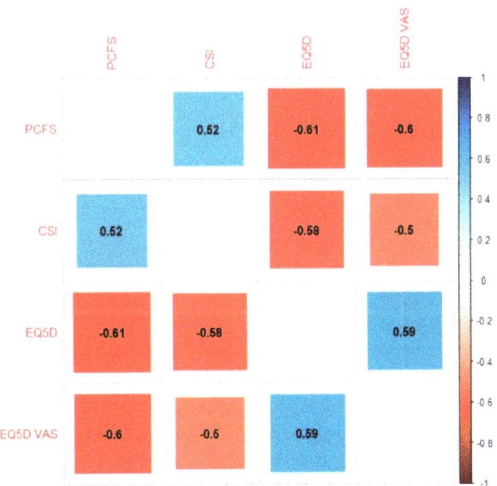

Figure 2. Correlation plot. Correlation coefficients range from −1 (red) to +1 (blue) and presented with the actual value on the plot. Abbreviations. CSI: Central Sensitization Inventory, PCFS: Post-COVID-19 Functional Status Scale, VAS: Visual Analogue Scale.

Based on a One-way ANOVA testing, there was a significant effect of PCFS group level on the total CSI score at the 5% level ($F(4,486) = 46.17$, $p < 0.001$). Post hoc comparison using the Tukey HSD test indicated that mean score for the PCFS group 0 was significantly lower than for PCFS 1 group (mean difference of 8.82 (95% CI from 1.87 to 15.76), $p = 0.005$). Additionally, the mean difference in CSI score between PCFS groups 1 and 2 (mean difference of 7.09 (95% CI from 1.95 to 12.22), $p = 0.002$), groups 2 and 3 (mean difference of 6.33 (95% CI from 3.24 to 9.42), $p < 0.001$), and groups 3 and 4 (mean difference of 10.60 (95% CI from 2.86 to 18.34), $p = 0.002$) were statistically significant. Similarly, there was a significant effect of PCFS group level on the EQ5D score at the 5% ($F(4,499) = 83.41$, $p < 0.001$). Post hoc comparison using the Tukey HSD test indicated a statistically significant difference in EQ5D scores for all level comparisons of the PCFS Scale. All post hoc tests can be found in Figure 3.

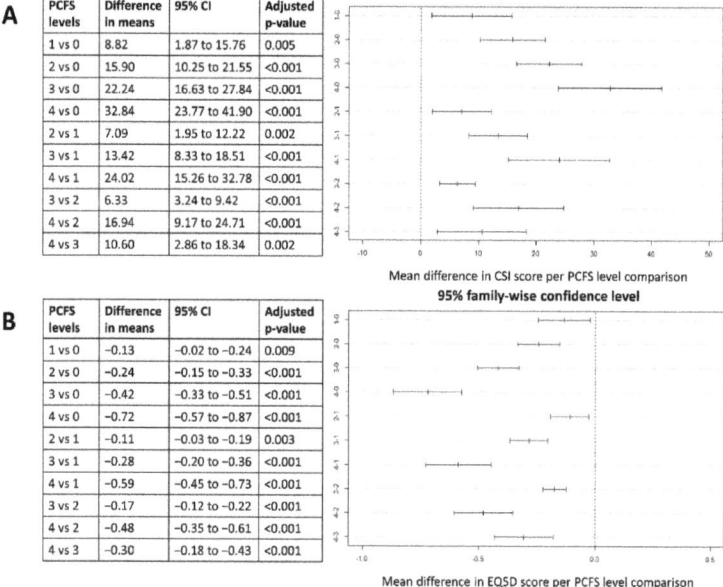

A

PCFS levels	Difference in means	95% CI	Adjusted p-value
1 vs 0	8.82	1.87 to 15.76	0.005
2 vs 0	15.90	10.25 to 21.55	<0.001
3 vs 0	22.24	16.63 to 27.84	<0.001
4 vs 0	32.84	23.77 to 41.90	<0.001
2 vs 1	7.09	1.95 to 12.22	0.002
3 vs 1	13.42	8.33 to 18.51	<0.001
4 vs 1	24.02	15.26 to 32.78	<0.001
3 vs 2	6.33	3.24 to 9.42	<0.001
4 vs 2	16.94	9.17 to 24.71	<0.001
4 vs 3	10.60	2.86 to 18.34	0.002

B

PCFS levels	Difference in means	95% CI	Adjusted p-value
1 vs 0	−0.13	−0.02 to −0.24	0.009
2 vs 0	−0.24	−0.15 to −0.33	<0.001
3 vs 0	−0.42	−0.33 to −0.51	<0.001
4 vs 0	−0.72	−0.57 to −0.87	<0.001
2 vs 1	−0.11	−0.03 to −0.19	0.003
3 vs 1	−0.28	−0.20 to −0.36	<0.001
4 vs 1	−0.59	−0.45 to −0.73	<0.001
3 vs 2	−0.17	−0.12 to −0.22	<0.001
4 vs 2	−0.48	−0.35 to −0.61	<0.001
4 vs 3	−0.30	−0.18 to −0.43	<0.001

Figure 3. Post hoc comparisons between CSI scores (**A**) and EQ5D scores (**B**) for the different PCFS Scale group levels with a visual presentation of the 95% family-wise confidence intervals for all group level comparisons. Abbreviations. CI: confidence interval, CSI: Central Sensitisation Inventory, PCFS: Post-COVID-19 Functional Status Scale, vs: versus.

4. Discussion

In 2017, the International Association for the Study of Pain (IASP) introduced the term nociplastic pain as mechanistic pain descriptor in addition to nociceptive and neuropathic pain [27]. The underlying mechanism of nociplastic pain is central sensitisation, whereby several dysfunctions within the central nervous system, including altered sensory processing in the brain, altered activity in brain-orchestrated nociceptive facilitatory pathways, and poor functioning of endogenous analgesia, can lead to an increased responsiveness to a variety of sensory inputs and/or hypersensitivity to external stimuli such as light, sound or chemical substances [14]. The aim of this study was to evaluate whether there were indications for symptoms of central sensitisation to explain persisting symptoms in patients post COVID-19 infection. Based on the CSI, a screening questionnaire to identify the presence of symptoms of central sensitisation, 70.26% of the respondents reported total CSI scores of ≥40/100, indicating the presence of central sensitisation in this population. Furthermore, when classifying patients according to the level of central sensitisation-related symptom severity, 4.28% were classified as low level, 30.96% as medium level and 64.76% as high level. Therefore, this online survey is suggestive for the presence of symptoms of central sensitisation in post COVID-19 patients. Mean values of 45.9 (SD: 13.1) on the CSI were revealed in this population, which was in line with values obtained in patients with chronic low back pain (total score of 41.6 (SD: 14.8)) [19] and a large group of 368 chronic pain patients (total score of 43.88 (SD: 17.67)) [20]. In healthy persons, mean values of 21.55 (SD: 10.92) [20] and 28.9 (SD: 13.5) [19] were reported in datasets of 49 and 40 persons, respectively. These reference data were observed in studies with other designs; therefore, they only provide a rough indication to better interpret the currently observed findings in post COVID-19 patients. Future studies could further explore the suggestion of central sensitisation as an underlying mechanism of persisting symptoms in post COVID-19 patients by a thorough evaluation of the underlying pain state. Quantitative sensory testing, i.e., a widely used method to measure patients' verbal and behavioural response to quantifiable sensory stimuli, may be used to assess detection and/or pain thresholds, temporal summation (as measure of imbalanced pain facilitation by controlling for increasing evoked pain by fixed repetitive stimuli) and conditioned pain modulation (as measure of imbalanced pain inhibition by controlling for the ability to reduce evoked pain by a second stimulus) [28], while offset analgesia and functional neuroimaging could evaluate cerebral pain processing [29]. In line with previous research in patients with chronic pain, less efficacious conditioned pain modulation, as an indirect measure for the functioning and efficiency of the endogenous descending nociceptive inhibitory systems in humans [30–32] (presumably due to a shift between nociceptive facilitation and nociceptive inhibition), increased nociceptive facilitation [33] and decreased pain thresholds [34,35] are expected if the stated hypothesis based on this online survey is valid.

The exact underlying pathogenetic mechanisms of central sensitisation are not yet fully unravelled; however, it is suggested that infectious agents play a role in, for example myalgic encephalomyelitis/chronic fatigue syndrome (ME/CFS) [36]. It was previously proposed that several viruses (Epstein-Barr virus [37,38], cytomegalovirus [39], human herpesvirus 6-8 [40–42] or bacteria such as mycoplasma [43]) trigger ME/CFS and may reactivate under various conditions, thereby inducing inflammation and immune dysregulation [36]. In comparison to healthy controls, patients who underwent a COVID-19 infection presented with dysregulated immune response (decreased T, B and NK cells and increased inflammatory cytokines) [44], indicating that immune dysfunction plays critical roles in disease progression [45]. Additionally, viral infections also lead to neuroinflammation with the activation of microglia and astrocytes, which leads to the release of proinflammatory cytokines and chemokines [46]. Central cytokines and chemokines play a role in inducing hyperalgesia and allodynia, while a sustained increase leads to chronic widespread pain at several body locations, suggesting that neuroinflammation drives widespread chronic pain through central sensitisation [47]. Therefore, neuroinflammation is expected to play a role in persisting symptoms after COVID-19 infection as well [48,49].

In this survey, it was also revealed that the degree of functional limitations was significantly associated with the degree of symptoms of central sensitisation. The PCFS Scale measured the impact of symptoms on the functional status of patients after COVID-19 infection, whereby previous research already revealed a gradual increase in impairment in work and usual activities and the intensity of symptoms from grade 2 to 4 on the PCFS Scale [50]. The current study demonstrated gradual increases in symptoms of central sensitisation in all grades (except death) of the PCFS Scale, ranging from no symptoms up to severe functional limitations. Thus, it seems that patient-reported consequences of COVID-19 and their effect on functional status are associated with symptoms of central sensitisation. Furthermore, statistically significant negative correlations were found between PCFS Scale score and EQ5D utility and VAS scores, indicating that a higher impact of symptoms on the functional status of patients after a COVID-19 infection was associated with lower health-related index scores and lower health-related quality of life. This correlation has also been reported in patients with lumbar degenerative disorders, whereby the authors evaluated whether the EQ5D score could be derived from other currently used questionnaires with negative (i.e., not accurate) results [51]. Therefore, it might be hypothesised that despite the association between the PCFS Scale and health-related quality of life in patients post COVID-19 infection, both questionnaires are evaluating different aspects and are not interchangeable. The PCFS Scale could be used at the time of hospital discharge, and to monitor functional status after hospital discharge [50], which could potentially help clinicians to determine an appropriate treatment strategy at the early stages after COVID-19 infection [52]. Nevertheless, this only provides an indication about the functional status of these patients, and not the health-related quality of life.

One of the limitations of this online survey is the unequal sex distribution with a higher response rate of females compared to males. Male patients have higher odds of requiring intensive treatment unit admission and higher odds of death compared to females, although there is no difference in the proportion of males and females with confirmed COVID-19 [53]. Nevertheless, it appeared that female post COVID-19 patients were more likely to respond to this online survey than males. Additionally, patients who were associated with a patient support group on social media and who were interested in post COVID sequelae were more likely to receive the link to the survey, which may have caused a selection bias. Moreover, the survey was only spread in the Flemish speaking part of Belgium. Therefore, the results cannot be generalised towards all patients who underwent a COVID-19 infection. Finally, in this survey, only one evaluation took place, namely after infection with COVID-19. Other study designs with a longitudinal aspect (for example a cohort study in 1000 respondents without symptoms) in which evaluations are performed at several time points could have provided information about causality. More information on existing comorbidities, medication use, the presence of structural dysfunctions, psychological factors or severity of COVID-19 infection in addition to pre-infection status should be recorded in future studies to evaluate their potential influence on the relation between symptoms of central sensitisation and COVID-19 infection.

5. Conclusions

This online survey indicated the presence of symptoms of central sensitisation in a sample of post COVID-19 infection patients. Moreover, the more functional limitations due to COVID-19 infection, the higher the degree of symptoms of central sensitisation. The results of this study suggest the need for multimodal rehabilitation and patient education in patients after COVID-19 infection.

Author Contributions: Conceptualization, L.G., A.D.S., M.M.; Formal analysis, L.G. and M.M.; Methodology, L.G., A.D.S., M.M.; Writing-original draft, L.G.; Writing-review and editing, M.N., A.D.S., M.M. All authors have read and agreed to the published version of the manuscript.

Funding: This research received no external funding.

Institutional Review Board Statement: The study was conducted according to the guidelines of the Declaration of Helsinki, and approved by the Institutional Review Board of Universitair Ziekenhuis Brussels (B.U.N. 1432021000484) on 26 May 2021.

Informed Consent Statement: Not applicable.

Data Availability Statement: The data presented in this study are available on motivated request from the corresponding author.

Conflicts of Interest: Maarten Moens has received speaker fees from Medtronic and Nevro. Lisa Goudman is a postdoctoral research fellow funded by the Research Foundation Flanders (FWO), Belgium (project number 12ZF622N). STIMULUS received independent research grants from Medtronic. There are no other conflicts of interest to declare.

References

1. Eliezer, M.; Eloit, C.; Hautefort, C. Olfactory Loss of Function as a Possible Symptom of COVID-19—Reply. *JAMA Otolaryngol. Head Neck Surg.* **2020**, *146*, 874–875. [CrossRef]
2. Joob, B.; Wiwanitkit, V. Arthralgia as an initial presentation of COVID-19: Observation. *Rheumatol. Int.* **2020**, *40*, 823. [CrossRef] [PubMed]
3. Zhao, H.; Shen, D.; Zhou, H.; Liu, J.; Chen, S. Guillain-Barre syndrome associated with SARS-CoV-2 infection: Causality or coincidence? *Lancet Neurol.* **2020**, *19*, 383–384. [CrossRef]
4. Sun, P.; Lu, X.; Xu, C.; Sun, W.; Pan, B. Understanding of COVID-19 based on current evidence. *J. Med. Virol.* **2020**, *92*, 548–551. [CrossRef]
5. Abdullahi, A.; Candan, S.A.; Abba, M.A.; Bello, A.H.; Alshehri, M.A.; Afamefuna Victor, E.; Umar, N.A.; Kundakci, B. Neurological and Musculoskeletal Features of COVID-19: A Systematic Review and Meta-Analysis. *Front. Neurol.* **2020**, *11*, 687. [CrossRef] [PubMed]
6. Pfortmueller, C.A.; Spinetti, T.; Urman, R.D.; Luedi, M.M.; Schefold, J.C. COVID-19-associated acute respiratory distress syndrome (CARDS): Current knowledge on pathophysiology and ICU treatment—A narrative review. *Best Pract. Res. Clin. Anaesthesiol.* **2021**, *35*, 351–368. [CrossRef] [PubMed]
7. Docherty, A.B.; Harrison, E.M.; Green, C.A.; Hardwick, H.E.; Pius, R.; Norman, L.; Holden, K.A.; Read, J.M.; Dondelinger, F.; Carson, G.; et al. Features of 20 133 UK patients in hospital with COVID-19 using the ISARIC WHO Clinical Characterisation Protocol: Prospective observational cohort study. *BMJ* **2020**, *369*, m1985. [CrossRef]
8. Bansal, M. Cardiovascular disease and COVID-19. *Diabetes Metab. Syndr.* **2020**, *14*, 247–250. [CrossRef]
9. Cheung, K.S.; Hung, I.F.N.; Chan, P.P.Y.; Lung, K.C.; Tso, E.; Liu, R.; Ng, Y.Y.; Chu, M.Y.; Chung, T.W.H.; Tam, A.R.; et al. Gastrointestinal Manifestations of SARS-CoV-2 Infection and Virus Load in Fecal Samples from a Hong Kong Cohort: Systematic Review and Meta-analysis. *Gastroenterology* **2020**, *159*, 81–95. [CrossRef]
10. Zhou, Y.; Li, W.; Wang, D.; Mao, L.; Jin, H.; Li, Y.; Hong, C.; Chen, S.; Chang, J.; He, Q.; et al. Clinical time course of COVID-19, its neurological manifestation and some thoughts on its management. *Stroke Vasc. Neurol.* **2020**, *5*, 177–179. [CrossRef]
11. Mao, L.; Jin, H.; Wang, M.; Hu, Y.; Chen, S.; He, Q.; Chang, J.; Hong, C.; Zhou, Y.; Wang, D.; et al. Neurologic Manifestations of Hospitalized Patients with Coronavirus Disease 2019 in Wuhan, China. *JAMA Neurol.* **2020**, *77*, 683–690. [CrossRef]
12. The, L. Understanding long COVID: A modern medical challenge. *Lancet* **2021**, *398*, 725. [CrossRef]
13. Woolf, C.J. Central sensitization: Implications for the diagnosis and treatment of pain. *Pain* **2011**, *152*, S2–S15. [CrossRef]
14. Nijs, J.; Lahousse, A.; Kapreli, E.; Bilika, P.; Saracoglu, I.; Malfliet, A.; Coppieters, I.; De Baets, L.; Leysen, L.; Roose, E.; et al. Nociplastic Pain Criteria or Recognition of Central Sensitization? Pain Phenotyping in the Past, Present and Future. *J. Clin. Med.* **2021**, *10*, 3203. [CrossRef]
15. Neblett, R.; Cohen, H.; Choi, Y.; Hartzell, M.M.; Williams, M.; Mayer, T.G.; Gatchel, R.J. The Central Sensitization Inventory (CSI): Establishing clinically significant values for identifying central sensitivity syndromes in an outpatient chronic pain sample. *J. Pain Off. J. Am. Pain Soc.* **2013**, *14*, 438–445. [CrossRef] [PubMed]
16. Candan, S.A.; Elibol, N.; Abdullahi, A. Consideration of prevention and management of long-term consequences of post-acute respiratory distress syndrome in patients with COVID-19. *Physiother. Theory Pract.* **2020**, *36*, 663–668. [CrossRef] [PubMed]
17. Carfi, A.; Bernabei, R.; Landi, F. Persistent Symptoms in Patients after Acute COVID-19. *JAMA* **2020**, *324*, 603–605. [CrossRef] [PubMed]
18. Aaron, L.A.; Buchwald, D. A review of the evidence for overlap among unexplained clinical conditions. *Ann. Intern. Med.* **2001**, *134*, 868–881. [CrossRef]
19. Mayer, T.G.; Neblett, R.; Cohen, H.; Howard, K.J.; Choi, Y.H.; Williams, M.J.; Perez, Y.; Gatchel, R.J. The development and psychometric validation of the central sensitization inventory. *Pain Pract.* **2012**, *12*, 276–285. [CrossRef]
20. Kregel, J.; Vuijk, P.J.; Descheemaeker, F.; Keizer, D.; van der Noord, R.; Nijs, J.; Cagnie, B.; Meeus, M.; van Wilgen, P. The Dutch Central Sensitization Inventory (CSI): Factor Analysis, Discriminative Power, and Test-Retest Reliability. *Clin. J. Pain* **2016**, *32*, 624–630. [CrossRef]
21. Cuesta-Vargas, A.I.; Neblett, R.; Nijs, J.; Chiarotto, A.; Kregel, J.; van Wilgen, C.P.; Pitance, L.; Knezevic, A.; Gatchel, R.J.; Mayer, T.G.; et al. Establishing Central Sensitization-Related Symptom Severity Subgroups: A Multicountry Study Using the Central Sensitization Inventory. *Pain Med.* **2020**, *21*, 2430–2440. [CrossRef]
22. Corsi, G.; Nava, S.; Barco, S. A novel tool to monitor the individual functional status after COVID-19: The Post-COVID-19 Functional Status (PCFS) scale. *G. Ital. Cardiol.* **2020**, *21*, 757. [CrossRef]
23. Klok, F.A.; Boon, G.; Barco, S.; Endres, M.; Geelhoed, J.J.M.; Knauss, S.; Rezek, S.A.; Spruit, M.A.; Vehreschild, J.; Siegerink, B. The Post-COVID-19 Functional Status scale: A tool to measure functional status over time after COVID-19. *Eur. Respir. J.* **2020**, *56*, 2001494. [CrossRef]
24. Rabin, R.; de Charro, F. EQ-5D: A measure of health status from the EuroQol Group. *Ann. Med.* **2001**, *33*, 337–343. [CrossRef] [PubMed]
25. The EuroQol Group. EuroQol—A new facility for the measurement of health-related quality of life. *Health Policy* **1990**, *16*, 199–208. [CrossRef]
26. EuroQol Group. *Self-Reported Population Health: An International Perspective Based on EQ-5D*; Springer: Dordrecht, The Netherlands, 2014. [CrossRef]

27. Aydede, M.; Shriver, A. Recently introduced definition of "nociplastic pain" by the International Association for the Study of Pain needs better formulation. *Pain* **2018**, *159*, 1176–1177. [CrossRef] [PubMed]
28. Fillingim, R.B.; Loeser, J.D.; Baron, R.; Edwards, R.R. Assessment of Chronic Pain: Domains, Methods, and Mechanisms. *J. Pain Off. J. Am. Pain Soc.* **2016**, *17*, T10–T20. [CrossRef]
29. Kosek, E.; Clauw, D.; Nijs, J.; Baron, R.; Gilron, I.; Harris, R.E.; Mico, J.A.; Rice, A.S.; Sterling, M. Chronic nociplastic pain affecting the musculoskeletal system: Clinical criteria and grading system. *Pain* **2021**, *162*, 2629–2634. [CrossRef] [PubMed]
30. Coppieters, I.; De Pauw, R.; Kregel, J.; Malfliet, A.; Goubert, D.; Lenoir, D.; Cagnie, B.; Meeus, M. Differences between Women with Traumatic and Idiopathic Chronic Neck Pain and Women without Neck Pain: Interrelationships among Disability, Cognitive Deficits, and Central Sensitization. *Phys. Ther.* **2017**, *97*, 338–353. [CrossRef]
31. Staud, R. Abnormal endogenous pain modulation is a shared characteristic of many chronic pain conditions. *Expert Rev. Neurother.* **2012**, *12*, 577–585. [CrossRef]
32. Kennedy, D.L.; Kemp, H.I.; Ridout, D.; Yarnitsky, D.; Rice, A.S. Reliability of conditioned pain modulation: A systematic review. *Pain* **2016**, *157*, 2410–2419. [CrossRef]
33. Soon, B.; Vicenzino, B.; Schmid, A.B.; Coppieters, M.W. Facilitatory and inhibitory pain mechanisms are altered in patients with carpal tunnel syndrome. *PLoS ONE* **2017**, *12*, e0183252. [CrossRef]
34. Imamura, M.; Chen, J.; Matsubayashi, S.R.; Targino, R.A.; Alfieri, F.M.; Bueno, D.K.; Hsing, W.T. Changes in pressure pain threshold in patients with chronic nonspecific low back pain. *Spine* **2013**, *38*, 2098–2107. [CrossRef]
35. Goubert, D.; Danneels, L.; Graven-Nielsen, T.; Descheemaeker, F.; Meeus, M. Differences in Pain Processing between Patients with Chronic Low Back Pain, Recurrent Low Back Pain, and Fibromyalgia. *Pain Physician* **2017**, *20*, 307–318.
36. Rasa, S.; Nora-Krukle, Z.; Henning, N.; Eliassen, E.; Shikova, E.; Harrer, T.; Scheibenbogen, C.; Murovska, M.; Prusty, B.K.; European Network on ME/CFS (EUROMENE). Chronic viral infections in myalgic encephalomyelitis/chronic fatigue syndrome (ME/CFS). *J. Transl. Med.* **2018**, *16*, 268. [CrossRef] [PubMed]
37. Straus, S.E.; Tosato, G.; Armstrong, G.; Lawley, T.; Preble, O.T.; Henle, W.; Davey, R.; Pearson, G.; Epstein, J.; Brus, I.; et al. Persisting illness and fatigue in adults with evidence of Epstein-Barr virus infection. *Ann. Intern. Med.* **1985**, *102*, 7–16. [CrossRef]
38. Holmes, G.P.; Kaplan, J.E.; Stewart, J.A.; Hunt, B.; Pinsky, P.F.; Schonberger, L.B. A cluster of patients with a chronic mononucleosis-like syndrome. Is Epstein-Barr virus the cause? *JAMA* **1987**, *257*, 2297–2302. [CrossRef] [PubMed]
39. Martin, W.J. Detection of RNA sequences in cultures of a stealth virus isolated from the cerebrospinal fluid of a health care worker with chronic fatigue syndrome. Case report. *Pathobiology* **1997**, *65*, 57–60. [CrossRef] [PubMed]
40. Buchwald, D.; Cheney, P.R.; Peterson, D.L.; Henry, B.; Wormsley, S.B.; Geiger, A.; Ablashi, D.V.; Salahuddin, S.Z.; Saxinger, C.; Biddle, R.; et al. A chronic illness characterized by fatigue, neurologic and immunologic disorders, and active human herpesvirus type 6 infection. *Ann. Intern. Med.* **1992**, *116*, 103–113. [CrossRef] [PubMed]
41. Yalcin, S.; Kuratsune, H.; Yamaguchi, K.; Kitani, T.; Yamanishi, K. Prevalence of human herpesvirus 6 variants A and B in patients with chronic fatigue syndrome. *Microbiol. Immunol.* **1994**, *38*, 587–590. [CrossRef] [PubMed]
42. Ablashi, D.V.; Eastman, H.B.; Owen, C.B.; Roman, M.M.; Friedman, J.; Zabriskie, J.B.; Peterson, D.L.; Pearson, G.R.; Whitman, J.E. Frequent HHV-6 reactivation in multiple sclerosis (MS) and chronic fatigue syndrome (CFS) patients. *J. Clin. Virol.* **2000**, *16*, 179–191. [CrossRef]
43. Nasralla, M.; Haier, J.; Nicolson, G.L. Multiple mycoplasmal infections detected in blood of patients with chronic fatigue syndrome and/or fibromyalgia syndrome. *Eur. J. Clin. Microbiol. Infect. Dis.* **1999**, *18*, 859–865. [CrossRef]
44. Song, C.-Y.; Xu, J.; He, J.-Q.; Lu, Y.-Q. Immune dysfunction following COVID-19, especially in severe patients. *Sci. Rep.* **2020**, *10*, 15838. [CrossRef]
45. Rendeiro, A.F.; Casano, J.; Vorkas, C.K.; Singh, H.; Morales, A.; DeSimone, R.A.; Ellsworth, G.B.; Soave, R.; Kapadia, S.N.; Saito, K.; et al. Profiling of immune dysfunction in COVID-19 patients allows early prediction of disease progression. *Life Sci. Alliance* **2021**, *4*, e202000955. [CrossRef]
46. Li, T.; Chen, X.; Zhang, C.; Zhang, Y.; Yao, W. An update on reactive astrocytes in chronic pain. *J. Neuroinflamm.* **2019**, *16*, 140. [CrossRef]
47. Ji, R.R.; Nackley, A.; Huh, Y.; Terrando, N.; Maixner, W. Neuroinflammation and Central Sensitization in Chronic and Widespread Pain. *Anesthesiology* **2018**, *129*, 343–366. [CrossRef] [PubMed]
48. Klein, R.; Soung, A.; Sissoko, C.; Nordvig, A.; Canoll, P.; Mariani, M.; Jiang, X.; Bricker, T.; Goldman, J.; Rosoklija, G.; et al. COVID-19 induces neuroinflammation and loss of hippocampal neurogenesis. *Res. Sq.* **2021**, *3*, 1031824. [CrossRef]
49. Chowdhury, B.; Sharma, A.; Satarker, S.; Mudgal, J.; Nampoothiri, M. Dialogue between Neuroinflammation and Neurodegenerative Diseases in COVID-19. *J. Environ. Pathol. Toxicol. Oncol.* **2021**, *40*, 37–49. [CrossRef]
50. Machado, F.V.C.; Meys, R.; Delbressine, J.M.; Vaes, A.W.; Goertz, Y.M.J.; van Herck, M.; Houben-Wilke, S.; Boon, G.; Barco, S.; Burtin, C.; et al. Construct validity of the Post-COVID-19 Functional Status Scale in adult subjects with COVID-19. *Health Qual. Life Outcomes* **2021**, *19*, 40. [CrossRef] [PubMed]
51. Carreon, L.Y.; Bratcher, K.R.; Das, N.; Nienhuis, J.B.; Glassman, S.D. Estimating EQ-5D values from the Oswestry Disability Index and numeric rating scales for back and leg pain. *Spine* **2014**, *39*, 678–682. [CrossRef]

52. Pant, P.; Joshi, A.; Basnet, B.; Shrestha, B.M.; Bista, N.R.; Bam, N.; Das, S.K. Prevalence of Functional Limitation in COVID-19 Recovered Patients Using the Post COVID-19 Functional Status Scale. *JNMA J. Nepal Med. Assoc.* **2021**, *59*, 7–11. [CrossRef] [PubMed]
53. Peckham, H.; de Gruijter, N.M.; Raine, C.; Radziszewska, A.; Ciurtin, C.; Wedderburn, L.R.; Rosser, E.C.; Webb, K.; Deakin, C.T. Male sex identified by global COVID-19 meta-analysis as a risk factor for death and ITU admission. *Nat. Commun.* **2020**, *11*, 6317. [CrossRef] [PubMed]

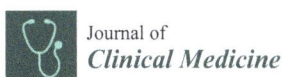

Article

Cross-Cultural Adaptation, Reliability, and Psychophysical Validation of the Pain and Sleep Questionnaire Three-Item Index in Finnish

Jani Mikkonen [1,2,*], Ville Leinonen [3,4], Hannu Luomajoki [5], Diego Kaski [6], Saana Kupari [7], Mika Tarvainen [7,8], Tuomas Selander [9] and Olavi Airaksinen [2,10]

1. Private Practice, Helsinki, Finland
2. Department of Surgery (Incl. Physiatry), Institute of Clinical Medicine, University of Eastern Finland, 70211 Kuopio, Finland; Olavi.Airaksinen@kuh.fi
3. Institute of Clinical Medicine-Neurosurgery, University of Eastern Finland, 70211 Kuopio, Finland; ville.leinonen@kuh.fi
4. Department of Neurosurgery, Kuopio University Hospital, 70211 Kuopio, Finland
5. ZHAW School of Health Professions, Zurich University of Applied Sciences, CH-8401 Winterthur, Switzerland; luom@zhaw.ch
6. Department of Clinical and Movement Neurosciences, University College London, London WC1E 6BT, UK; d.kaski@ucl.ac.uk
7. Department of Applied Physics, University of Eastern Finland, 70211 Kuopio, Finland; saanaku@uef.fi (S.K.); mika.tarvainen@uef.fi (M.T.)
8. Department of Clinical Physiology and Nuclear Medicine, Kuopio University Hospital, 70211 Kuopio, Finland
9. Science Service Center, Kuopio University Hospital, 70211 Kuopio, Finland; tuomas.selander@kuh.fi
10. Department of Physical and Rehabilitation Medicine, Kuopio University Hospital, 70211 Kuopio, Finland
* Correspondence: jani@selkakuntoutus.fi

Citation: Mikkonen, J.; Leinonen, V.; Luomajoki, H.; Kaski, D.; Kupari, S.; Tarvainen, M.; Selander, T.; Airaksinen, O. Cross-Cultural Adaptation, Reliability, and Psychophysical Validation of the Pain and Sleep Questionnaire Three-Item Index in Finnish. *J. Clin. Med.* **2021**, *10*, 4887. https://doi.org/10.3390/jcm10214887

Academic Editor: Jo Nijs

Received: 6 September 2021
Accepted: 20 October 2021
Published: 23 October 2021

Publisher's Note: MDPI stays neutral with regard to jurisdictional claims in published maps and institutional affiliations.

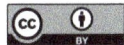

Copyright: © 2021 by the authors. Licensee MDPI, Basel, Switzerland. This article is an open access article distributed under the terms and conditions of the Creative Commons Attribution (CC BY) license (https://creativecommons.org/licenses/by/4.0/).

Abstract: Reciprocal relationships between chronic musculoskeletal pain and various sleep disturbances are well established. The Pain and Sleep Questionnaire three-item index (PSQ-3) is a concise, valid, and reliable patient-reported outcome measure (PROM) that directly evaluates how sleep is affected by chronic low back pain (CLBP). Translation and cross-cultural validation of The Pain and Sleep Questionnaire three-item index Finnish version (PSQ-3-FI) were conducted according to established guidelines. The validation sample was 229 subjects, including 42 pain-free controls and 187 subjects with chronic musculoskeletal pain. Our aims were to evaluate internal consistency, test–retest reliability, measurement error, structural validity, convergent validity, and discriminative validity and, furthermore, to study the relationships between dizziness, postural control on a force plate, and objective sleep quality metrics and total PSQ-3-FI score. The PSQ-3-FI demonstrated good internal consistency, excellent test–retest reliability, and small measurement error. Confirmatory factor analysis confirmed acceptable fit indices to a one-factor model. Convergent validity indicated fair to good correlation with pain history and well-established pain-related PROMs. The PSQ-3-FI total score successfully distinguished between the groups with no pain, single-site pain, and multisite pain. A higher prevalence of dizziness, more impaired postural control, and a general trend towards poorer sleep quality were observed among subjects with higher PSQ-3-FI scores. Postural control instability was more evident in eyes-open tests. The Finnish PSQ-3 translation was successfully cross-culturally adapted and validated. The PSQ-3-FI appears to be a valid and reliable PROM for the Finnish-speaking CLBP population. More widespread implementation of PSQ-3 would lead to better understanding of the direct effects of pain on sleep.

Keywords: pain; chronic low back pain; sleep; questionnaire; cross-cultural validation; patient-reported outcome measure; postural control; dizziness; actigraphy; sleep quality

1. Introduction

Chronic low back pain (CLBP) is the leading disability globally [1]. More than half of patients with CLBP experience various sleep disturbances, such as problems falling asleep and staying asleep, waking up because of pain, difficulties getting back to sleep after awakening, restless sleep, fatigue after sleeping, insomnia, and/or restless legs syndrome [2,3]. Sleep disturbances have a fundamental effect on health and are associated with mental disorders such as anxiety; depression; numerous chronic systemic metabolic, cardiovascular, respiratory, and neurological diseases; and increased risk of certain types of cancer [4–6], as well as negative effects on short-term, day-to-day function, and well-being [7,8]. Reciprocal relationships between sleep disturbances and different chronic musculoskeletal pain conditions have also been well-established [9–11]; thus, there is a need for a concise, reliable, and valid patient-reported outcome measure (PROM) for clinical assessments and research to measure the direct effects of pain on sleep.

The Pain and Sleep Questionnaire three-item index (PSQ-3), a three-question questionnaire, was developed in 2012 [12] to directly assess the impact of pain on sleep during a one-week period. The three items are "1. How often have you had trouble falling asleep because of pain?", "2. How often have you been awakened by pain during the night?", and "3. How often have you been awakened by pain in the morning?". The possible answers range on a scale from 0 indicating "never" to 100 representing "always". Previous validation of the PSQ-3 demonstrated good internal consistency and good structural validity for a one-factor model, but doubtful convergence validity [12,13].

A 2018 systematic review of PROMs for clinical assessment of sleep quality among patients with chronic pain reviewed twelve different questionnaires assessing sleep on six different pain populations [13]. The PSQ-3 has been validated for the CLBP population [12] and the Chronic Pain Sleep Inventory for patients with hip osteoarthritis [14]. Interestingly, these PROMs appear essentially identical, as the Chronic Pain Sleep Inventory includes three questions that are the same as the questions in the PSQ-3. There have been no previous cross-cultural validations of the PSQ-3 or Chronic Pain Sleep Inventory. Overall, only one cross-cultural validation has previously been performed for the twelve PROMs for the effect of pain on sleep [13].

Sleep quality and disturbances have several significant effects on daytime functions, such as increased postural control instability [15–17] and subjective symptoms such as dizziness [18]. Postural control instability can be objectively studied using a force plate, which is a mechanical sensing system designed to measure the ground reaction forces and moments involved in postural control [19]. Diagnosis of dizziness is mostly based on patient-reported symptoms, and there is no single objective clinical test to diagnose or classify dizziness into different subtypes [20,21]. Due to previous studies showing associations between sleep disturbances and postural control instability and dizziness, we hypothesized that there may be potential relationships between higher PSQ-3 scores and postural instability and an increased prevalence of subjective dizziness. Despite the known effects of poor sleep on balance and vestibular function, the relationships between PSQ-3 scores and postural stability and subjective dizziness have never been formally explored.

Objective sleep quality can be directly assessed via actigraphy, which monitors activity and rest cycles based on movement (accelerometer) data [22]. Sleep-wake patterns are evaluated by determining activity counts using scoring algorithms [22,23]. Frequently used measures of the continuity of sleep in various conditions include the total sleep time, sleep efficiency, and amount and duration of awakenings [24]. Previous studies have reported associations between various other pain–sleep questionnaires and actigraphy measurements among subjects with chronic musculoskeletal pain [2,25,26]; however, the relationship between actigraphy measurements and the PSQ-3 has not yet been studied. Hence, actigraphy measurements were also included in this study.

The study aimed to translate and cross-culturally adapt the PSQ-3 into Finnish (PSQ-3-FI) and to evaluate its reliability (internal consistency, test–retest reliability, and measurement error), structural validity for a one-factor model, convergence validity (based on its correlation with pain history, prevalence of dizziness history, The Central Sensitization Inventory (CSI), The Tampa Scale of Kinesiophobia (TSK), The Depression Scale (DEPS), the 5-level EQ-5D version of the EuroQol (EQ-5D-5L), and The Roland–Morris Disability Questionnaire (RMDQ)), and discriminative validity. We also investigated the relationships between the PSQ-3-FI and subjective dizziness, postural control on a force plate and objective sleep quality.

2. Materials and Methods

Ethical approval for this study was obtained from the Research Ethics Committee of the Northern Savo Hospital District (identification number, 1106/13.02.00/2018). Written informed consent was obtained from all subjects before the study began, and the study was conducted in accordance with the Declaration of Helsinki. This validation study adhered, where applicable, to the Consensus-based Standards for the selection of health Measurement Instruments (COSMIN) checklist to ensure the methodological quality of studies on measurement instruments [27,28].

2.1. Study Subjects

The subjects for this study were recruited via advertisements on the website of the private chiropractic practice where this study was performed, as well as the websites and social media accounts of a variety of national Finnish musculoskeletal pain and spine-related organizations and colleagues involved in healthcare. All subjects from the general population who met the study inclusion criteria were invited to participate, regardless of whether they experienced pain or not. The inclusion criteria were: (1) age 18 to 65 years old and (2) proficient in written and spoken Finnish. The exclusion criteria were: (1) a history of cancer or (2) a history of trauma or conditions involving the central nervous system, including dementia, Alzheimer's disease, and multiple sclerosis. A total of 257 subjects provided informed consent to participate in the study and booked a clinical appointment using the online booking system.

2.2. Translation and Cross-Cultural Adaptation of the PSQ-3

Translation and cross-cultural validation of the Finnish CSI were conducted following standard guidelines and included forward–backward translation [29]. Permission to translate the PSQ-3 into Finnish was granted by the first author of the study, who identified the one-factor structure of the PSQ-3 [12]. The PSQ-3 was initially translated from English into Finnish by the first author (JM; completed undergraduate and postgraduate degrees in English-speaking countries) and a professional translator specializing in medical and healthcare texts, both of whom are native Finnish speakers and were blinded to the other's translations. Then, an expert panel composed of the second (VL) and third (HL) authors independently reviewed the initial translations, selected the most appropriate translations, and suggested and discussed changes for one item with the first author. A small number of minor changes in wording were made. Next, the translated version was back-translated by another native English-speaking professional translator who is fluent in Finnish; this translator was naïve to the purpose of this study and the PSQ-3. The backtranslation was assessed and approved by the author of the original English version of the PSQ-3, who is a native English speaker, and some final changes in the wording of the content were made.

Finally, the face validity of the provisional PSQ-3-FI was assessed among twenty subjects with chronic musculoskeletal pain, who were informed of the purpose of this study and were requested to provide non-structured verbal or written feedback on each item on the provisional PSQ-3-FI. All subjects provided positive feedback on their comprehension of each of the items of the PSQ-3-FI and completed the questionnaire without difficulties. The Finnish version of PSQ-3 can be found in Appendix A.

2.3. Data Collection

Data were collected from May 2019 until March 2020 at a single private chiropractic practice. During each individual's clinical visit, objective clinical measurements of postural control were obtained using a force plate. After returning home, subjects were instructed to complete an online web-based form to collect demographic information (age, gender, weight, height, and pain history) and to fill in clinical questionnaires, including the PSQ-3-FI. During the data analysis phase, body mass index was calculated for each subject based on their self-reported height and weight. The total sample size for PSQ-3-FI validation was determined by the ratio of the number of items in each measure, which was 76.7 and hence exceeded recommended range from 2 to 20 items in each measure [30]. To assess test–retest reliability, the subjects were emailed and invited to complete the PSQ-3-FI again 7 ± 1 days after completing the initial questionnaires. The email invitations were stopped after 104 subjects had completed the PSQ-3-FI twice. The ratio of the number of items in each measure to the sample size for evaluating test–retest reliability was 1:34.7. Therefore, the recommended 1:5 ratio was satisfied [31]. All test–retest participants were asked to avoid starting any new types of pain medication and/or physical treatment, when ethically possible, during the 7 ± 1-day gap between administration of the tests. Actigraphy data were collected between December 2019 to March 2020 and August 2020 to November 2020; 24 h actigraphy data were always collected from a Tuesday afternoon until the next Wednesday. The break in actigraphy data collection was due to the COVID-19 outbreak in Finland.

2.3.1. Subject-Reported Pain History Questions

Each subject completed a structured web-based pain history, which asked dichotomous (yes/no) questions related to the presence of chronic low back pain, referred pain to leg or leg pain (if "yes" to chronic low back), presence of other chronic musculoskeletal pain, chronic headaches, and history of a rheumatic disease previously diagnosed by a physician. Subjects who reported pain were also asked to rate the severity of their pain on a numerical pain scale ranging from 0–10 and to indicate the duration of pain in months.

2.3.2. Patient-Reported Clinical Outcome Measures

The three-item PSQ-3 sleep questionnaire was designed to measure the impact of chronic pain on sleep over the previous seven days [12]. The three questions are "1. How often have you had trouble falling asleep because of pain?", "2. How often have you been awakened by pain during the night?", and "3. How often have you been awakened by pain in the morning?". We translated these items into Finnish for this study. The original PSQ-3 employed a visual analog scale that ranges from 0 to 100 mm. However, due to the difficulty of representing a visual analog scale in a universal digital format, we adopted a numerical eleven-point rating scale (NRPS) from 0 to 10 for the Finnish version. In both the original and Finnish versions, 0 indicates "never" and 100 mm or 10 on the numerical scale represents "always." Thus, the final score for the PSQ-3-FI ranges from 0 to 30 rather than 0 to 300.

The eleven-point numerical pain scale (NPRS) assesses pain on a scale ranging from 0 (no pain at all) to 10 (worst pain imaginable) [32]. Chronic pain was defined as more than three days of pain every week for more than three months.

The Central Sensitization Inventory (CSI) questionnaire contains two parts [33]. Part A is composed of 25 questions in which the frequency of CS-related symptomology is rated on a Likert-like scale from 0 (never) to 4 (always). The total score ranges from 0 to 100; higher scores indicate a higher frequency and number of CS-related symptoms. [34]. Part B includes "No/Yes" and "year diagnosed" questions about previous diagnoses of ten central sensitization syndromes or related diagnoses; Part B is not scored [35]. The CSI was previously translated into Finnish and validated in the Finnish population [36].

The 17-item Tampa Scale of Kinesiophobia (TSK) is used to assess subjective kinesiophobia (fear of movement). Each item is rated as: 1 = strongly disagree, 2 = disagree,

3 = agree, or 4 = strongly agree. The possible scores range from 17 to 68; higher scores indicate more severe kinesiophobia [37]. The TSK was previously translated into Finnish and validated in the Finnish population [38].

The 10-item Depression Scale (DEPS) was designed to assess depressive symptoms. Each item response is rated on a four-point Likert scale as: 0 = not at all, 1 = a little, 2 = quite a lot, or 3 = extremely. Higher scores (range, 0 and 30) indicate a higher possibility of a diagnosis of a major depressive disorder [39]. The DEPS has been validated for patients with CLBP [40].

Health-related quality of life was assessed using the Finnish translation of the 5-level EQ-5D version of the EuroQol (EQ-5D-5L) questionnaire [41], which provides a simple descriptive profile of a respondent's health status over five dimensions: mobility, self-care, usual activities, pain/discomfort, and anxiety/depression. Each dimension is rated as: 0 = no problems, 1 = slight problems, 2 = moderate problems, 3 = severe problems, or 4 = unable to/extreme problems. The EQ-5D-5L also includes the EQ visual analog scale (EQ VAS), which assesses the respondent's current overall health status using a visual, vertical analog scale that ranges from 0 (dead) to 1 (full health) [41]. The index value between 0 and 1 is calculated. A standard value set has not yet been defined for the Finnish population; therefore, as recommended by the EuroQol EQ-5D-5L User Guide, the index values for this study were calculated using a Danish value set [42].

The 24-item Roland–Morris Disability Questionnaire (RMDQ) is an extensively validated questionnaire of disability among patients with chronic low back pain [43]. The RMDQ score is obtained by summing up the number of low-back-pain-related daily activity disabilities to which the respondents check "yes". A higher total score (range, 0 to 24) suggests a higher extent of low back pain related-disability [44].

2.3.3. Subjective Dizziness Structured Interview

In agreement with the literature, where dizziness is based on symptoms rather than a clinical diagnosis of a specific vestibular or neuromusculoskeletal condition [45], structured interviews were conducted during the clinical visit to assess the subject's history of dizziness in the previous year. The questions were "Do you suffer dizziness at the moment? Have you suffered dizziness during the last 12 months? Dizziness means an abnormal sensation causing disability for more than one day, which is not the same as normal brief light-headedness when standing up quickly". We asked further questions to all subjects who had experienced dizziness resulting in disability that had persisted for more than 24 h (n = 52; 23%) to classify the symptoms of dizziness into seven categories: 1. off balance or unsteadiness, 2. Light-headedness, 3. feeling as if passing out, 4. spinning or vertigo, 5. floating or tilting sensation, 6. blurring of vision when moving the head, or 7. other types. This classification was based on recent dizziness subtype research [45].

2.3.4. Clinical Tests of Postural Control Using a Force Plate

The cohort of subjects who reported pain was divided into two groups according to their PSQ-3-FI score. As there are no established PSQ-3 cut-off scores for different severity classes of the effect of pain on sleep, we classified the subjects on two groups based on a PSQ-3-FI score of 4 or less (cumulative 48%; n = 110) or a score of 5 or more (cumulative 52%; n = 119).

Postural stability was measured with a four-channel portable computerized force plate (BT4; HUR Labs Oy, Tampere, Finland). As the subjects completed the questionnaires after their clinical visit, the assessor was blinded to the participants' pain history and questionnaire scores. Postural control measurements included length, area, and velocity of center of pressure (COP) displacement, which are the most commonly used parameters for postural control in previous quality of sleep and postural control-related studies [15,16]. Various postural control parameters describe the neuromuscular response to shifts in the body's center of mass measured on the force plate [19].

The postural control tests were carried out in the same room under identical conditions for all subjects, including the distance to the opposite wall and lighting. The force plate was calibrated before each individual's measurement. All subjects were instructed to stand barefoot, with their feet as close together as comfortably possible. If the subjects found this stance unnatural, they were instructed to place their feet farther apart to create a more stable and natural-feeling standing stance. Small variations in foot stance should not affect the results of bipedal balance tests [46]. The subjects were instructed to look straight ahead and try to maintain a steady posture in a relaxed manner, with their arms at their sides in a relaxed position. There was no clear fixation point for gaze, and the opposite wall was more than three meters away.

Four postural control tests were carried out in the same non-randomized order: eyes open on a stable surface (EOS), eyes closed on a stable surface (ECS), eyes open on an unstable foam surface (EOU), and eyes closed on an unstable foam surface (ECU). The protocol for the bipedal standing tests was similar to the Modified Clinical Test of Sensory Interaction in balance (CTSIB-M) protocol, except each test lasted 60 s and was conducted once. Sixty seconds is the most commonly used measurement time for the bipedal standing test for the CLBP population [47]. The CTSIB-M has been shown to be a reliable, valid test in adults with vestibular disorders [48]. No similar protocol has been recommended or validated for the CLBP population [49]. A five-second pre-phase period was employed before the actual COP measurement of 60 s. Additionally, there was a short designated resting period between each test, when the instructions for the next test were repeated, and the subjects had to step off the postural plate between the second and third tests to allow the balance pad to be placed on the plate. The sampling frequency was set to 50 Hz, as recommended by the manufacturer, to obtain a balance between consistent data acquisition and manageable data size. A rectangular, high-density (50 kg/m^3) closed-cell Airex Balance Pad (delivered by the manufacturer with the force plate) was used in all tests requiring a foam surface to provide an unstable surface.

2.3.5. Sleep Quality Recordings

Sleep activity was measured with a ActiGraph GT9X link research-grade activity bracelet (ActiGraph LLC., Pensacola, FL, USA) over 24 h and the data were analyzed with Actilife 6.0 analysis software (ActiGraph LLC., USA). The following five parameters were selected to represent sleep quality: 1. total sleep time, 2. sleep efficiency, i.e., the ratio between the total sleep time and time spent in bed, 3. the number of awakenings lasting more than one minute, 4. average awakening length, and 5. the number of awakenings greater than or equal to five minutes.

PSQ-3 validation data were collected simultaneously with data for validation of the Finnish version of the CSI. The subjects with the lowest and highest CSI and PSQ-3-FI scores were also invited to participate in this study. The recruitment process was stopped when the required 40 subjects were recruited and both groups included an almost equal number of subjects. The recruited subjects were divided into two groups based on their PSQ-3 scores: (1) a group with PSQ-3 scores ≤ 4 ($n = 19$) and (2) a group with scores ≥ 5 ($n = 21$). Similar numbers of subjects were assessed in previous studies of comparable subject cohorts to compare activity measures between two groups [50,51].

2.4. Statistical Methods

Statistical analysis was performed using SPSS version 25 (IBM SPSS Statistics for Windows, Version 25.0. IBM Corp., Armonk, NY, USA), R statistical software version 4.0.4 was used for factor analysis, and sleep quality analysis was conducted using MATLAB (R2019b, MathWorks, Natick, MA, USA). Statistical significance was defined as $p < 0.05$. Data are reported as percentages or means with standard deviations (mean ± SD). Cronbach's alpha was used to assess internal consistency; an alpha value between 0.70 and 0.90 was considered good, and higher than 0.90 was considered excellent. Test–retest reliability was calculated by determining the intraclass correlation coefficient (ICC) for the second

PSQ-3-FI administration 7 ± 1 days later. ICC values ≤ 0.40 are considered to indicate fair reliability; 0.41–0.60, moderate reliability; 0.61–0.80, substantial reliability; and ≥0.81, excellent reliability. ICCs are reported with 95% confidence intervals (CI). Standard error of measurement (SEM) was calculated using the formula standard deviation × square root (1-ICC), where SD = the standard deviation for the change in PSQ-3 score from baseline to second administration. The smallest detectable change (SDC) was calculated using the formula SEM × 2. Confirmatory factor analysis (CFA) with ordinal variables in a one-factor model was used to investigate the validity of five variables with appropriate goodness-of-fit indices. Spearman's correlation coefficients were used to investigate the convergent validity of the PSQ-3-FI by calculating the associations between total PSQ-3-FI scores and the scores on the CSI, TSK, DEPS, EQ-5D-5L, RMDQ, and pain history questions. The strengths of the correlations were interpreted as little or no correlation (Rs < 0.25), fair (0.25 > Rs ≤ 0.50), moderate to good (0.50 > Rs ≤ 0.75), or good to excellent (Rs > 0.75). The normality of the data was assessed using the Shapiro–Wilks and Kolmogorov–Smirnov tests. Group comparisons for normally distributed variables were performed using two-sample t-tests or repeated-measures ANOVA followed by the post hoc least significant difference (LSD) test. Categorical variables were compared using Fisher's exact tests. The minimum required sample size for postural control comparison between groups was calculated with average means and estimated standard deviation from the review comparing pain-free controls and subjects with low back pain [47]. The two-tailed hypothesis was calculated on two independent study groups with 0.05 probability of type I error, 0.80 effect size, and 0.8 statistical power. The calculation revealed that at least 25 subjects had to be included in each group.

3. Results

3.1. Total Sample

There were no missing items in the data, as the electronic questionnaires automatically reminded the respondents if any items were missing.

Three subjects were excluded because they did not complete the study questionnaires as instructed during the clinical appointments. Five additional subjects were excluded as they had clear signs and symptoms of undiagnosed neurological pathological conditions affecting the central nervous system. Thus, the total number of participants included in this study was 249 (67 males and 162 females). Twenty of these participants only provided feedback on the face validity of the Finnish translation of the PSQ-3, and 229 subjects completed the psychometric validation portion of the study. The age range of the subjects was 20 to 65 years old (mean ± SD; 44.5 ± 11.7), and body mass index ranged from 25.6 to 45.2 (mean ± SD; 25.6 ± 4.8). The total cohort was divided into different subsamples for various analyses to test discriminative ability, postural control on the force plate, and sleep quality via actigraphy. The flow chart of subject recruitment and assessment is shown in Figure 1.

3.2. Reliability

Internal consistency (Cronbach's alpha) was good (0.83 and ICC 0.61; 95% CI 0.55–0.68) and the ICC indicated test–retest reliability was excellent (0.91 and ICC 0.62; 95% CI 0.54–0.70). The inter-item correlation was 0.56 between items one and two, 0.73 between items two and three, and 0.53 between items one and three. The SEM for the change in PSQ-3 score between baseline and the second administration was calculated to be 1.28 and the SDC was 2.56. Details of the PSQ-3 scores and reliability data are presented in Table 1.

3.3. Structure Validation

The Kaiser–Meyer–Olkin measure (0.68) and Bartlett's test of sphericity ($p < 0.001$) indicated that factor analysis was appropriate for this study sample. CFA analysis was carried out with ordinal variables to evaluate the fit of the indices to a one-factor model. As the PSQ-3 is a three-item PROM, the minimum number of items required for a one-factor model, no other factor model was considered. Additionally, the ratio of items per subject (1:76) exceeded the minimum ratio required (1:10) [52,53]. The recommended values for the fit indices and the CFA values for the one-factor model are presented in Table 2.

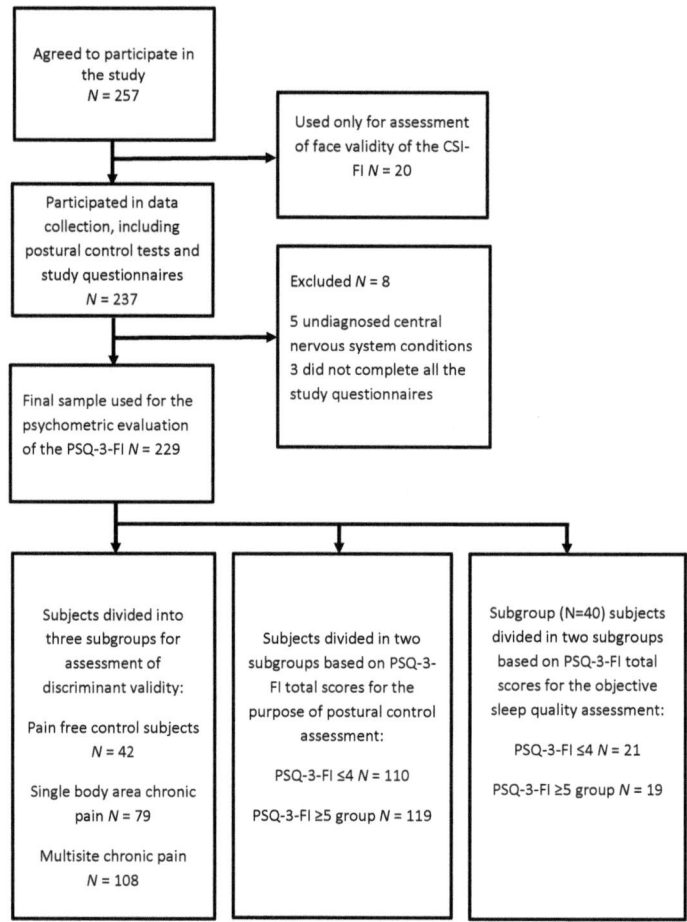

Figure 1. Flow chart of subjects.

Table 1. Mean Pain and Sleep Questionnaire three-item index (PSQ-3-FI) scores.

Question	Item	Mean (95% CI)	Range	ICC
1	How often have you had trouble falling asleep because of pain?	2.5 (2.1–2.8)	0–9	0.55
2	How often have you been awakened by pain during the night?	2.4 (2.0–2.8)	0–10	0.52
3	How often have you been awakened by pain in the morning?	2.0 (1.7–2.4)	0–10	0.74
Total		6.9 (6.0–7.8)	0–32	0.61

Confidence interval (CI); Intraclass correlation (ICC).

Table 2. Confirmatory factor analysis fit indices for the one-factor model.

Fit Index	Recommended Value	Value	Not Acceptable/Acceptable
Chi-Square	>0.05	p-value, 0.041	Not acceptable
CFI	>0.95	0.985	Acceptable
TLI	>0.95	0.978	Acceptable
RMSEA	<0.05	ICC 0.098; 95% CI 0.017–0.188; p-value 0.127	Acceptable
SRMR	<0.08	0.07	Acceptable

Comparative fit index (CFI); Tucker–Lewis index (TLI); Root mean square error of approximation (RMSEA); Standardized Root Mean Square Residual (SRMR).

3.4. Convergent Validity of the PSQ-3-FI

As shown in Table 3, fair to good correlations were observed between the PSQ-3-FI and the Tampa Scale of Kinesiophobia, the Depression scale, and the 5-level EQ-5D. Moderate to good correlations were obtained between the PSQ-3-FI and the Roland–Morris disability questionnaire and Central Sensitization Inventory.

Table 3. Correlations between total PSQ-3-FI scores and subject-reported outcome measures, history, and postural control test parameters (n = 229).

Clinical Variables	Correlation (ρ) with PSQ-3 Total Score
Subject-reported outcome measures	
Tampa scale of kinesiophobia (TSK)	0.41 *
Depression scale (DEPS)	0.305 *
The Roland–Morris disability questionnaire (RMDQ)	0.54 **
The Central Sensitization Inventory (CSI)	0.51 **
EuroQol The 5-level EQ-5D version (EQ-5D-5L)	−0.44 *
History	
Chronic low back pain	0.39 *
Pain referral to leg	0.32 *
Other chronic musculoskeletal pain	0.31 *
Numerical pain scale	0.50 *
Pain duration in months	0.33 *
Chronic headache	0.18
Dizziness in past 12 months	0.16
Postural control EOS	
Length of sway	0.13
Area of sway	0.13
Velocity of sway	0.13
Postural control ECS	
Length of sway	0.08
Area of sway	0.20
Velocity of sway	0.08

Table 3. Cont.

Clinical Variables	Correlation (ρ) with PSQ-3 Total Score
Postural control EOU	
Length of sway	0.12
Area of sway	0.19
Velocity of sway	0.12
Postural control ECU	
Length of sway	0.02
Area of sway	0.14
Velocity of sway	0.02

The Spearman's rank correlation coefficient (ρ). Little or no correlation (ρ < 0.25), fair correlation (0.25 > ρ ≤ 0.50) *, moderate to good correlation (0.50 > ρ ≤ 0.75) **. Eyes open on a stable surface (EOS); eyes closed on a stable surface (ECS); eyes open on an unstable foam surface (EOU); eyes closed on an unstable foam surface (ECU).

3.5. Discriminative Validity of the PSQ-3-FI

Of the total of 229 subjects, 42 (18.7%) reported no pain and were categorized as a control group. Specifically, the pain-free control subjects reported no CLBP, no radicular pain, a score of 0/10 on the pain scale, 0 months of pain history, no other chronic musculoskeletal pain, and no chronic headaches. The remainder of the subjects (187; 81.3%) reported chronic pain, of whom 161 (86%) reported CLBP. No subjects reported acute or subacute pain. Of the 187 subjects with chronic pain, 79 (34%) reported pain in a single body area only (CLBP group without leg referral or other chronic musculoskeletal pain or chronic headaches), and 108 (47%) reported multisite chronic pain (two or more of the following: CLBP with or without radiculopathy, other chronic musculoskeletal pain, and/or chronic headaches).

The comparisons of the demographics and clinical features of the groups presented in Table 4 revealed statistically significant differences in the PSQ-3-FI score between the pain-free control group, single chronic pain group, and multisite chronic pain group.

Table 4. Demographics and discriminative validity of the PSQ-3 among the three subgroups (n = 229).

	Pain-Free Control Group (n = 42)	Chronic Pain in a Single Body Area (n = 79)	Multisite Pain (Two or More Chronic Pain Locations) (n = 108)	p-Value One-Way ANOVA	Comparison between Three Groups; Post Hoc LSD
Age (years)	40.2 ± 10.6	44.5 ± 11.6	46.1 ± 12.0	0.02 *	b (0.005 *)
Male/female (n/n)	13/29	31/48	23/85	0.03 *	c (0.008 *)
Height (cm)	171.3 ± 8.2	172.6 ± 9.9	170.1 ± 9.2	0.18	
Weight (kg)	76.6 ± 15.9	76.1 ± 19.3	74.4 ± 15.4	0.71	
BMI	26.0 ± 4.8	25.2 ± 4.8	25.8 ± 4.9	0.66	
PSQ-3-FI	2.0 ± 3.6	6.2 ± 6.6	9.3 ± 7.4	<0.001 *	a (0.01 *) b (<0.001 *) c (0.01 *)

One-Way ANOVA post hoc comparison based on Fisher's Least Significant Difference (LSD). Statistical significance, $p < 0.05$ *. Comparison between control group without pain and single body area pain (a), between the control group without pain and multisite pain (b), and between single body area pain and multisite pain (c). Body mass index (BMI).

3.6. PSQ-3-FI Score Subgroups

The total cohort was divided into two subgroups according to PSQ-3-FI score, namely ≤4 (48%; n = 110) or ≥5 (52%; n = 119). The only significant demographic difference between these groups was age, with the ≥5 subgroup being older (mean ± SD; 42.6 ± 10.9 vs. mean ± SD; 46.2 ± 12.2; $p = 0.03$). None of the subjects reported dizziness at the same time the postural control tests were carried out.

In the PSQ-3-FI score ≤ 4 group, 18 subjects reported dizziness and 92 reported no dizziness (dizziness:no dizziness ratio: 1:5.1) over the previous 12 months. In the PSQ-3-FI score ≥ 5 group, 34 subjects reported dizziness and 84 reported no dizziness (ratio: 1:2.4) over the previous 12 months. Group comparisons showed the prevalence of dizziness was significantly higher ($p = 0.03$) in the higher PSQ-3-FI score group. The subtypes of dizziness were classified into seven classifications (Table 5).

Table 5. Comparison of the PSQ-3-FI score ≤ 4 and ≥ 5 groups ($n = 229$).

	PSQ-3-FI ≤ 4 ($n = 110$)	PSQ-3-FI ≥ 5 ($n = 119$)	p-Value
Age (years)	42.6 ± 11.0	46.2 ± 12.2	0.02 *
Height (cm)	171.1 ± 8.8	171.3 ± 9.8	0.85
Weight (kg)	74.3 ± 15.3	76.4 ± 18.3	0.34
BMI	25.3 ± 4.7	25.9 ± 5.0	0.33
PSQ-3-FI	1.22 ± 1.4	12.1 ± 6.1	0.001 *
Male/female (n/n)	35/75	32/87	0.47
Dizziness in past 12 months, no/yes	92/18	85/34	0.03 *
Dizziness subtypes, n (%)			
1. Off balance or unsteadiness	4 (22%)	2 (6%)	
2. Light-headedness	7 (40%)	5 (15%)	
3. Feeling as if passing out	0	8 (24%)	
4. Spinning or vertigo	2 (10%)	4 (12%)	
5. Floating or tilting sensation	5 (28%)	12 (34%)	
6. Blurring of vision when moving the head	0	3 (9%)	
7. Other	0	0	

One-Way ANOVA and Fisher's exact tests; statistical significance, $p < 0.05$ *. Body mass index (BMI).

The results of postural control tests on the force plate for the PSQ-3-FI score ≤ 4 or ≥ 5 groups are compared in Table 6. The higher-score PSQ-3-FI group consistently exhibited (in 12 out of 12 tests) greater postural control impairment, with significant differences observed between the two PSQ-3 groups in the majority (7/12; 58%) of tests. Significant differences were observed between groups for all tests performed with eyes open (6/6; 100%). The only significant difference between groups in eyes-closed tests was observed on the stable surface (Figure 2).

Table 6. Postural control on the force plate for the PSQ-3-FI score ≤ 4 and ≥ 5 groups ($n = 229$).

Test	PSQ-3 Group	Mean ± SD	p-Value
Length of sway (mm)			
EOS	≤ 4	547 ± 150	0.048 *
	≥ 5	592 ± 186	
ECS	≤ 4	891 ± 452	0.34
	≥ 5	940 ± 349	
EOU	≤ 4	826 ± 220	0.04 *
	≥ 5	860 ± 240	
ECU	≤ 4	1794 ± 645	0.80
	≥ 5	1805 ± 638	

Table 6. Cont.

Test	PSQ-3 Group	Mean ± SD	p-Value
Area of sway (mm^2)			
EOS	≤4	258 ± 138	0.04 *
	≥5	303 ± 178	
ECS	≤4	364 ± 253	0.002 *
	≥5	503 ± 383	
EOU	≤4	438 ± 218	0.012 *
	≥5	518 ± 260	
ECU	≤4	1029 ± 540	0.08
	≥5	1170 ± 659	
Velocity of sway (mm/s)			
EOS	≤4	9.1 ± 2.5	0.048 *
	≥5	9.9 ± 3.1	
ECS	≤4	14.9 ± 7.5	0.35
	≥5	15.7 ± 5.8	
EOU	≤4	13.8 ± 3.7	0.036 *
	≥5	14.9 ± 4.2	
ECU	≤4	29.9 ± 10.7	0.802
	≥5	30.3 ± 10.6	

Eyes open on a stable surface (EOS); eyes closed on a stable surface (ECS); eyes open on an unstable foam surface (EOU); eyes closed on an unstable foam surface (ECU). Repeated measures ANOVA and post hoc Least Significant Difference (LSD); statistical significance, $p < 0.05$ *.

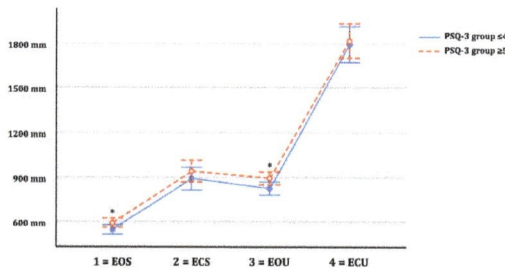

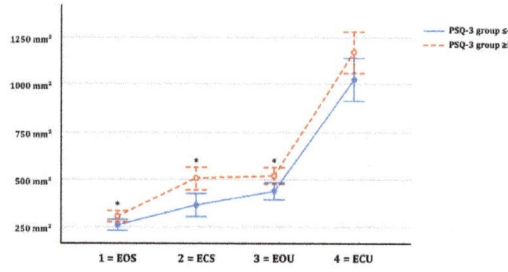

Figure 2. Cont.

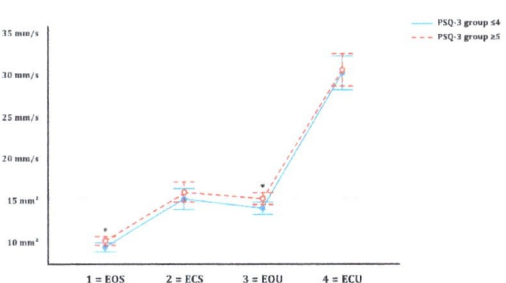

Figure 2. Postural control on PSQ-3-FI groups score ≤4 or ≥5 groups (n = 229).

3.7. Objective Sleep Quality

The parameters representing sleep quality are presented in Table 7 for the lower and higher PSQ-3-FI score groups. The average awakening length was longer in the group with higher PSQ-3-FI score (PSQ-3-FI ≥ 5) compared to the group with lower PSQ-3-FI score. The other four sleep quality parameters, total sleep time, sleep efficiency, and number of awakenings lasting more than one of five minutes, were not significantly different between the groups with higher and lower PSQ-3 scores.

Table 7. Sleep quality measures based on actigraphy for the PSQ-3-FI score ≤ 4 and ≥ 5 groups (n = 40).

	PSQ-3-FI ≤ 4 (n = 21)	PSQ-3-FI ≥ 5 (n = 19)	p-Value
Age (years)	41.6 ± 12.2	51.9 ± 10.8	0.008 *
Height (cm)	170.5 ± 8.23	169.7 ± 7.6	0.77
Weight (kg)	74.6 ± 14.1	74.2 ± 12.5	0.93
BMI	25.6 ± 3.8	25.8 ± 4.2	0.87
PSQ-3-FI	1.6 ± 1.9	12.6 ± 7.1	0.001 *
Male/female (n/n)	6/15	0/19	0.02 *
Total sleep time (min)	401.8 ± 58.7	393.4 ± 77.7	0.70
Sleep efficiency (%)	86.1 ± 4.1	83.5 ± 7.4	0.18
Number of Awakenings > 1 min	22.8 ± 8.0	22.6 ± 10.6	0.94
Average awakening length (min)	2.6 ± 0.7	3.3 ± 1.2	0.03 *
Number of awakenings > 5 min	4.3 ± 3.0	5.8 ± 3.6	0.16

Statistical significance, $p < 0.05$ *.

4. Discussion

The reciprocal relationship between pain affecting sleep—and disturbances to sleep affecting pain—is well-established [2–5,9–11]. However, the PSQ-3 is the only PROM for directly assessing pain–sleep interactions in the CLBP population [13]. It appears that the study of the direct sleep–pain interaction is neglected in almost all clinical musculoskeletal chronic pain studies, and the short, reliable, valid PSQ-3 has not been widely used in clinical assessment or research. This might be because there are quite a large number of similar, but improperly validated pain–sleep PROMs [13]. Additionally, clinical studies on CLBP over the last decades have paid little attention to the assessment and outcome measurements for sleep [54,55].

The results of this validation reveal the acceptable measurement properties of the PSQ-3 for the CLBP population; therefore, we propose a more widespread implementation of the PSQ-3 for clinical assessments, and research will enable the measurement of the direct effect of pain on sleep. Moreover, a meta-analysis published in 2018 lends further clinical validity to the items of the PSQ-3, as gold-standard objective polysomnographic measures of sleep among a population with chronic musculoskeletal pain syndromes concluded these individuals "experience significant sleep disturbances, particularly concerning sleep initiation and maintenance" [3], which are the exact features measured by the PSQ-3 [12].

4.1. Reliability

Internal consistency (Cronbach's alpha) indicates how well PROM items correlate with and predict each other. The total inter-item correlation and prediction for the PSQ-3-FI were rated as good (0.83) and single inter-item correlations were moderate to good. The highest correlation was observed between items "2. How often have you been awakened by pain during the night?" and "3. How often have you been awakened by pain in the morning?". Moreover, test–retest reliability was excellent (0.91). Interestingly, the PSQ-3 questions consider symptoms over the previous week, which is identical to the test–retest evaluation timeframe (7 ± 1 days). Hence, we conclude that symptom recall over one week appears to be a reliable timeframe for the majority of the subjects in this study. The inter-item correlation between items one and two was 0.56, 0.73 between items two and three, and 0.53 between items one and three; these values compare well with the English version, for which the inter-item correlations were 0.65, 0.73, and 0.58, respectively [12]. The SEM value indicates the likelihood of a "true" score that represents a reliable score without any fluctuations due to systematic and random factors related to the measurement process. The general rule is that lower SEM values indicate higher reliability and more confidence that the score has been measured accurately. The SDC is defined as the change in the instrument's score beyond measurement error [56]. The SEM value of 1.28 and SDC value of 2.56 indicate that the results were measured fairly accurately, without fluctuations due to systemic or random factors related to the measurement process. Based on the SDC, we can be confident that the observed change is real, as a minimum change of 2.56 on a scale from 0 to 10 needs to be observed. Internal consistency was 0.87 in the previous PSQ-3 validation [12], in line with our value of 0.83. Test–retest reliability, SEM, and SDC were not calculated in the previous validation [12]; hence, comparison of these values is not possible.

4.2. Structure Validation

Model fit indices with CFA can be used for test to accept or refute the proposed factor model [57]. Chi-Square, CFI, TLI, RMSEA, and SRMR are the most commonly reported fit indices of CFA [58]. In our results, model fit indices showed acceptable fit indices for a one-factor model, except for the Chi-Square test. However, it is well known that the larger the sample size, the greater the chances of obtaining a statistically significant Chi-square result [59]. Hence, rejection of the Chi-Square is probably due to the Chi-Square test being insensitive to larger sample sizes as in this study. Overall, fit indices indicated an acceptable fit for the one-factor model. CFI and TLI indicated a perfect fit compared to the PSQ-3 English version, though the Chi-Square and RMSEA tests showed non-acceptable fits. Overall, one-factor model also represented the best fit for the original version, where the PSQ-3 was shortened to only include three items [12].

4.3. Convergent Validity

The relationship of PSQ-3-FI total score with PROMs showed a fair correlation of TSK, EQ-5D-5L, and DEPS and moderate to good correlation with RMDQ and CSI. The DEPS and CSI include questions that directly assess the quality of sleep [32,38]. In the previous validation of the PSQ-3, the Pain and Disability Index, Pain Intensity Questionnaire, and SF-36 Short Form Health Survey pain-related questionnaires exhibited very similar correlations with the total PSQ-3 score [12]. The total PSQ-3-FI scores showed a fair correlation with pain duration in months and dichotomous yes/no answers on chronic low back pain, pain referring to leg, other chronic musculoskeletal pain, and pain duration in months. Chronic headache and dizziness in the past 12 months showed little or no correlation with PSQ-3-FI total score. The numerical pain scale was the only dichotomous variable that showed moderate to good correlation with the total PSQ-3 score. The tight correlation between sleep quality and next-day pain intensity is well established, with previous studies showing a clear relationship between poorer sleep and short-term increases in pain intensity in patients with chronic pain [60,61]. The correlations with pain and disability PROMs were generally at the same level in this study and the English version; however, quality of life was better in this study. It must be noted that such comparisons are not reliable due to the variability across the measurement properties of different PROMs.

4.4. Discriminative Validity

There are no previous studies of the discriminative validity of any PROMs that assess the effect of pain on sleep [13]. However, the total PSQ-3-FI score could distinguish pain-free controls, subjects with chronic pain in a single body area, and subjects with multisite chronic pain. The factors leading to chronic pain are complex, with multiple contributors leading to persistent symptoms [1]. Sleep quality and disturbances are one of the main contributors to chronic musculoskeletal pain [10,11]. The significant discriminative ability of the total PSQ-3-FI score to identify controls with no pain and the -ite and multisite chronic pain groups is in line with previous research that showed clear relationships between multisite pain and various sleep disturbances [62,63].

4.5. Relationships of PSQ-3-FI Score with Subjective Dizziness, Postural Control, and Sleep Quality

We observed a higher prevalence of dizziness in the higher PSQ-3-FI score group. A single study that explored the relationship between sleep disturbances and dizziness reported an increase in the prevalence of dizziness symptoms among subjects with a variety of sleep disturbances (16).

We also found little total sample correlation but consistent relationships between the PSQ-3-FI score and a range of postural control parameters, indicating poorer postural control among the group with higher PSQ-3-FI score. Overall, greater postural instability was observed during the more challenging eyes-closed rather than eyes-open conditions, and more so on an unstable surface. These statistically significant intergroup differences (PSQ-3-FI ≤ 4 vs. PSQ-3-FI ≥ 5) were observed in the majority of tests. Perhaps surprisingly, significant differences between groups were observed for all eyes open tests, but in only one of the six eyes-closed tests. This is especially surprising, as the majority of subjects in our study were suffering from CLBP. Previous studies of the CLBP population have shown a clear relationship between postural control impairments that are most marked when the subject's eyes are closed [64–66]. This clinical phenomenon is explained by the sensory weighting theory of postural control, which suggests that somatosensory, vestibular, and visual sensory information have mutual effects on postural control and are weighted as a sum of parts [67]. Subjects with CLBP exhibit impaired somatosensory information processing (the ability to feel through muscle, joint, and fascia-based sensory receptors) and hence this sensory channel is "down-weighted" due to pain and associated physical disabilities. Moreover, this altered sensory weighting causes increased postural sway in eyes-closed tests due to an inability to compensate for impaired somatosensory information using visual cues. Naturally, postural control is not simply just the sum of the weighting of sensory information. Sensorimotor integration in the central nervous system acts in conjunction with these raw sensory signals to ultimately govern postural control in a context-dependent manner [68,69]. Sleep disturbances, such as sleep deprivation, are well-known to negatively influence central nervous system processes across multiple cognitive [8], emotional [6], and motor functions [7], and in turn, vestibular pathologies can induce sleep disturbances [17]. The reciprocal effect of sleep disturbances upon such motor and cognitive processes may be one explanation for this seemingly paradoxical finding. In contrast, there was just one significant difference between groups out of the six parameters assessed under eyes-closed conditions. The fact that the higher PSQ-3 score group reported significantly more dizziness symptoms argues in favor of such a reciprocal relationship between vestibular dysfunction and sleep disturbances. Unfortunately, the mixed results obtained after subgrouping dizziness into seven subtypes did not help to further elaborate our findings.

Regarding sleep quality, the average awakening length was longer in the higher total PSQ-3 score group than the lower total PSQ-3 score group. Only minor differences were observed for the other sleep quality measurements, though there was a general trend towards poorer sleep quality among the higher PSQ-3 score group. These differences between groups (PSQ-3-FI ≤ 4 vs. PSQ-3-FI ≥ 5) may be affected to at least some degree by the long administration period between the PSQ-3 and actigraphy, which could have been up to 18 months. This was partly due to the COVID-19 outbreak in Finland, when data collection was stopped for five months. PSQ-3 test–retest reliability was excellent over one week; however, reliability may obviously vary after more than one year. Gender differences may also evidently affect the group comparisons, as females generally exhibit better sleep parameters in actigraphy [70]. The lower PSQ-3 score group contained 40% males and the higher PSQ-3 score group did not include any males. Moreover, the group with higher PSQ-3 score was, on average, more than ten years older than the lower-score group, which can be theorized to have a counter-intergroup effect on the results, as sleep quality parameters generally correlate negatively with aging [71]. Despite some limitations in relation to the long administration time and gender differences between groups, actigraphy may represent a relevant component of future pain–sleep PROM validations. Indeed, previous studies reported similar general trends between higher PROM scores and poorer sleep quality with other pain–sleep-related questionnaires (25, 26). We therefore conclude that there is an evident trend towards poorer sleep quality among individuals with higher PSQ-3-FI scores.

4.6. Strengths and Limitations

4.6.1. Strengths

Some strengths of this study include the very thorough validation of different measurement properties of the PSQ-3, including cross-cultural validity, face validity, internal consistency, test–retest reliability, measurement error, discriminant validity, and convergent validity, as well as the adequate size of the subject cohort and control group. Furthermore, the relationships between three novel measurements and PSQ-3 scores were investigated: subjective symptoms of dizziness, postural control testing, and sleep quality by actigraphy. Moreover, this is the first study to assess the exact effect of pain on sleep in relation to postural control between two groups of subjects. As far as we are aware, this study is the most comprehensive validation of any of the existing twelve PROMs that assess the effect of pain on sleep [13].

4.6.2. Limitations

As with other studies of this kind, our results are based on a single cohort assessed at a single clinic, so generalization to other subject populations should be made with caution. All symptoms were self-reported, and pain reporting was limited by the items on a single questionnaire. Actual medical diagnoses by a trained clinician were lacking. However, the self-reported data from our subject sample showed no discrepancies or illogical patterns of answers to suggest the results were invalid or had any considerable negative effects on our findings. Furthermore, it should also be noted that diagnoses of different types of musculoskeletal pain by trained clinicians are mostly based on patient self-reporting [72].

The most notable data collection limitation was the rather long time period between PSQ-3 administration and actigraphy.

4.6.3. Suggestions for Further Research

Future studies could validate the PSQ-3 in different musculoskeletal pain populations, such as individuals with neck pain and central sensitization syndromes such as fibromyalgia. Due to the high acceptable objective reliability of actigraphy for sleep parameters, actigraphy could be more extensively implemented in future validations of the PSQ-3 among larger cohorts of subjects and over longer time periods. Naturally, the only path towards more universal use of PSQ-3 is following cross-cultural validations.

5. Conclusions

The Finnish translation of the PSQ-3 was successfully cross-culturally adapted and validated. The measurement properties of the PSQ-3-FI were all acceptable for the Finnish-speaking CLBP population. Additional studies that implement the PSQ-3 as a short, valid, reliable instrument for screening assessments and outcome measurements could lead to the development of a better understanding of the direct effect of multifactorial musculoskeletal pain on sleep.

Author Contributions: Conceptualization and methodology, J.M., V.L., H.L, S.K., M.T. and O.A.; software and validation, J.M., V.L., H.L., S.K., M.T., T.S. and O.A.; formal analysis, J.M., V.L., D.K., S.K., M.T. and T.S.; investigation, J.M., V.L.; resources, and data curation, J.M., V.L. and O.A; writing—original draft preparation, J.M. and V.L.; writing—review and editing, J.M., V.L., H.L., D.K, S.K., M.T., T.S. and O.A.; visualization, J.M. and V.L.; supervision, V.L., H.L. and O.A.; project administration, J.M., V.L. and O.A.; All authors have read and agreed to the published version of the manuscript.

Funding: This research received no external funding.

Institutional Review Board Statement: Ethical approval for this study was obtained from the Research Ethics Committee of the Northern Savo Hospital District (identification number, 1106/13.02.00/2018). The study was conducted in accordance with the Declaration of Helsinki.

Informed Consent Statement: Written informed consent was obtained from all subjects before study entry.

Data Availability Statement: The data presented in this study are available on request from the corresponding author. The data are not publicly available due to containing information that could compromise the privacy of research participants.

Acknowledgments: The authors would like to thank all of the study participants who volunteered to participate in this study. Moreover, the authors would like to thank Lindsay Ayearst for help with backtranslation and data analysis, Nicole Oliver for advice on postural control analysis, and Pauli Ohukainen, Jon Haglund, Tuomo Ahola, Kristian Ekström, Mia Jokiniva and Emma Honkonen for their contributions to data collection.

Conflicts of Interest: The authors declare no conflict of interest.

Appendix A. Finnish Version of the Pain and Sleep Questionnaire Three-Item Index (PSQ-3-FI)

Kolmen Kohdan Kipu ja Uni -Kysely (PSQ-3)

Muistellessasi viime viikkoa, kuinka kipu on vaikuttanut nukkumiseesi?

Vastaukset tulevat numeroasteikolla 0-10, jossa 0 = ei ikinä ja 10 = aina. Merkitse rastilla.

1. Kuinka usein sinulla on ollut vaikeuksia nukahtaa kivun vuoksi?

ei ikinä | 0 | 1 | 2 | 3 | 4 | 5 | 6 | 7 | 8 | 9 | 10 | aina

2. Kuinka usein heräsit kivun vuoksi yön aikana?

ei ikinä | 0 | 1 | 2 | 3 | 4 | 5 | 6 | 7 | 8 | 9 | 10 | aina

3. Kuinka usein heräsit kivun vuoksi aamulla?

ei ikinä | 0 | 1 | 2 | 3 | 4 | 5 | 6 | 7 | 8 | 9 | 10 | aina

Pistemäärä: _____ / 30

References

1. Hartvigsen, J.; Hancock, M.J.; Kongsted, A.; Louw, Q.; Ferreira, M.L.; Genevay, S.; Hoy, D.; Karppinen, J.; Pransky, G.; Sieper, J.; et al. What low back pain is and why we need to pay attention. *Lancet* **2018**, *391*, 2356–2367. [CrossRef]
2. Kelly, G.A.; Blake, C.; Power, C.K.; O'keeffe, D.; Fullen, B.M. The association between chronic low back pain and sleep: A systematic review. *Clin. J. Pain* **2011**, *27*, 169–181. [CrossRef]
3. Mathias, J.L.; Cant, M.L.; Burke, A.L.J. Sleep disturbances and sleep disorders in adults living with chronic pain: A meta-analysis. *Sleep Med.* **2018**, *52*, 198–210. [CrossRef]
4. Zaki, N.F.W.; Spence, D.W.; Subramanian, P.; Bharti, V.K.; Karthikeyan, R.; BaHammam, A.S.; Pandi-Perumal, S.R. Basic chronobiology: What do sleep physicians need to know? *Sleep Sci.* **2020**, *13*, 256–266.
5. Brzecka, A.; Sarul, K.; Dyła, T.; Avila-Rodriguez, M.; Cabezas-Perez, R.; Chubarev, V.N.; Minyaeva, N.N.; Klochkov, S.G.; Neganova, M.E.; Mikhaleva, L.M.; et al. The Association of Sleep Disorders, Obesity and Sleep-Related Hypoxia with Cancer. *Curr. Genom.* **2020**, *21*, 444–453. [CrossRef]
6. Pires, G.N.; Bezerra, A.G.; Tufik, S.; Andersen, M.L. Effects of acute sleep deprivation on state anxiety levels: A systematic review and meta-analysis. *Sleep Med.* **2016**, *24*, 109–118. [CrossRef]
7. Dawson, D.; Reid, K. Fatigue, alcohol and performance impairment. *Nature* **1997**, *388*, 235. [CrossRef] [PubMed]
8. Killgore, W.D. Effects of sleep deprivation on cognition. *Prog. Brain Res.* **2010**, *185*, 105–129. [PubMed]
9. Moldofsky, H. Sleep and pain. *Sleep Med. Rev.* **2001**, *5*, 385–396. [CrossRef] [PubMed]
10. Othman, R.; Dassanayake, S.; Jayakaran, P.; Tumilty, S.; Swain, N.; Mani, R. Relationships Between Psychological, Social, Physical Activity, and Sleep Measures and Somatosensory Function in Individuals With Spinal Pain: A Systematic Review and Meta-analysis. *Clin. J. Pain* **2020**, *36*, 124–134. [CrossRef]

11. Othman, R.; Jayakaran, P.; Swain, N.; Dassanayake, S.; Tumilty, S.; Mani, R. Relationships Between Psychological, Sleep, and Physical Activity Measures and Somatosensory Function in People with Peripheral Joint Pain: A Systematic Review and Meta-Analysis. *Pain Pract.* **2021**, *21*, 226–261. [CrossRef] [PubMed]
12. Ayearst, L.; Harsanyi, Z.; Michalko, K.J. The Pain and Sleep Questionnaire three-item index (PSQ-3): A reliable and valid measure of the impact of pain on sleep in chronic nonmalignant pain of various etiologies. *Pain Res. Manag.* **2012**, *17*, 281–290. [CrossRef]
13. Phelps, C.; Bellon, S.; Hinkey, M.; Nash, A.; Boyd, J.; Cook, C.E.; Garcia, A.N. Measurement properties of Patient-Reported Outcome Measures used to assess the sleep quality in adults with high prevalence chronic pain conditions: A systematic review. *Sleep Med.* **2020**, *74*, 315–331. [CrossRef] [PubMed]
14. Kosinski, M.; Janagap, C.C.; Gajria, K.; Schein, J. Psychometric testing and validation of the Chronic Pain Sleep Inventory. *Clin. Ther.* **2007**, *29*, 2562–2577. [CrossRef]
15. Furtado, F.; Gonçalves, B.D.; Abranches, I.L.; Abrantes, A.F.; Forner-Cordero, A. Chronic Low Quality Sleep Impairs Postural Control in Healthy Adults. *PLoS ONE* **2016**, *11*, e0163310. [CrossRef]
16. Degache, F.; Goy, Y.; Vat, S.; Haba Rubio, J.; Contal, O.; Heinzer, R. Sleep-disordered breathing and daytime postural stability. *Thorax* **2016**, *71*, 543–548. [CrossRef] [PubMed]
17. Besnard, S.; Tighilet, B.; Chabbert, C.; Hitier, M.; Toulouse, J.; Le Gall, A.; Machado, M.L.; Smith, P.F. The balance of sleep: Role of the vestibular sensory system. *Sleep Med. Rev.* **2018**, *42*, 220–228. [CrossRef]
18. Kim, S.K.; Kim, J.H.; Jeon, S.S.; Hong, S.M. Relationship between sleep quality and dizziness. *PLoS ONE* **2018**, *13*, e0192705. [CrossRef]
19. Błaszczyk, J.W. The use of force-plate posturography in the assessment of postural instability. *Gait Posture* **2016**, *44*, 1–6. [CrossRef]
20. Meldrum, D.; Burrows, L.; Cakrt, O.; Kerkeni, H.; Lopez, C.; Tjernstrom, F.; Vereeck, L.; Zur, O.; Jahn, K. Vestibular rehabilitation in Europe: A survey of clinical and research practice. *J. Neurol.* **2020**, *267* (Suppl. 1), 24–35. [CrossRef]
21. Whitman, G.T. Dizziness. *Am. J. Med.* **2018**, *131*, 1431–1437. [CrossRef]
22. Sadeh, A. The role and validity of actigraphy in sleep medicine: An update. *Sleep Med. Rev.* **2011**, *15*, 259–267. [CrossRef] [PubMed]
23. Girschik, J.; Fritschi, L.; Heyworth, J.; Waters, F. Validation of self-reported sleep against actigraphy. *J. Epidemiol.* **2012**, *22*, 462–468. [CrossRef]
24. Ohayon, M.; Wickwire, E.M.; Hirshkowitz, M.; Albert, S.M.; Avidan, A.; Daly, F.J.; Dauvilliers, Y.; Ferri, R.; Fung, C.; Gozal, D.; et al. National Sleep Foundation's sleep quality recommendations: First report. *Sleep Health* **2017**, *3*, 6–19. [CrossRef] [PubMed]
25. Abeler, K.; Friborg, O.; Engstrøm, M.; Sand, T.; Bergvik, S. Sleep Characteristics in Adults with and Without Chronic Musculoskeletal Pain: The Role of Mental Distress and Pain Catastrophizing. *Clin. J. Pain* **2020**, *36*, 707–715. [CrossRef]
26. Eadie, J.; van de Water, A.T.; Lonsdale, C.; Tully, M.A.; van Mechelen, W.; Boreham, C.A.; Daly, L.; McDonough, S.M.; Hurley, D.A. Physiotherapy for sleep disturbance in people with chronic low back pain: Results of a feasibility randomized controlled trial. *Arch. Phys. Med. Rehabil.* **2013**, *94*, 2083–2092. [CrossRef]
27. Mokkink, L.B.; Terwee, C.B.; Knol, D.L.; Stratford, P.W.; Alonso, J.; Patrick, D.L.; Bouter, L.M.; de Vet, H.C. The COSMIN checklist for evaluating the methodological quality of studies on measurement properties: A clarification of its content. *BMC Med. Res. Methodol.* **2010**, *10*, 22. [CrossRef]
28. Mokkink, L.B.; Terwee, C.B.; Patrick, D.L.; Alonso, J.; Stratford, P.W.; Knol, D.L.; Bouter, L.M.; de Vet, H.C. The COSMIN checklist for assessing the methodological quality of studies on measurement properties of health status measurement instruments: An international Delphi study. *Qual. Life Res.* **2010**, *19*, 539–549. [CrossRef]
29. Beaton, D.E.; Bombardier, C.; Guillemin, F.; Ferraz, M.B. Guidelines for the process of cross-cultural adaptation of self-report measures. *Spine* **2000**, *25*, 3186–3191. [CrossRef]
30. Anthoine, E.; Moret, L.; Regnault, A.; Sébille, V.; Hardouin, J.B. Sample size used to validate a scale: A review of publications on newly-developed patient reported outcomes measures. *Health Qual. Life Outcomes* **2014**, *12*, 176. [CrossRef] [PubMed]
31. Costello, A.B.; Osborne, J. Best practices in exploratory factor analysis: Four recommendations for getting th e most from your analysis. *Pract. Assess. Res. Eval.* **2005**, *10*, 7.
32. Haefeli, M.; Elfering, A. Pain assessment. *Eur. Spine J.* **2006**, *15* (Suppl. 1), S17–S24. [CrossRef]
33. Mayer, T.G.; Neblett, R.; Cohen, H.; Howard, K.J.; Choi, Y.H.; Williams, M.J.; Perez, Y.; Gatchel, R.J. The development and psychometric validation of the central sensitization inventory. *Pain Pract.* **2012**, *12*, 276–285. [CrossRef]
34. Neblett, R.; Cohen, H.; Choi, Y.; Hartzell, M.M.; Williams, M.; Mayer, T.G.; Gatchel, R.J. The Central Sensitization Inventory (CSI): Establishing clinically significant values for identifying central sensitivity syndromes in an outpatient chronic pain sample. *J. Pain* **2013**, *14*, 438–445. [CrossRef]
35. Neblett, R. The central sensitization inventory: A user's manual. *J. Appl. Behav. Res.* **2018**, *23*, e12123. [CrossRef]
36. Mikkonen, J.; Luomajoki, H.; Airaksinen, O.; Neblett, R.; Selander, T.; Leinonen, V. Cross-cultural adaptation and validation of the Finnish version of the central sensitization inventory and its relationship with dizziness and postural control. *BMC Neurol.* **2021**, *21*, 141. [CrossRef] [PubMed]
37. Miller, R.P.; Kori, S.H.; Todd, D.D. The Tampa Scale. A Measure of Kinesiophobia. *Clin. J. Pain* **1991**, *7*, 51–52. [CrossRef]
38. Koho, P.; Borodulin, K.; Kautiainen, H.; Kujala, U.; Pohjolainen, T.; Hurri, H. Finnish version of the Tampa Scale of Kinesiophobia: Reference values in the Finnish general population and associations with leisure-time physical activity. *J. Rehabil. Med.* **2015**, *47*, 249–255. [CrossRef]

39. Poutanen, O.; Koivisto, A.M.; Kaaria, S.; Salokangas, R.K. The validity of the Depression Scale (DEPS) to assess the severity of depression in primary care patients. *Fam. Pract.* **2010**, *27*, 527–534. [CrossRef] [PubMed]
40. Kyrölä, K.; Häkkinen, A.H.; Ylinen, J.; Repo, J.P. Rasch validation of the Depression Scale among patients with low back pain. *J. Back Musculoskelet. Rehabil.* **2021**, *34*, 261–267.
41. Janssen, M.F.; Pickard, A.S.; Golicki, D.; Gudex, C.; Niewada, M.; Scalone, L.; Swinburn, P.; Busschbach, J. Measurement properties of the EQ-5D-5L compared to the EQ-5D-3L across eight patient groups: A multi-country study. *Qual. Life Res.* **2013**, *22*, 1717–1727. [CrossRef] [PubMed]
42. Van Hout, B.; Janssen, M.F.; Feng, Y.S.; Kohlmann, T.; Busschbach, J.; Golicki, D.; Lloyd, A.; Scalone, L.; Kind, P.; Pickard, A.S. Interim scoring for the EQ-5D-5L: Mapping the EQ-5D-5L to EQ-5D-3L value sets. *Value Health* **2012**, *15*, 708–715. [CrossRef] [PubMed]
43. Roland, M.; Fairbank, J. The Roland-Morris Disability Questionnaire and the Oswestry Disability Questionnaire. *Spine* **2000**, *25*, 3115–3124. [CrossRef] [PubMed]
44. Stevens, M.L.; Lin, C.C.; Maher, C.G. The Roland Morris Disability Questionnaire. *J. Physiother.* **2016**, *62*, 116. [CrossRef]
45. Kerber, K.A.; Callaghan, B.C.; Telian, S.A.; Meurer, W.J.; Skolarus, L.E.; Carender, W.; Burke, J.F. Dizziness Symptom Type Prevalence and Overlap: A US Nationally Representative Survey. *Am. J. Med.* **2017**, *130*, 1465.e1–1465.e9. [CrossRef]
46. Wrisley, D.M.; Whitney, S.L. The effect of foot position on the modified clinical test of sensory interaction and balance. *Arch. Phys. Med. Rehabil.* **2004**, *85*, 335–338. [CrossRef]
47. Ruhe, A.; Fejer, R.; Walker, B. Center of pressure excursion as a measure of balance performance in patients with non-specific low back pain compared to healthy controls: A systematic review of the literature. *Eur. Spine J.* **2011**, *20*, 358–368. [CrossRef]
48. Horn, L.B.; Rice, T.; Stoskus, J.L.; Lambert, K.H.; Dannenbaum, E.; Scherer, M.R. Measurement Characteristics and Clinical Utility of the Clinical Test of Sensory Interaction on Balance (CTSIB) and Modified CTSIB in Individuals With Vestibular Dysfunction. *Arch. Phys. Med. Rehabil.* **2015**, *96*, 1747–1748. [CrossRef]
49. Ruhe, A.; Fejer, R.; Walker, B. The test-retest reliability of centre of pressure measures in bipedal static task conditions—A systematic review of the literature. *Gait Posture* **2010**, *32*, 436–445. [CrossRef]
50. Van de Water, A.T.; Eadie, J.; Hurley, D.A. Investigation of sleep disturbance in chronic low back pain: An age- and gender-matched case-control study over a 7-night period. *Man. Ther.* **2011**, *16*, 550–556. [CrossRef] [PubMed]
51. O'Donoghue, G.M.; Fox, N.; Heneghan, C.; Hurley, D.A. Objective and subjective assessment of sleep in chronic low back pain patients compared with healthy age and gender matched controls: A pilot study. *BMC Musculoskelet. Disord.* **2009**, *10*, 122. [CrossRef] [PubMed]
52. Norris, M.; Lecavalier, L. Evaluating the use of exploratory factor analysis in developmental disability psychological research. *J. Autism. Dev. Disord.* **2010**, *40*, 8–20. [CrossRef] [PubMed]
53. El-Den, S.; Schneider, C.; Mirzaei, A.; Carter, S. How to measure a latent construct: Psychometric principles for the development and validation of measurement instruments. *Int. J. Pharm. Pract.* **2020**, *28*, 326–336. [CrossRef]
54. Ramasamy, A.; Martin, M.L.; Blum, S.I.; Liedgens, H.; Argoff, C.; Freynhagen, R.; Wallace, M.; McCarrier, K.P.; Bushnell, D.M.; Hatley, N.V.; et al. Assessment of Patient-Reported Outcome Instruments to Assess Chronic Low Back Pain. *Pain Med.* **2017**, *18*, 1098–1110. [CrossRef] [PubMed]
55. Chapman, J.R.; Norvell, D.C.; Hermsmeyer, J.T.; Bransford, R.J.; DeVine, J.; McGirt, M.J.; Lee, M.J. Evaluating common outcomes for measuring treatment success for chronic low back pain. *Spine* **2011**, *36* (Suppl. 21), S54–S68. [CrossRef]
56. Geerinck, A.; Alekna, V.; Beaudart, C.; Bautmans, I.; Cooper, C.; De Souza Orlandi, F.; Konstantynowicz, J.; Montero-Errasquín, B.; Topinková, E.; Tsekoura, M.; et al. Standard error of measurement and smallest detectable change of the Sarcopenia Quality of Life (SarQoL) questionnaire: An analysis of subjects from 9 validation studies. *PLoS ONE* **2019**, *14*, e0216065. [CrossRef] [PubMed]
57. Babyak, M.A.; Green, S.B. Confirmatory factor analysis: An introduction for psychosomatic medicine researchers. *Psychosom. Med.* **2010**, *72*, 587–597. [CrossRef]
58. Jackson, D.L.; Gillaspy, J.A.; Purc-Stephenson, R. Reporting practices in confirmatory factor analysis: An overview and some recommendations. *Psychol. Methods* **2009**, *14*, 6–23. [CrossRef] [PubMed]
59. Alavi, M.; Visentin, D.C.; Thapa, D.K.; Hunt, G.E.; Watson, R.; Cleary, M. Chi-square for model fit in confirmatory factor analysis. *J. Adv. Nurs.* **2020**, *76*, 2209–2211. [CrossRef]
60. Costa, N.; Smits, E.; Kasza, J.; Salomoni, S.; Ferreira, M.; Sullivan, M.; Hodges, P.W. ISSLS PRIZE IN CLINICAL SCIENCE 2021: What are the risk factors for low back pain flares and does this depend on how flare is defined? *Eur. Spine J.* **2021**, *30*, 1089–1097. [CrossRef]
61. Gerhart, J.I.; Burns, J.W.; Post, K.M.; Smith, D.A.; Porter, L.S.; Burgess, H.J.; Schuster, E.; Buvanendran, A.; Fras, A.M.; Keefe, F.J. Relationships Between Sleep Quality and Pain-Related Factors for People with Chronic Low Back Pain: Tests of Reciprocal and Time of Day Effects. *Ann. Behav. Med.* **2017**, *51*, 365–375. [CrossRef]
62. Davies, K.A.; Macfarlane, G.J.; Nicholl, B.I.; Dickens, C.; Morriss, R.; Ray, D.; McBeth, J. Restorative sleep predicts the resolution of chronic widespread pain: Results from the EPIFUND study. *Rheumatology* **2008**, *47*, 1809–1813. [CrossRef] [PubMed]
63. McBeth, J.; Wilkie, R.; Bedson, J.; Chew-Graham, C.; Lacey, R.J. Sleep disturbance and chronic widespread pain. *Curr. Rheumatol. Rep.* **2015**, *17*, 469. [CrossRef] [PubMed]

64. Koch, C.; Hänsel, F. Non-specific Low Back Pain and Postural Control during Quiet Standing-A Systematic Review. *Front. Psychol.* **2019**, *10*, 586. [CrossRef] [PubMed]
65. Mazaheri, M.; Coenen, P.; Parnianpour, M.; Kiers, H.; van Dieën, J.H. Low back pain and postural sway during quiet standing with and without sensory manipulation: A systematic review. *Gait Posture* **2013**, *37*, 12–22. [CrossRef]
66. Berenshteyn, Y.; Gibson, K.; Hackett, G.C.; Trem, A.B.; Wilhelm, M. Is standing balance altered in individuals with chronic low back pain? A systematic review. *Disabil. Rehabil.* **2019**, *41*, 1514–1523. [CrossRef] [PubMed]
67. Assländer, L.; Peterka, R.J. Sensory reweighting dynamics in human postural control. *J. Neurophysiol.* **2014**, *111*, 1852–1864. [CrossRef]
68. Roemmich, R.T.; Bastian, A.J. Closing the Loop: From Motor Neuroscience to Neurorehabilitation. *Annu. Rev. Neurosci.* **2018**, *41*, 415–429. [CrossRef]
69. Ivanenko, Y.; Gurfinkel, V.S. Human Postural Control. *Front. Neurosci.* **2018**, *12*, 171. [CrossRef]
70. Kocevska, D.; Lysen, T.S.; Dotinga, A.; Koopman-Verhoeff, M.E.; Luijk, M.P.C.M.; Antypa, N.; Biermasz, N.R.; Blokstra, A.; Brug, J.; Burk, W.J.; et al. Sleep characteristics across the lifespan in 1.1 million people from the Netherlands, United Kingdom and United States: A systematic review and meta-analysis. *Nat. Hum. Behav.* **2021**, *5*, 113–122. [CrossRef]
71. Ohayon, M.M.; Carskadon, M.A.; Guilleminault, C.; Vitiello, M.V. Meta-analysis of quantitative sleep parameters from childhood to old age in healthy individuals: Developing normative sleep values across the human lifespan. *Sleep* **2004**, *27*, 1255–1273. [CrossRef] [PubMed]
72. Breivik, H.; Borchgrevink, P.C.; Allen, S.M.; Rosseland, L.A.; Romundstad, L.; Hals, E.K.; Kvarstein, G.; Stubhaug, A. Assessment of pain. *Br. J. Anaesth.* **2008**, *101*, 17–24. [CrossRef] [PubMed]

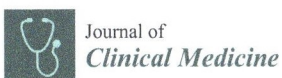

Article

Neck Active Movements Assessment in Women with Episodic and Chronic Migraine

Carina F. Pinheiro [1], Anamaria S. Oliveira [1], Tenysson Will-Lemos [1], Lidiane L. Florencio [2], César Fernández-de-las-Peñas [2], Fabiola Dach [3] and Débora Bevilaqua-Grossi [1,*]

1 Department of Health Sciences, Ribeirão Preto Medical School, University of Sao Paulo, Ribeirão Preto 14049-900, Brazil; carinafp@usp.br (C.F.P.); siriani@fmrp.usp.br (A.S.O.); tenysson@fmrp.usp.br (T.W.-L.)
2 Department of Physical Therapy, Occupational Therapy, Rehabilitation and Physical Medicine, King Juan Carlos University, Alcorcón, 28922 Madrid, Spain; lidiane.florencio@urjc.es (L.L.F.); cesar.fernandez@urjc.es (C.F.-d.-l.-P.)
3 Department of Neurosciences and Behavioral Sciences, Ribeirão Preto Medical School, University of São Paulo, Ribeirão Preto 14049-900, Brazil; fabioladach@usp.br
* Correspondence: deborabg@fmrp.usp.br

Abstract: We aimed to compare movement parameters and muscle activity during active cervical spine movements between women with episodic or chronic migraine and asymptomatic control. We also assessed the correlations between cervical movement measures with neck-related disability and kinesiophobia. Women with episodic (n = 27; EM) or chronic (n = 27; CM) migraine and headache-free controls (n = 27; CG) performed active cervical movements. Cervical range of motion, angular velocity, and percentage of muscular activation were calculated in a blinded fashion. Compared to CG, the EM and CM groups presented a reduced total range of motion ($p < 0.05$). Reduced mean angular velocity of cervical movement was also observed in both EM and CM compared to CG ($p < 0.05$). Total cervical range of motion and mean angular velocity showed weak correlations with disability (r = −0.25 and −0.30, respectively; $p < 0.05$) and weak-to-moderate correlations with kinesiophobia (r = −0.30 and −0.40, respectively; $p < 0.05$). No significant correlation was observed between headache features and total cervical range of motion or mean angular velocity ($p > 0.05$). No differences in the percentage of activation of both flexors and extensors cervical muscles during active neck movements were seen ($p > 0.05$). In conclusion, episodic and chronic migraines were associated with less mobility and less velocity of neck movements, without differences within muscle activity. Neck disability and kinesiophobia are negative and weakly associated with cervical movement.

Keywords: headache; cervical spine; motion; chronic pain; musculoskeletal pain

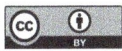

1. Introduction

Migraine is a primary headache ranked as the second world cause of disability when considered years living with disability [1]. Migraine diagnostic criteria are defined by recurrent attacks lasting 4–72 h with headaches that are typically unilateral, pulsating, moderate or severe intensity, aggravated by routine physical activity, and also associated with nausea and/or photophobia and phonophobia [2].

Migraine is recognized as a complex clinical condition considering its variety of symptoms and its range of comorbidities [3–5]. The association of migraine with neck pain or with pain on manual examination of the upper cervical joints is one of these interactions that might contribute to its clinical complexity, negatively influencing the impact, treatment, and prognosis of migraine [4,6–8].

Reduced cervical range of motion (ROM) has been confirmed in patients with migraines by the most updated meta-analyses [9,10]. The relationship of this reduced ROM with the frequency of migraine attacks is still under debate. Some reports suggest that cervical ROM is only impaired in patients with chronic migraines [11,12], while others do not support this [13–15]. Further, cervical ROM may also be affected by kinesiophobia reported by patients with migraines [16,17], especially considering that individuals with migraines frequently experience pain aggravation due to head movements during migraine attacks [17]. Although it has not been previously analyzed in migraineurs, angular velocity during cervical ROM is also a parameter for movement analysis that could contribute to detecting sensorimotor alterations of the neck [18]. Previous studies have revealed a reduced velocity of cervical movements in individuals with neck pain compared with asymptomatic subjects [18–20].

Individuals with migraines also exhibit altered superficial muscle activity during isometric contractions. Benatto et al. observed reduced extensor/flexor muscle activity ratio during maximal voluntary isometric contractions in flexion in migraineurs compared to healthy controls [21]. Furthermore, patients with chronic migraine also present higher coactivation of neck extensors during isometric contraction in cervical flexion [22] and a craniocervical flexion test [23] than healthy controls. However, to date, no study has assessed cervical muscle activity during active neck movements in patients with migraines.

The current study aimed to assess kinematic data (cervical range of motion and angular velocity) and muscle activity during active cervical ROM (flexion, extension, lateral flexions, and rotations) comparing asymptomatic women with episodic or chronic migraine sufferers. We also aimed to determine the correlation of the kinematic data with neck-related disability and kinesiophobia. We hypothesized that women with migraines would exhibit different kinematic patterns and muscle activity than headache-free controls. A secondary hypothesis was that kinematic patterns would be associated with related-disability and kinesiophobia in migraine women.

2. Materials and Methods

2.1. Participants Selection

Women aged between 18 and 55 were recruited from the local population between January 2018 and August 2019 through advertisements via social media (Instagram®, Facebook®) and local university radio. Potential participants were diagnosed by a neurologist of a headache clinic for both migraine groups according to the third edition of the International Headache Society criteria [2]. The episodic migraine group consisted of women presenting 2 to 12 days of migraine attacks for at least three months [2]. Participants who presented ≥15 days of headache attacks/month, which, on at least eight days/month, had the features of migraine headache for more than three months, composed the chronic migraine group [2]. Women without a history of frequent headaches composed the control headache-free group. The previous history of neck pain was permitted in the control group.

Participants were excluded if they underwent anesthetic nerve block or received physical therapy the previous year, history of degenerative cervical conditions, history of trauma at the neck and face, or pregnancy. For participants within both migraine groups, we also excluded those presenting with a second concomitant headache diagnosis (i.e., cervicogenic headache or tension-type headache) or those treated with botulinum toxin or anesthetic blocks. The local ethics committee approved this study protocol (protocol number 12145/2016), and all participants signed the written informed consent before their inclusion.

2.2. Instrumentation

The Multi-Cervical Rehabilitation Unit (MCU) (BTE Technologies, Inc.™, Hanover, USA) was used to assess active ROM. It is a fixed-frame device with a head assembly system (movable inner and outer head brace). It also contains an adjustable parameter at the seat to stabilize the individual and avoid compensations (Figure 1). The potentiometer was calibrated daily by first setting the outer brace (transverse plane) at 0°, 90° rotation to the left, and 90° to the right, and then by setting the inner brace (sagittal plane) at 0°, 100° flexion, and 100° extension. Measurement of the active ROM using this device has shown excellent reliability in people with neck pain and healthy participants (intraclass correlation coefficient ranging from 0.81 to 0.96) [24].

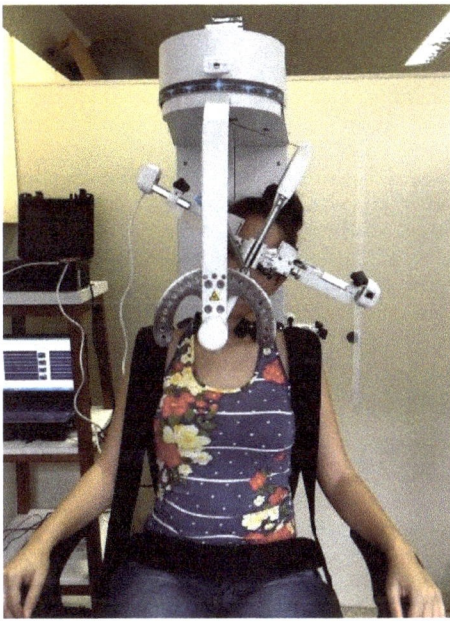

Figure 1. Representation of a participant's position and stabilization on the Multi-Cervical Rehabilitation Unit (MCU).

Surface EMG was acquired using the Trigno^{TM} Wireless System (CMRR of 80 dB, input impedance exceeding 1000 Ω, Delsys Inc. Boston, MA, USA). Each Trigno sensor comprises two parallel groups with two bars, each one (Ag-AgCl), with a fixed inter-electrode distance of 10 mm. Myoelectric signals were acquired, digitalized, amplified (gain = 300), band-pass filtered (20–450 Hz with 40 and 80 dB/dec), and sampled at 4 kHz per channel with a 16-bit resolution A/D by software EMGworks Acquisition (Delsys Inc. Boston, MA, USA).

An A/D converter board (USB-1616HS-BNC; Measurement Computer Corporation, Norton, MA, USA) was used to synchronize MCU and EMG data. The A/D converter board digitalized the electrical signals from the potentiometer previously amplified (MKTC5-10; MK Controle e Instrumentação, São Paulo, Brazil). It also received inputs from the Transistor-Transistor Logic (TTL) Trigger Module (Delsys Trigno; Delsys Inc. Boston, MA, USA). The digitalized data from MCU and Trigger Module were relayed to a customized MATLAB script and sampled at 2 kHz. The TrignoTM Wireless System and A/D converter board were connected to an external power supply (12 V, 9 Ah, rechargeable, GetPower) to avoid power grid noise.

2.3. Procedures

Clinical features of migraine, such as frequency of migraine episodes (days per month), the intensity of migraine attacks (numerical pain rate scale (NPRS), 0–10), and years with migraine were collected. Participants were also questioned about the self-rated presence of neck pain and its characteristics, including frequency, intensity, and time of onset. Finally, participants fulfilled the questionnaires Neck Disability Index (NDI) [25] and Tampa Scale for Kinesiophobia (TSK) [26]. The NDI is a 10-item questionnaire widely used to assess neck pain-related disability. Individual items are scored, and the total score can range from 0% to 100% [27]. The NDI has excellent reliability (intraclass correlation coefficient 0.86) [28] and internal consistency (Cronbach alpha 0.87 to 0.92) [29]. The TSK is a questionnaire with 17-items to assess kinesiophobia, with a total score ranging from 17 to 68 points [30]. This tool has suitable reliability (intraclass correlation coefficient 0.93) [26] and a suitable correlation with depressive and catastrophic symptoms [30]. Subjects with TSK scores >37 points are considered subjects with high fear [30].

Participants were assessed in a pain-free period for movement analysis by a trained examiner blinded to the individual's condition. The Trigno sensors were firmly fixed with adhesive tape bilaterally after proper skin cleaning (cleaned with alcohol/trichotomized when necessary). Electrodes were placed according to the standard instructions at the sternocleidomastoid [31], anterior scalene [31], splenius capitis [32], and upper trapezius [33] muscles. Participants were seated at MCU and fixed firmly with belts. They were asked to perform three repetitions for each cervical movement: flexion, extension, left/right lateral flexions, and left/right rotations in a random sequence. They were instructed to complete the total movement in about 4 s, following audio feedback, in order to obtain similar intervals and velocities to analyze EMG amplitude data. There was a 15 s interval between the repetitions and a one-minute interval between each neck movement. The presence of pain in the neck or the head was assessed using the NPRS immediately after each measurement.

2.4. Data Processing

Data were analyzed using a custom MATLAB code (MathWorks, Natick, MA, USA). Kinematic data were filtered with a 4th order low-pass filter with a cutoff frequency of 10 Hz. The peak angle determined maximal cervical ROM, and the angular velocity was calculated based on the mean angular velocity from the beginning to peak angle. ROM and mean angular velocity were reported for each movement separately to be consistent with the EMG data report. However, we do not have biological plausibility to assume a specific laterality restriction in patients with migraines. Moreover, reduced ROM has been inconsistently reported for patients with migraines in all planes [9,10]. So, to provide a reasonable variable for clinical application, we also reported: the sum of the six cervical ROM, which will be named as total cervical ROM, and the average between the six angular velocities named as the mean angular velocity of cervical movement.

Despite the time constraint to perform the active movements, there were still differences among groups at the mean angular velocity. Consequently, we were not able to calculate the signal amplitude of the EMG [19,34]. EMG data were filtered with a 4th order with band-pass filtering 10–950 Hz [35]. Onset muscles were determined when the EMG signal exceeded a 2SD threshold from more than a 25 ms window. These thresholds were determined visually after pilot trials based on recommendations of Hodges et al. [35]. A few trials in which we observed signal interference due to electrode movement were excluded. Detection of the onset and offset of muscle activities during each movement was then quantified in terms of percentage of activation duration to represent temporal characteristics of the muscle activity [20]. A 100% activation indicates that the muscle was active all the time [20].

2.5. Statistical Analysis

Normality of data was verified using the Shapiro–Wilk test and observation of residuals distribution on histograms. Means, standard deviations, and frequencies were calculated to describe the variables. Clinical and demographic data, cervical ROM, and angular velocity were compared among the three groups using a one-way analysis of variance (ANOVA) with a Bonferroni post hoc test. The frequency of self-reported neck pain was compared among groups using the chi-square test. Pearson's correlation was used to verify the association of mean angular velocity of cervical movement and total cervical ROM with headache features (years with migraine, frequency, and intensity), NDI, and TSK scores. Correlation values less than 0.40 indicated a weak correlation, 0.40 to 0.69, moderate, and more than 0.70, strong correlation [36].

Comparison among control, episodic migraine, and chronic migraine groups were performed first. In the case of any significant difference, analysis of subgroups considered by the history of neck pain and the presence of pain during the active movements were also carried out as covariates. For that, a two-way ANOVA with a Bonferroni post hoc test was used.

Multivariate ANOVA was used to compare the percentage of activation duration of all cervical muscles during each movement among groups.

SPSS software (version 20.0, SPSS Inc, Chicago, IL, USA) was used for all statistical analyses adopting a significance level of 0.05.

3. Results

3.1. Demographics

Of 103 potential eligible individuals, 6 were excluded due to comorbid headache diagnosis, 4 had a history of neck trauma, 2 had received recent anesthetic blocks, and 10 were unavailable to attend the evaluation. Accordingly, the final sample consisted of 27 women with episodic migraine, 27 women with chronic migraine, and 27 headache-free women as controls.

All groups presented similar age ($F_{(2,80)} = 1.39$ $p = 0.26$) and body mass index ($F_{(2,80)} = 0.94$, $p = 0.40$). Both episodic and chronic migraine groups exhibited greater prevalence of self-reported neck pain ($X^2 = 16.40$, $p < 0.001$) than control group. Significant differences among groups were observed for frequency of neck pain ($F_{(2,45)} = 3.42$, $p = 0.04$), NDI ($F_{(2,44)} = 9.22$, $p < 0.001$), and TSK ($F_{(2,80)} = 8.48$, $p < 0.001$) scores. The chronic migraine group exhibited higher frequency of neck pain than the episodic migraine group ($p = 0.04$), and higher related disability than the control group ($p < 0.001$). The TSK scores were higher in both episodic ($p = 0.001$) and chronic migraine groups ($p = 0.004$) when compared with the control group (Table 1). High fear was identified in 15% of the control group ($n = 4$), 48% of the episodic migraine group ($n = 13$) and 52% of the chronic migraine group ($n = 14$).

Table 1. Mean, standard deviation, and frequency of sample sociodemographic characteristics and clinical features.

	Control Group (n = 27)	Episodic Migraine (n = 27)	Chronic Migraine (n = 27)
Age (years)	31.2 (9.17)	33.0 (9.05)	35.5 (10.27)
BMI (kg/cm^2)	25.0 (4.00)	23.7 (3.89)	23.9 (2.95)
Years with migraine	-	14.1 (8.33)	18.1 (11.55)
Migraine frequency (days/month)	-	6.7 (3.29)	24.5 (5.66)
Migraine intensity (NPRS)	-	7.6 (1.49)	8.0 (1.57)
Self-report of neck pain †	7 (25.9%)	18 (66.7%)	21 (77.8%)
Years with neck pain	3.6 (2.17)	9.2 (4.58)	8.4 (6.82)
Neck pain frequency (days/month)	13.9 (11.34)	12.5 (10.70)	20.5 (8.64) **
Neck pain intensity (NPRS)	4.4 (1.27)	5.5 (2.01)	5.8 (2.18)
NDI score	11.1 (11.65)	24.9 (11.58)	35.1 (14.66) *
TSK score	28.7 (7.53)	36.1 (8.05) *	37.2 (9.14) *

* $p < 0.05$ vs. control group; ** $p < 0.05$ vs. episodic migraine group; † chi-square test $p < 0.05$; BMI: body mass index; NPRS: numeric pain rating scale; NDI: Neck Disability Index; TSK: Tampa Scale for Kinesiophobia.

3.2. Cervical ROM and Angular Velocity

Total cervical ROM differed among groups ($F_{(2,80)} = 5.61$, $p < 0.01$). Lower ROM could be observed for both episodic (mean difference: 30.52°, $p = 0.01$) and chronic migraine (mean difference: 30.07°, $p = 0.02$) groups compared to controls. When the movements were analyzed separately, differences were observed for left lateral flexion ($F_{(2,80)} = 5.05$, $p = 0.009$), and right rotation. ($F_{(2,80)} = 4.24$, $p = 0.02$): chronic migraine women showed less left lateral flexion than controls ($p = 0.007$), whereas episodic migraine women showed less right rotation ($p = 0.03$, Table 2). Differences in right lateral flexion ($F_{(2,80)} = 3.26$, $p = 0.04$), and left rotation ($F_{(2,80)} = 3.14$. $p = 0.04$) were observed, but with no significant pairwise comparisons after the adjustments for multiple comparisons were seen ($p > 0.05$, Table 2).

No differences for flexion ($F_{(2,80)}$ = 1.38, p = 0.25), and extension ($F_{(2,80)}$ = 3.11, p = 0.05, Table 2) among the groups were observed.

Table 2. Mean and standard deviation of cervical range of motion angle and angular velocity.

	Control Group (n = 27)	Episodic Migraine (n = 27)	Chronic Migraine (n = 27)
Cervical range of motion (degrees)			
Total range of motion	310.7 (28.39)	280.21 (37.01) *	280.65 (47.39) *
Flexion	58.0 (6.91)	53.8 (7.68)	55.5 (12.68)
Extension	59.7 (7.49)	53.9 (9.71)	55.2 (9.59)
Right lateral flexion	51.6 (8.26)	46.3 (7.42)	46.6 (9.80)
Left lateral flexion	51.0 (7.68)	46.1 (8.26)	43.4 (10.53) *
Right rotation	73.0 (8.50)	65.1 (9.29) *	65.9 (14.40)
Left rotation	68.9 (11.93)	61.3 (12.21)	60.7 (15.81)
Angular velocity (degrees/s)			
Mean angular velocity of cervical moviment	26.60 (4.62)	22.67 (4.72) *	22.09 (5.84) *
Flexion	27.17 (5.43)	23.2 (5.07)	23.0 (7.34) *
Extension	25.33 (5.51)	22.7 (5.78)	22.2 (4.57)
Right lateral flexion	23.07 (5.31)	19.7 (4.90)	19.2 (5.80) *
Left lateral flexion	22.9 (5.77)	19.2 (5.10)	18.8 (6.13) *
Right rotation	30.4 (5.82)	26.2 (6.48)	26.4 (9.44)
Left rotation	30.7 (5.86)	25.0 (6.57) *	25.3 (8.04) *

* p < 0.05 vs. control group.

Subgroup analysis considering the history of neck pain revealed a main effect of group for the total range of motion ($F_{(2,80)}$ = 4.19, p = 0.02), but no significant differences for the history of neck pain or the interaction between group and neck pain (p > 0.05, Table S1). When groups were stratified by the presence of neck pain during active movement, a group * neck pain interaction was verified for neck flexion ($F_{(2,75)}$ = 3.18, p = 0.047, Table S2): women with chronic migraine and neck pain during cervical motion present lower cervical ROM than those with chronic migraine but without pain during cervical ROM (p = 0.02). The chronic migraine group with neck pain during cervical ROM exhibited lower cervical ROM than the control group with neck pain during cervical flexion (p = 0.04).

Mean angular velocity of cervical movement was different among groups ($F_{(2,80)}$ = 6.28, p = 0.003). Both groups with migraine presented lower angular velocity than controls, with a mean difference of 3.93°/s for episodic migraine (p = 0.02) and 4.51°/s for chronic migraine (p < 0.01). When the movements were analyzed separately, angular velocity was different in flexion ($F_{(2,80)}$ = 4.06, p = 0.02), right lateral flexion ($F_{(2,80)}$ = 4.66, p = 0.01), left lateral flexion ($F_{(2,80)}$ = 4.75, p = 0.01), and left rotation ($F_{(2,80)}$ = 6.19, p = 0.003). Angular velocity was reduced in chronic migraine as compared to controls for flexion (p = 0.04), right (p = 0.01) and left (p = 0.01) lateral flexion (Table 2). Episodic (p = 0.01) and chronic (p = 0.006) migraine groups showed lower angular velocity than controls for left rotation (Table 2). No differences were found for extension ($F_{(2,75)}$ = 2.75, p = 0.07) and right rotation ($F_{(2,80)}$ = 2.66, p = 0.07).

The subgroups analysis of history of neck pain showed a main effect of group for right lateral flexion ($F_{(2,80)}$ = 4.78, p = 0.01) and right rotation ($F_{(2,80)}$ = 5.19, p = 0.008) but no difference related to the history of neck pain neither the interaction of them (p > 0.05, Table S3). Similar findings were obtained from the subgroup analysis considering neck pain experienced during cervical ROM. We only found the main effects of the group for flexion ($F_{(2,80)}$ = 4.71, p = 0.01, Table S4) without any significant differences for neck pain during the test or the interaction between these two factors (p > 0.05).

3.3. Percentage of Activation

Figure 2 displays the mean percentage of activation of all cervical muscles assessed during active cervical ROM. No differences among groups for any muscle, regardless of being agonist/antagonist, during flexion ($F_{(16,34)} = 0.744$; $p = 0.73$), extension ($F_{(16,58)} = 0.949$; $p = 0.52$), right lateral flexion ($F_{(16,46)} = 1.324$; $p = 0.22$), left lateral flexion ($F_{(16,42)} = 1.089$; $p = 0.39$), right rotation ($F_{(16,34)} = 1.314$; $p = 0.25$), or left rotation ($F_{(16,56)} = 0.472$; $p = 0.95$).

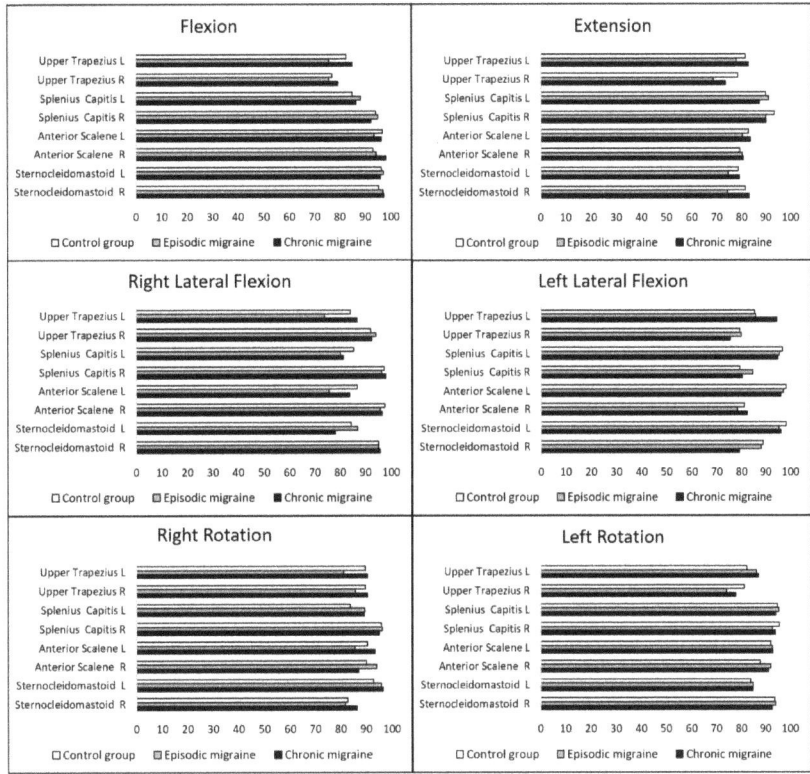

Figure 2. Mean percentage of activation of cervical muscles during active neck movements. R: **right**; L: **left**.

3.4. Correlations

Table 3 presents the correlation analysis. Weak negative correlations were observed between total cervical ROM and NDI and TSK scores ($p < 0.05$). Weak-to-moderate negative correlations were observed between mean angular velocity of cervical movement and NDI and TSK scores ($p < 0.05$). No significant correlation was observed between headache features and total cervical ROM or mean angular velocity of cervical movements ($p < 0.05$).

Table 3. Pearson's correlations (r) and 95% confidence intervals of angular velocity and cervical range of motion angle with both Neck Disability Index (NDI) and Tampa Scale for Kinesiophobia (TSK) scores and with headache features.

	Total Cervical Range of Motion (°)	Angular Velocity (°/s)
Total sample (n = 81)		
NDI scores	−0.25 * (−0.48 to −0.04)	−0.28 (−0.50 to −0.06) *
TSK scores	−0.30 * (−0.51 to −0.08)	−0.40 (−0.60 to −0.19) **
Participants with migraine (n = 54)		
Years with migraine	−0.003 (−0.32 to 0.32)	0.01 (−0.28 to 0.31)
Migraine frequency (days/month)	0.14 (−0.16 to 0.47)	0.04 (−0.25 to 0.34)
Migraine intensity (NPRS)	0.13 (−0.39 to 1.07)	0.02 (−0.64 to 0.74)

* $p < 0.05$; ** $p < 0.01$.

4. Discussion

The current study revealed that women with migraines present reduced total cervical ROM and angular velocity during neck active movements compared to controls. In general, those variables were not influenced by the history of neck pain or pain evoked with movement. Differences in the angular velocity were more frequently observed in those with chronic migraines. Cervical ROM and angular velocity were weakly correlated with neck-related disability and kinesiophobia in women with migraines but not with headache features. Finally, the duration of neck muscle activation did not differ between groups for any active movements, regardless of whether agonist or antagonist. These results partially confirmed the study hypotheses.

Our total cervical ROM results agree with a previous study [15], showing reduced total mobility in migraine patients compared to controls, but no differences between episodic and chronic migraineurs. The results of the separate movements may be misinterpreted as a preferred directional restriction. However, currently, there is no plausibility to assume any lateral preference. Moreover, data from two recent systematic reviews with meta-analyses reinforce that any specific side or plane restriction might be random. Liang et al. revealed a reduction in cervical ROM in the sagittal and frontal planes [9], whereas Szikszay et al. observed lower ROM in sagittal and transverse planes, comparing migraineurs and controls [10].

This is the first study analyzing neck angular velocity in migraineurs, revealing a significant reduction in patients with migraine, especially those with the chronic form. However, we should recognize that the mean angular velocity observed in this study does not represent a self-paced velocity that subjects use during their daily activity. The time constraint of our experiment may have forced the participants to adopt a slow movement. Nevertheless, even under the same experimental circumstances, the migraine groups performed the active neck movements more slowly than the controls. It agrees with the lower velocity (peak or average) observed for patients with neck pain when performing self-paced active neck movements [18,37]. Vikne et al. [19] assessed patients with chronic whiplash-associated disorders adopting slow, preferred, and maximal speed to move their head and neck. Lower average velocity was also observed for the patients compared to controls to perform cervical extension and flexion back to the neutral position regardless of the speed assessed [19]. For the cervical flexion, differences were observed only at the maximal speed [19]. Future studies may expand the knowledge about kinematic variables of active neck movements in migraineurs using preferred speed, as maximal speed would not be appropriate for these patients considering the high frequency of vestibular symptoms [38].

Several hypotheses can be raised to speculate the mechanisms behind the lower angular velocity observed in the migraine groups, including the possibility of a combination of them. Subjects with migraines avoid moving their head during a migraine attack [17], so if they perpetuate their behavior even during interictal phases (out of migraine attack), it could facilitate kinematic alterations. Indeed, half of our migraine groups were classified as high fear subjects according to TKS scores, which is the proportion expected among migraineurs [16]. In individuals with neck pain, kinesiophobia presented negative weak-to-moderate associations with kinematic variables [39]. However, the correlations observed in our sample between TKS scores and angular velocity were too low to be clinically highlighted and justify our findings.

Another aspect that could contribute would be the higher frequency of migraine, as the chronic migraine group seems to be more affected when we consider the movements separately. However, the absence of a significant correlation between the frequency of headache and the mean angular velocity suggests that this relationship may not have a significant role in our findings.

In addition to the behavioral and headache frequency hypotheses, there is also the potential contribution of a cervical mechanoreceptor dysfunction to the impairment of kinematic performance [18]. In this context, Meise et al. observed that patients with chronic migraine presented altered cervical proprioception, and the presence of neck pain did not modify it [40]. As no data regarding cervical proprioception were collected, we cannot confirm nor discard this hypothesis. It might be a subject to be explored in further studies.

The combination of lesser active ROM with low velocity might point toward a change in motor control strategies by increasing coactivation of neck muscles to avoid pain or maintain cervical stability [41]. In contrast to our findings, altered superficial muscle activity has been previously reported in patients with migraines [21,23] through a higher activity of extensor muscles during the flexion when compared to healthy controls. However, in those studies, electromyographic activity was assessed during isometric contractions or low-load craniocervical flexion movement. In addition, in the current study, we could not analyze muscle coactivation due to the between-group differences in angular velocity, making a direct comparison between studies difficult. Therefore, our data suggest that the performance of active neck movements is not associated with an altered muscle activation time. It may be justified by the low effort demanded during the task or by its similarity to cervical movements performed frequently during daily routine. Similarly, individuals with migraines did not also differ from controls on muscle activity during the endurance test with submaximal contractions [42]. Current and previous data suggest a complex adaptation of motor control patterns of the cervical musculature in patients with migraines.

The analysis of movement and muscle pattern recruitment during active cervical movements has been analyzed in individuals with chronic neck pain. Previous studies have revealed a reduced range of motion, lower velocity, and increased co-contraction ratio in cervical muscles [18,20,41]. Despite a higher prevalence of neck pain in migraine groups in contrast to the control group, our results were not altered by the history of neck pain or neck pain induced during movement. These findings support the hypothesis that one of the migraine characteristics might be an alteration in the efferent system that affects motor control and mobility of the craniocervical area since some symptoms and signs of cervical dysfunction are related to the migraine itself and not dependent on the presence of neck pain [43].

Nevertheless, the role of neck pain in cervical mobility cannot be totally excluded, whereas we observed in those individuals with self-reported neck pain weak correlations between neck-related disability with cervical ROM and angular velocity. Similar results were previously observed in individuals with migraines [14] and neck pain [39]. For clinicians, we reinforce the importance of cervical assessment in patients with migraines, regardless of the presence of neck pain and the assessment of psychosocial aspects, since they could be negative factors in treatment success. From a scientific perspective, cervical motor control in patients with migraines should be investigated during functional tasks to understand the impact of symptoms or signs of musculoskeletal dysfunction in daily activities. The role of kinesiophobia on musculoskeletal deficits associated with migraine also needs to be better explored since it could be an anticipatory behavior of fear-avoidance to potential pain. Future studies may also investigate a potential relationship between hypervigilance and angular velocity in patients with migraines.

Finally, we recognize some limitations of the current study. Since our sample consisted of only women, the results should not be generalized to men with migraines. In addition, due to the study design, we cannot infer any causal relationship between the factors. Head and neck postures were not assessed, and the altered spine alignment could influence the motor strategies to perform the active cervical movement. Finally, although the TSK had revealed differences in kinesiophobia between patients with migraine and controls, it is not a validated tool in the migraine population. Despite these limitations, this is the first study investigating muscle activity during active neck movements and neck kinematic aspects in patients with migraines, adding that the velocity of the active cervical movement may be as affected as its range of motion. Moreover, it highlights that the history of neck pain or the presence of neck pain during the task seems to exhibit little or no influence on these reduced parameters. However, psychosocial aspects may also contribute to them.

5. Conclusions

Women with episodic and chronic migraines presented lower total cervical ROM and mean angular velocity during neck active movements when compared with headache-free controls. Total cervical ROM and mean angular velocity were negative and weakly correlated to neck disability and kinesiophobia, but not to headache features. No differences were observed for the percentage of activation of both neck flexors and extensors acting as antagonists or as agonists during active neck movements.

Supplementary Materials: The following are available online at https://www.mdpi.com/article/10.3390/jcm10173805/s1, Table S1: Cervical range of motion (degrees) of the three groups stratified according to the history of neck pain (mean and standard deviation), Table S2: Cervical range of motion (degrees) of the three groups stratified according to the presence of neck pain during active movement (mean and standard deviation, Table S3: Angular velocity (degrees/s) of the three groups stratified according to the history of neck pain (mean and standard deviation), Table S4: Angular velocity (°/s) of the three groups stratified according to the presence of neck pain during active movement (mean and standard deviation).

Author Contributions: Conceptualization, C.F.P., A.S.O., L.L.F., F.D. and D.B.-G.; methodology, C.F.P., A.S.O., T.W.-L. and L.L.F.; formal analysis, C.F.P. and L.L.F.; investigation, C.F.P., A.S.O., T.W.-L., C.F.-d.-l.-P. and L.L.F.; data curation, C.F.P., T.W.-L. and L.L.F.; writing—original draft preparation, C.F.P. and L.L.F.; writing—review and editing, C.F.P., A.S.O., T.W.-L., L.L.F., C.F.-d.-l.-P.; F.D. and D.B.-G.; supervision, A.S.O. and D.B.-G.; project administration, D.B.-G.; funding acquisition, C.F.P. and D.B.-G. All authors have read and agreed to the published version of the manuscript.

Funding: This research was funded by São Paulo Research Foundation (FAPESP), grant numbers 2018/23832-5 and 2015/18031-5, and in part by the Coordenação de Aperfeiçoamento de Pessoal de Nível Superior—Brasil (CAPES)—Finance Code 001.

Institutional Review Board Statement: The study was conducted according to the guidelines of the Declaration of Helsinki and approved by the Ethics Committee of Ribeirão Preto Medical School of the University of São Paulo (protocol code 12145/2016, approved 23 November 2016).

Informed Consent Statement: Informed consent was obtained from all subjects involved in the study.

Data Availability Statement: The data presented in this study are available on request from the corresponding author. The data are not publicly available due to containing information that could compromise the privacy of research participants.

Conflicts of Interest: The authors declare no conflict of interest. The funders had no role in the design of the study, in the collection, analyses, or interpretation of data, in the writing of the manuscript, or in the decision to publish the results.

References

1. Steiner, T.J.; Stovner, L.J.; Jensen, R.; Uluduz, D.; Katsarava, Z. Lifting The Burden: The Global Campaign against Headache. Migraine remains second among the world's causes of disability, and first among young women: Findings from GBD2019. *J. Headache Pain* **2020**, *21*, 137. [CrossRef] [PubMed]
2. Headache Classification Committee of the International Headache Society (IHS). The International Classification of Headache Disorders, 3rd ed. *Cephalalgia* **2018**, *38*, 1–211. [CrossRef]
3. Burch, R.C.; Buse, D.C.; Lipton, R.B. Migraine: Epidemiology, Burden, and Comorbidity. *Neurol. Clin.* **2019**, *37*, 631–649. [CrossRef] [PubMed]
4. Lipton, R.B.; Fanning, K.M.; Buse, D.C.; Martin, V.T.; Reed, M.L.; Adams, A.M.; Goadsby, P.J. Identifying Natural Subgroups of Migraine Based on Comorbidity and Concomitant Condition Profiles: Results of the Chronic Migraine Epidemiology and Outcomes (CaMEO) Study. *Headache* **2018**, *58*, 933–947. [CrossRef]
5. Goadsby, P.J.; Holland, P.R.; Martins-Oliveira, M.; Hoffmann, J.; Schankin, C.; Akerman, S. Pathophysiology of Migraine: A Disorder of Sensory Processing. *Physiol. Rev.* **2017**, *97*, 553–622. [CrossRef] [PubMed]
6. Aguila, M.R.; Rebbeck, T.; Pope, A.; Ng, K.; Leaver, A.M. Six-month clinical course and factors associated with non-improvement in migraine and non-migraine headaches. *Cephalalgia* **2018**, *38*, 1672–1686. [CrossRef] [PubMed]
7. Ford, S.; Calhoun, A.; Kahn, K.; Mann, J.; Finkel, A. Predictors of disability in migraineurs referred to a tertiary clinic: Neck pain, headache characteristics, and coping behaviors. *Headache* **2008**, *48*, 523–528. [CrossRef]
8. Charles, A. The pathophysiology of migraine: Implications for clinical management. *Lancet Neurol.* **2018**, *17*, 174–182. [CrossRef]
9. Liang, Z.; Galea, O.; Thomas, L.; Jull, G.; Treleaven, J. Cervical musculoskeletal impairments in migraine and tension type headache: A systematic review and meta-analysis. *Musculoskelet. Sci. Pract.* **2019**, *42*, 67–83. [CrossRef]
10. Szikszay, T.M.; Hoenick, S.; von Korn, K.; Meise, R.; Schwarz, A.; Starke, W.; Luedtke, K. Which Examination Tests Detect Differences in Cervical Musculoskeletal Impairments in People With Migraine? A Systematic Review and Meta-Analysis. *Phys. Ther.* **2019**, *99*, 549–569. [CrossRef]
11. Oliveira-Souza, A.I.S.; Florencio, L.L.; Carvalho, G.F.; Fernández-de-Las-Peñas, C.; Dach, F.; Bevilaqua-Grossi, D. Reduced flexion rotation test in women with chronic and episodic migraine. *Braz. J. Phys. Ther.* **2019**, *23*, 387–394. [CrossRef]
12. Bevilaqua-Grossi, D.; Pegoretti, K.S.; Goncalves, M.C.; Speciali, J.G.; Bordini, C.A.; Bigal, M.E. Cervical mobility in women with migraine. *Headache* **2009**, *49*, 726–731. [CrossRef]
13. Ferracini, G.N.; Florencio, L.L.; Dach, F.; Bevilaqua-Grossi, D.; Palacios-Ceña, M.; Ordás-Bandera, C.; Chaves, T.C.; Speciali, J.G.; Fernández-de-las-Peñas, C. Musculoskeletal disorders of the upper cervical spine in women with episodic or chronic migraine. *Eur. J. Phys. Rehabil. Med.* **2017**, *53*, 342–350. [CrossRef]
14. Carvalho, G.F.; Chaves, T.C.; Gonçalves, M.C.; Florencio, L.L.; Braz, C.A.; Dach, F.; Fernández-de-las-Peñas, C.; Bevilaqua-Grossi, D. Comparison between neck pain disability and cervical range of motion in patients with episodic and chronic migraine: A cross-sectional study. *J. Manip. Physiol. Ther.* **2014**, *37*, 641–646. [CrossRef] [PubMed]
15. Luedtke, K.; Starke, W.; May, A. Musculoskeletal dysfunction in migraine patients. *Cephalalgia* **2018**, *38*, 865–875. [CrossRef] [PubMed]
16. Benatto, M.T.; Bevilaqua-Grossi, D.; Carvalho, G.F.; Bragatto, M.M.; Pinheiro, C.F.; Lodovichi, S.S.; Dach, F.; Fernández-de-las-Peñas, C.; Florencio, L.L. Kinesiophobia Is Associated with Migraine. *Pain Med.* **2019**, *20*, 846–851. [CrossRef] [PubMed]
17. Martins, I.P.; Gouveia, R.G.; Parreira, E. Kinesiophobia in migraine. *J. Pain* **2006**, *7*, 445–451. [CrossRef] [PubMed]
18. Salehi, R.; Rasouli, O.; Saadat, M.; Mehravar, M.; Negahban, H.; Shaterzadeh, M.J. Cervical movement kinematic analysis in patients with chronic neck pain: A comparative study with healthy subjects. *Musculoskelet. Sci. Pract.* **2021**, *53*, 102377. [CrossRef]
19. Vikne, H.; Bakke, E.S.; Liestøl, K.; Engen, S.R.; Vøllestad, N. Muscle activity and head kinematics in unconstrained movements in subjects with chronic neck pain; cervical motor dysfunction or low exertion motor output? *BMC Musculoskelet. Disord.* **2013**, *4*, 314. [CrossRef]
20. Tsang, S.M.; Szeto, G.P.; Lee, R.Y. Altered spinal kinematics and muscle recruitment pattern of the cervical and thoracic spine in people with chronic neck pain during functional task. *J. Electromyogr. Kinesiol.* **2014**, *24*, 104–113. [CrossRef] [PubMed]
21. Benatto, M.T.; Florencio, L.L.; Bragatto, M.M.; Lodovichi, S.S.; Dach, F.; Bevilaqua-Grossi, D. Extensor/flexor ratio of neck muscle strength and electromyographic activity of individuals with migraine: A cross-sectional study. *Eur. Spine J.* **2019**, *28*, 2311–2318. [CrossRef] [PubMed]
22. Florencio, L.L.; Oliveira, A.S.; Lemos, T.W.; Carvalho, G.F.; Dach, F.; Bigal, M.E.; Falla, D.; Fernández-de-las-Peñas, C.; Bevilaqua-Grossi, D. Patients with chronic, but not episodic, migraine display altered activity of their neck extensor muscles. *J. Electromyogr. Kinesiol.* **2016**, *30*, 66–72. [CrossRef]
23. Florencio, L.L.; Oliveira, A.S.; Carvalho, G.F.; Tolentino, G.A.; Dach, F.; Bigal, M.E.; Fernández-de-las-Peñas, C.; Bevilaqua-Grossi, D. Cervical Muscle Strength and Muscle Coactivation During Isometric Contractions in Patients With Migraine: A Cross-Sectional Study. *Headache* **2015**, *55*, 1312–1322. [CrossRef]
24. Chiu, T.T.; Sing, K.L. Evaluation of cervical range of motion and isometric neck muscle strength: Reliability and validity. *Clin. Rehabil.* **2002**, *16*, 851–858. [CrossRef] [PubMed]
25. Cook, C.; Richardson, J.K.; Braga, L.; Menezes, A.; Soler, X.; Kume, P.; Zaninelli, M.; Socolows, F.; Pietrobon, R. Cross-cultural adaptation and validation of the Brazilian Portuguese version of the Neck Disability Index and Neck Pain and Disability Scale. *Spine (Phila Pa 1976)* **2006**, *31*, 1621–1627. [CrossRef] [PubMed]

26. Souza, F.S.; Marinho, C.S.; Siqueira, F.B.; Maher, C.G.; Costa, L.O. Psychometric testing confirms that the Brazilian-Portuguese adaptations, the original versions of the Fear-Avoidance Beliefs Questionnaire, and the Tampa Scale of Kinesiophobia have similar measurement properties. *Spine (Phila Pa 1976)* **2008**, *33*, 1028–1033. [CrossRef]
27. Vernon, H. The Neck Disability Index: State-of-the-art, 1991-2008. *J. Manip. Physiol. Ther.* **2008**, *31*, 491–502. [CrossRef]
28. Jorritsma, W.; Dijkstra, P.U.; de Vries, G.E.; Geertzen, J.H.; Reneman, M.F. Detecting relevant changes and responsiveness of Neck Pain and Disability Scale and Neck Disability Index. *Eur. Spine J.* **2012**, *21*, 2550–2557. [CrossRef]
29. Schellingerhout, J.M.; Verhagen, A.P.; Heymans, M.W.; Koes, B.W.; de Vet, H.C.; Terwee, C.B. Measurement properties of disease-specific questionnaires in patients with neck pain: A systematic review. *Qual. Life Res.* **2012**, *21*, 659–670. [CrossRef] [PubMed]
30. Vlaeyen, J.W.; Kole-Snijders, A.M.; Rotteveel, A.M.; Ruesink, R.; Heuts, P.H. The role of fear of movement/(re)injury in pain disability. *J. Occup. Rehabil.* **1995**, *5*, 235–252. [CrossRef]
31. Falla, D.; Dall'Alba, P.; Rainoldi, A.; Merletti, R.; Jull, G. Location of innervation zones of sternocleidomastoid and scalene muscles–a basis for clinical and research electromyography applications. *Clin. Neurophysiol.* **2002**, *113*, 57–63. [CrossRef]
32. Joines, S.M.; Sommerich, C.M.; Mirka, G.A.; Wilson, J.R.; Moon, S.D. Low-level exertions of the neck musculature: A study of research methods. *J. Electromyogr. Kinesiol.* **2006**, *16*, 485–497. [CrossRef]
33. Surface ElectroMyoGraphy for the Non-Invasive Assessment of Muscles. Available online: http://www.seniam.org (accessed on 2 June 2014).
34. Tsang, S.M.; Szeto, G.P.; Lee, R.Y. Relationship between neck acceleration and muscle activation in people with chronic neck pain: Implications for functional disability. *Clin. Biomech.* **2016**, *35*, 27–36. [CrossRef]
35. Hodges, P.W.; Bui, B.H. A comparison of computer-based methods for the determination of onset of muscle contraction using electromyography. *Electroencephalogr. Clin. Neurophysiol.* **1996**, *101*, 511–519. [CrossRef]
36. Domholdt, E. *Physical Therapy Research: Principles and Applications*, 2nd ed.; WB Saunders Co.: Philadelphia, PA, USA, 2000.
37. Sarig Bahat, H.; Chen, X.; Reznik, D.; Kodesh, E.; Treleaven, J. Interactive cervical motion kinematics: Sensitivity, specificity and clinically significant values for identifying kinematic impairments in patients with chronic neck pain. *Man. Ther.* **2015**, *20*, 295–302. [CrossRef]
38. Carvalho, G.F.; Vianna-Bell, F.H.; Florencio, L.L.; Pinheiro, C.F.; Dach, F.; Bigal, M.E.; Bevilaqua-Grossi, D. Presence of vestibular symptoms and related disability in migraine with and without aura and chronic migraine. *Cephalalgia* **2019**, *39*, 29–37. [CrossRef] [PubMed]
39. Sarig Bahat, H.; Weiss, P.L.; Sprecher, E.; Krasovsky, A.; Laufer, Y. Do neck kinematics correlate with pain intensity, neck disability or with fear of motion? *Man. Ther.* **2014**, *19*, 252–258. [CrossRef] [PubMed]
40. Meise, R.; Lüdtke, K.; Probst, A.; Stude, P.; Schöttker-Königer, T. Zervikaler "joint position error" bei Kopfschmerzen: Systematische Literaturübersicht und empirische Daten bei chronischer Migräne [Joint position error in patients with headache: Systematic review of the literature and experimental data for patients with chronic migraine]. *Schmerz* **2019**, *33*, 204–211. (In German) [CrossRef]
41. Sjölander, P.; Michaelson, P.; Jaric, S.; Djupsjöbacka, M. Sensorimotor disturbances in chronic neck pain–range of motion, peak velocity, smoothness of movement, and repositioning acuity. *Man. Ther.* **2008**, *13*, 122–131. [CrossRef] [PubMed]
42. Florencio, L.L.; Oliveira, A.S.; Will-Lemos, T.; Pinheiro, C.F.; Marçal, J.C.D.S.; Dach, F.; Fernández-de-Las-Peñas, C.; Bevilaqua-Grossi, D. Muscle endurance and cervical electromyographic activity during submaximal efforts in women with and without migraine. *Clin. Biomech.* **2021**, *82*, 105276. [CrossRef] [PubMed]
43. Bragatto, M.M.; Bevilaqua-Grossi, D.; Benatto, M.T.; Lodovichi, S.S.; Pinheiro, C.F.; Carvalho, G.F.; Dach, F.; Fernández-de-las-Peñas, C.; Florencio, L.L. Is the presence of neck pain associated with more severe clinical presentation in patients with migraine? A cross-sectional study. *Cephalalgia* **2019**, *39*, 1500–1508. [CrossRef] [PubMed]

MDPI
St. Alban-Anlage 66
4052 Basel
Switzerland
Tel. +41 61 683 77 34
Fax +41 61 302 89 18
www.mdpi.com

Journal of Clinical Medicine Editorial Office
E-mail: jcm@mdpi.com
www.mdpi.com/journal/jcm

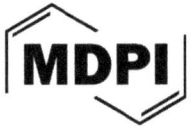